Spinal Disorders: Assessment, Treatment and New Pathways

Spinal Disorders: Assessment, Treatment and New Pathways

Edited by Rickon Hamill

hayle
medical

New York

Hayle Medical,
750 Third Avenue, 9th Floor,
New York, NY 10017, USA

Visit us on the World Wide Web at:
www.haylemedical.com

ISBN: 978-1-63241-718-3

Cataloging-in-Publication Data

Spinal disorders : assessment, treatment and new pathways / edited by Rickon Hamill.
    p. cm.
Includes bibliographical references and index.
ISBN 978-1-63241-718-3
1. Spine--Diseases. 2. Spine--Diseases--Diagnosis. 3. Spine--Diseases--Treatment.
4. Spine--Instability. 5. Spine--Puncture. I. Hamill, Rickon.
RD768 .S65 2019
616.73--dc23

Table of Contents

Preface

In my initial years as a student, I used to run to the library at every possible instance to grab a book and learn something new. Books were my primary source of knowledge and I would not have come such a long way without all that I learnt from them. Thus, when I was approached to edit this book; I became understandably nostalgic. It was an absolute honor to be considered worthy of guiding the current generation as well as those to come. I put all my knowledge and hard work into making this book most beneficial for its readers.

Spinal disease is a condition characterized by the impairment of the backbone, and includes diseases of the spine or back, such as kyphosis. Some spinal diseases are spinal tumors, spinal muscular atrophy, lumbar spinal stenosis, ankylosing spondylitis, spina bifida, etc. Spinal cord disorders can also include spinal fracture, burst fracture, anterior spinal artery syndrome, central cord syndrome, myelopathy, Morvan's syndrome, vascular myelopathy, syringomyelia, etc. This book covers in detail some existing theories and innovative concepts revolving around spinal disorders. It aims to give a general view of the different types of spine disorders, and their medical and surgical treatments, methodologies and pathways. This book will help the readers in keeping pace with the rapid changes in this field.

I wish to thank my publisher for supporting me at every step. I would also like to thank all the authors who have contributed their researches in this book. I hope this book will be a valuable contribution to the progress of the field.

Editor

Brace technology thematic series: the 3D Rigo Chêneau-type brace

Manuel Rigo[1*] and Mina Jelačić[2]

Abstract

Background: Chêneau and Matthias introduced in 1979 a brace concept inspired in casting. The brace was initially named "CTM" from Chêneau-Toulouse-Münster. The name "CTM" is still popular in France but "Chêneau-type brace" is its common name in the rest of the world. Principles to construct this brace were originally based on anatomical descriptions rather than biomechanics, and its standard is poor.

Methods: This paper follows the format of the "Brace technology thematic series." The Chêneau-type brace has been versioned by many authors. The contribution of the present authors is about to the description of the principles based on biomechanics and a specific classification created to help to standardize the brace design and construction. The classification also correlates with specific exercises (PSSE) according to the Barcelona School, using Schroth principles (BSPTS). This current authors' version has been named "3D Rigo Chêneau-type brace." The 3D principles are related to a detorsional mechanism created by forces and counterforces to bring the trunk into the best possible correction: (1) three-point system; (2) regional derotation; (3) sagittal alignment and balance. A custom-made TLS brace (thoracolumbosacral) is built in order to provide highly defined contact areas, which are located, shaped, and oriented in the space to generate the necessary vectors of force to correct in 3D. Expansion areas are also essential for tissue migration, growth, and breathing movements, although body reactions depend basically on how well designed are the contact areas. The brace is open in front and can be considered rigid and dynamic at the same time.

Results: Blueprints for construction of the brace according to the revisited Rigo classification are fully described in this paper.

Conclusions: Different independent teams have published comparable outcomes by using Chêneau-type braces and versions in combination with specific exercises and following a similar scoliosis comprehensive care model. This present version is also supported by scientific results from several independent teams.

Keywords: Idiopathic scoliosis, Non-operative treatment, Bracing, Rigo-Chêneau brace, Scoliosis classification

Background

This paper, which is about the author's custom-made version of the popular Chêneau brace, follows the format for the "*Scoliosis* brace thematic series."

The effectiveness of bracing in the treatment of adolescent idiopathic scoliosis is no longer a controversial issue. In a systematic review of the effectiveness of bracing treatment, Maruyama et al. [1] concluded that, although the quality of the evidence is limited due to the low methodological quality of the studies, "the available data suggest that, compared with observation, bracing is more potent in preventing the progression of scoliosis and may not have a negative impact on patients' quality of life." A previous Cochrane systematic review had showed low-quality evidence in favor of using braces [2]. However, a recent multicenter study about the effects of bracing on adolescents with idiopathic scoliosis, enrolling both a randomized cohort and a preference cohort, concluded that bracing significantly decreased the progression of high-risk curves to the threshold requiring surgery [3]. Corroborating the results of previous

* Correspondence: rigoquera@gmail.com
[1]Elena Salvá Institute (Rigo Quera Salvá S.L.P.), Vía Augusta 185, 08021 Barcelona, Spain
Full list of author information is available at the end of the article

prospective observational studies, this study showed a strong brace dose-response relationship, with increased benefits from longer hours of brace wear. However, the statement about the effectiveness of bracing is too general, which raises questions regarding the relevance of such a statement for each individual patient. First, the indications, limitations, and contra-indications are not universally established. Second, the amount of brace concepts with different principles of correction is too extensive to encompass in "a standard." More so, few principles of correction have achieved the desired consensus among experts [4]. Third, according to SOSORT guidelines (International *Society on Scoliosis Orthopaedic and Rehabilitation Treatment*), independent of the prescribed brace concept, the multidisciplinary treatment team seems to play a contributing role in the success or failure of bracing treatment [5]. Nevertheless, two well-defined factors have been associated with positive results and bracing success: (1) short-term in-brace correction of the Cobb angle and (2) compliance. However, since the reasons behind bracing success are extremely complex, using these two factors as the key points of bracing treatment and scoliosis management is obviously a simplification. In-brace correction depends on several factors, such as the correction principles of the prescribed brace, brace design according to curve pattern, specific quality of design achieved by a particular orthotist, brace fitting, and patient's characteristics. These combined factors determine how much Cobb angle correction will be achieved; however, ideally, the correction of the Cobb angle should be achieved through a 3-dimensional (3D) correction of the trunk and spine. Historically, the Chêneau-type brace was designed to oppose the spinal torsion and correct scoliosis in three dimensions. The original Chêneau-type brace has been defined and described in several books, primarily published in French and German [6–9] by Jacques Chêneau and his collaborators (Fig. 1), and many European doctors have used the brace since its presentation in 1979. The first author of this paper (MR) initially collaborated with Jacques Chêneau and Hans Rudolf Weiss to develop the technical evolution of the brace and is basically responsible for the re-definition of brace principles using biomechanical descriptions instead of the original anatomical descriptions provided by Jacques Chêneau. The author (MR) is also responsible for the additional brace designs that use a specific classification according to the scoliosis curve pattern [10]. This paper will provide a complete description of the correction principles according to the 3D nature of idiopathic scoliosis. The classification will be revisited with the introduction of some minor changes, and complete descriptions of specific brace designs for each curve pattern will be provided. Finally, indications, limitations, protocols, results, and case reports will be presented

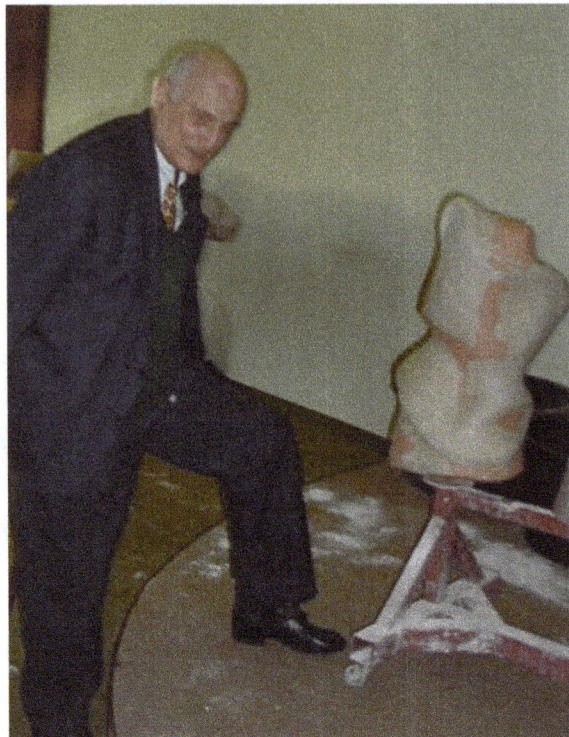

Fig. 1 Jacques Chêneau in Bad Sobernheim (Germany) circa 1998. Photo by Sanomed

according to the recommended format of the brace thematic series introduced by Negrini S and Grivas TB in *Scoliosis* [11].

The original brace, which was presented for the first time by Dr. Jacques Chêneau (Toulouse) and Prof. Matthias (Münster) around 1979, was initially called the Chêneau-Toulouse-Münster (CTM) brace by French physiatrists. The CTM brace was defined as a custom TLSO brace made from a corrected positive mould from a patient's negative mould. The correction of the positive mould consisted of a complicated process of removing plaster to build a series of pad areas that coincide with prominent regions of the patient's body in combination with an even more extensive process of adding plaster to build large expansion spaces that coincide with sunken regions of the patient's body. The pad areas were located, shaped, and oriented to provide a combined deflection-derotation effect, while the expansions had to provide the necessary room for tissue migration, growth, and breathing movements. Chêneau was inspired by Abbot's plaster cast. Abbot used this same deflection-derotation principle, putting the patient in the best possible corrective position by pushing the humps and decollapsing the sunken regions of the trunk, keeping the correction with a plaster cast that basically contacted the body on the humps.

Chêneau made a highly detailed description of the prominent and sunken regions of the scoliotic body in order to explain where to build pads and where to place expansion rooms when performing the correction on the positive mould. All the regions (prominent and sunken) where numbered, forming a numerical map with the purpose of helping the orthotists in their correction task. He also used the concept of "correction of the flat back." Some French masters used this concept in the 1950s when applying corrective plaster casts. The original mechanism proposed by Chêneau was "to build a strong pad region in the front at the level of the anterior rib hump and the sternum, leaving room on the back to create a kyphosant effect at the thoracic spine region." Some pictures and descriptions from the abovementioned masters suggest that Chêneau used their concept of overcorrection in the frontal plane for most effectively decollapsing all the concavities. In accordance with the teachings of Christa Lehnert-Schroth, Chêneau also introduced the simple classification of the 3- and 4-curve pattern (Fig. 2) into the field. It is evident that Chêneau was always open to his European colleagues' opinions and suggestions when improving the brace design. The number of people who contributed to the evolution of the brace is too numerous to list. The benefit of these myriad contributions is that it enhanced the logical evolution of the brace; however, it conversely produced an endless supply of Chêneau-type versions that lacked the high standards associated with the originals. In addition, Chêneau's classical anatomical descriptions and explanations about where and how to make

the corrections to the mould, while easy to interpret by some orthotists, were confusing to most, which has been associated with a very poor bracing standard, resulting in the serious consequence of brace failures and worsened prognosis (Fig. 3). Therefore, we should ask ourselves: What is a Chêneau brace? There is only a possible answer: A Chêneau brace is a brace made by Chêneau himself or made following his direct instructions. Any other brace could be called a "TLSO custom-made brace constructed according to Chêneau's principles" or, to simplify, a "Chêneau-type brace," where every prescribing doctor and constructing orthotist has the final responsibility of the brace design and manufacture, the fitting, and, consequently, the end result. In other words, the Chêneau-type brace should not be considered to be simply an "orthopedic product" that can be prescribed by any doctor and built by any orthotist, but a very complex corrective device that must be applied by highly experienced doctors and orthotists. To successfully and safely use this technique, both the MD and orthotist need a relatively long learning curve before reaching the desired standard; therefore, nobody should attempt this technique without being extensively and thoroughly supervised by a recognized master.

The main author (MR) has been intermittently in contact with Jacques Chêneau since 1989 and has been correcting the moulds of patients being treated at the Institut Elena Salvá in Barcelona since 1991. The observed poor standard, with totally different Chêneau-type brace designs for the same curve pattern, was the main impetus behind this author's proposition of a standardized treatment method in the late 1990s. The standardized treatment method consisted of redefining the theoretical principles, brace construction, and classification. Since 2002, the results of this proposition have been shared with many orthotists, MDs, and PTs during a yearly course offered at the Bundesfaschule für Orthopadie Technik (BUFA) under the name of "Chêneau Korsett nach Rigo," and have been partially published in two papers [9, 10]. In the next section, the authors describe in detail the theoretical principles of the Chêneau-type brace according to their own interpretation of how the brace should work. Consequently, the following principles would be better called "principles and recommendations from Rigo and Jelačić to construct a Chêneau-type brace or Rigo-Chêneau-type brace." Classical anatomical descriptions, such as the region map (i.e., pads and expansions) published by Chêneau in the past, shall not be reproduced here. To clarify, some orthotists improperly use the name RSC when building their own Chêneau-type braces following these current principles; it exists in a CAD CAM version—a commercial product with the registered name of Rigo System Chêneau or RSC®—which uses a German company to reproduce

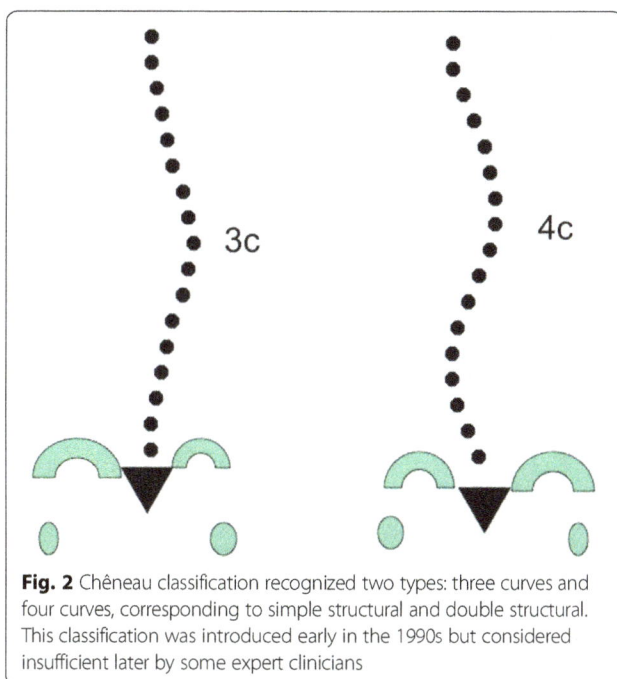

Fig. 2 Chêneau classification recognized two types: three curves and four curves, corresponding to simple structural and double structural. This classification was introduced early in the 1990s but considered insufficient later by some expert clinicians

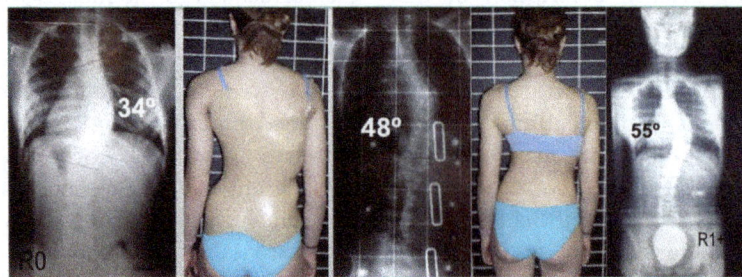

Fig. 3 This adolescent was first seen with a right thoracic curve measuring 35°. She was recommend wearing a Chêneau-type brace and received a totally wrong designed brace (deficient four-curve design for her three-curve pattern). The X-ray in brace showed an increased angle of 48° with a change in the curve pattern, adding on the curve some lumbar vertebrae due to the inexplicably strong left thoracolumbar pad. The girl was recommended to continue wearing the wrong brace with no modifications. One year later, a new X-ray out-brace showed a curve progression to 55° Cobb. The persistence of the original curve pattern, demonstrated the improper action of the left thoracolumbar pad, real cause of a temporary in-brace adding on phenomenon

braces from a library of original plaster moulds designed by the main author (MR), so the name RSC should not be used by those creating their own custom-made versions of the Rigo-Chêneau-type brace.

Methods

The 3D TLSO Rigo-Chêneau-type brace is a corrective device uniquely constructed to bring the trunk and spine into the best possible postural and morphological 3D corrected alignment by using a combination of forces applied to the trunk surface by specifically designed pads, facilitated by expansion or escaping spaces. As such, this is not a full-contact or almost-full-contact plastic, anatomic, and symmetric brace with pads inside to push the humps. All the pads are located, shaped, and oriented in a highly specific manner to push on selected regions of the trunk to bring the patient into the best possible 3D correction, while the remaining areas are not touched by the brace (i.e., areas of expansion or escaping spaces). The corrective reaction of the body depends on the level, shape, and orientation of the pads.

The authors have been following the general principle of correction defined in 1992 by Jean Dubousset during his amazing lecture about the importance of the 3D concept in the treatment of scoliotic deformities [12]. Dubousset defined the scoliotic deformity as "a combination of torsional regions joined by junctions; every torsional region formed by a variable number of vertebrae in anatomical lordosis, rotated and translated to the same side." In the section about practical considerations on cast and brace treatment, Dubousset remarked that "efforts at reducing a scoliotic curve had to be directed toward reduction of the structural lordosis and application of a detorsional force rather than the previous distraction force." Thus, by applying a detorsional mechanism, the objective is to achieve maximum derotation with the best possible alignment in the frontal as well as the sagittal planes.

The necessary detorsional forces to achieve the desirable 3D correction can be produced with a static brace by combining the following three mechanisms or systems:

1) Three-point systems in the frontal plane
2) Pair-of-force for regional and local derotation
3) Correct balance and physiological alignment in the sagittal plane

It is important to note that these principles do not work in isolation but rather in combination and, consequently, the isolated description of one principle after the other will always be imperfect. However, to maintain a logical format, the principles are explained separately below.

Three-point systems

In scoliosis, the lateral curvature of the spine produces a collapse of all the tissues on the concavity, ribs included, when referred to the thoracic region. Alternatively, on the convexity, tissues are expanded. The application of a single three-point system serves to correct single spinal curvature in the frontal plane. The correction of the lateral curvature, which we will refer to as deflection, frees up space on the collapsed concavity and releases tension on the convexity. This correction is essential to allow for derotation. A three-point system is formed by a force and two counterforces applied proximally and distally to the first one (Fig. 4). The direction of the forces and counterforces are always from lateral to medial, but the pads—mainly lumbar and thoracic—providing the vector forces are oriented in an oblique plane rather than in a single frontal plane, so they will also provide the forces for derotation in the transversal plane. The efficiency of the three-point system depends on the level and distance between the three pads designed to create this effect, as well as its orientation in the space

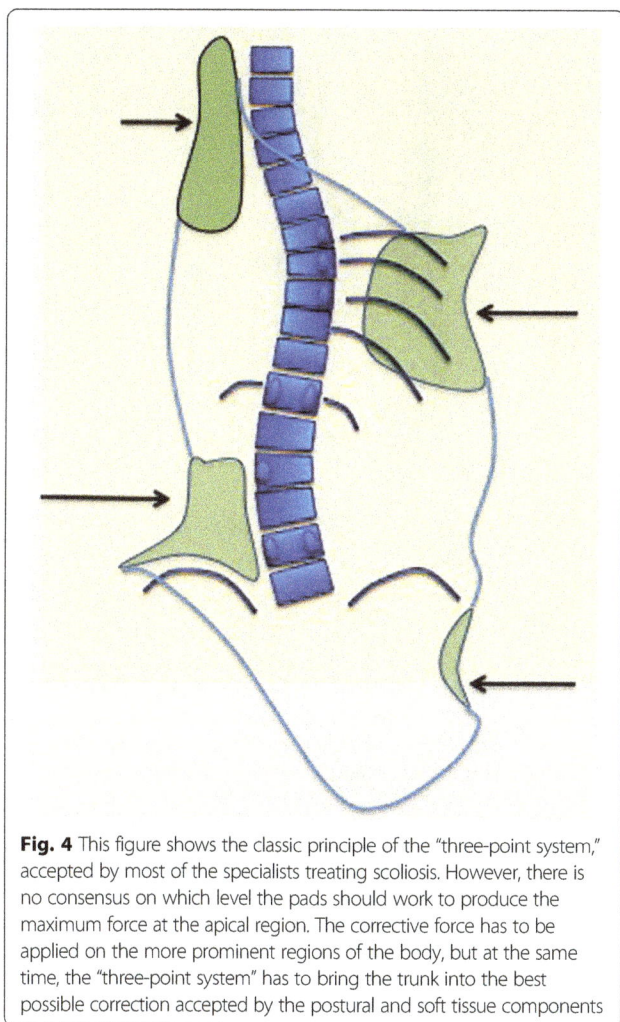

Fig. 4 This figure shows the classic principle of the "three-point system," accepted by most of the specialists treating scoliosis. However, there is no consensus on which level the pads should work to produce the maximum force at the apical region. The corrective force has to be applied on the more prominent regions of the body, but at the same time, the "three-point system" has to bring the trunk into the best possible correction accepted by the postural and soft tissue components

(Fig. 5). Thus, the shape and orientation of most of the pads allow them to work as part of a specific three-point system and simultaneously as a pair-of-force system working on the transversal plane to derotate, as explained below. Our speculative theory is that the sum of forces could be producing a detorsional mechanism, to the extent it is associated with an automatic effect of axial elongation, in absence of any traction force. The spatial location (level), distance, shape, and orientation are important not only in both the frontal and transverse planes but also in the sagittal plane to achieve the best sagittal alignment of the trunk and normalization of the sagittal geometry of the spine (in the sense of the physiological profile).

The observed curve pattern determines the specific design of the pads and expansion spaces. Therefore, it is necessary to use a specific and reliable classification to ensure a good standard. This classification has been described in a previous paper [10] and will be revisited later in this section.

Pair-of-force system

The pair-of-force system consists of two contrary forces in different directions applied on a somewhat wide section of the trunk at the same level in order to derotate the section (i.e., regional derotation). The pair-of-force system has to apply the highest force at the apical level, where the vertebra is more rotated (i.e., local derotation).

To simplify, let us imagine a quite rare case of a right convex single structural curve staring at T5 and finishing at L2 (apex at T9–10), where a relatively wide section of the trunk has to be derotated against the two proximal and distal adjacent regions. In order to get the best correction effect, the proximal and distal adjacent regions can be fixed in the frontal plane of reference (0° of rotation in the transversal plane), while the region affected by the main structural single curve can be over-derotated to the left. Thus, a big region of the trunk, from T5 to L2 is over-derotated against the two adjacent proximal and distal regions, fixed in the frontal plane of reference. The proximal region involves the proximal thoracic region (T1 to T4 in this case) and the distal involves the pelvic and low lumbosacral regions (L4—sacrum and pelvis). The distal section of the brace included a very short low lumbosacral support on the left to ensure that the lowest lumbar vertebrae will remain unrotated, while its immediate proximal region receives an over-derotation force to the left (Fig. 6). This mechanism of regional derotation provides the required detorsional force.

The pair-of-force system also has a special function in the main thoracic region: the correction of structural or anatomical lordosis of the main thoracic curve. This does not refer to the global or regional geometry of the scoliotic spine observed in the lateral projection on the X-ray. The structural or anatomical flat back is related to the torsional phenomena. It has also been defined as relative anterior spinal overgrowth (RASO) [13–23], and although it has been shown to be secondary to the torsion of the spine (Stokes' vicious cycle modified by Burwell [24, 25]), it could hypothetically be primary [26]. The objective is to achieve the best possible correction of this anatomical lordosis using only the detorsional mechanism while keeping the trunk in a correct sagittal alignment without forward flexion or backward extension. This is the hypothesis of the main author (MR) against the proposal of some colleagues promoting a forced forward flexion applied on the thoracic region in order to correct the flat back. The experience of the author is that, by following this proposal, the anatomical flat back does not attain a better correction, but the proximal and distal regions become more kyphotic. In any case, it must be accepted that, in scoliosis cases with significant potential for progression from a rapid and strong lordotization of the thoracic spine, no

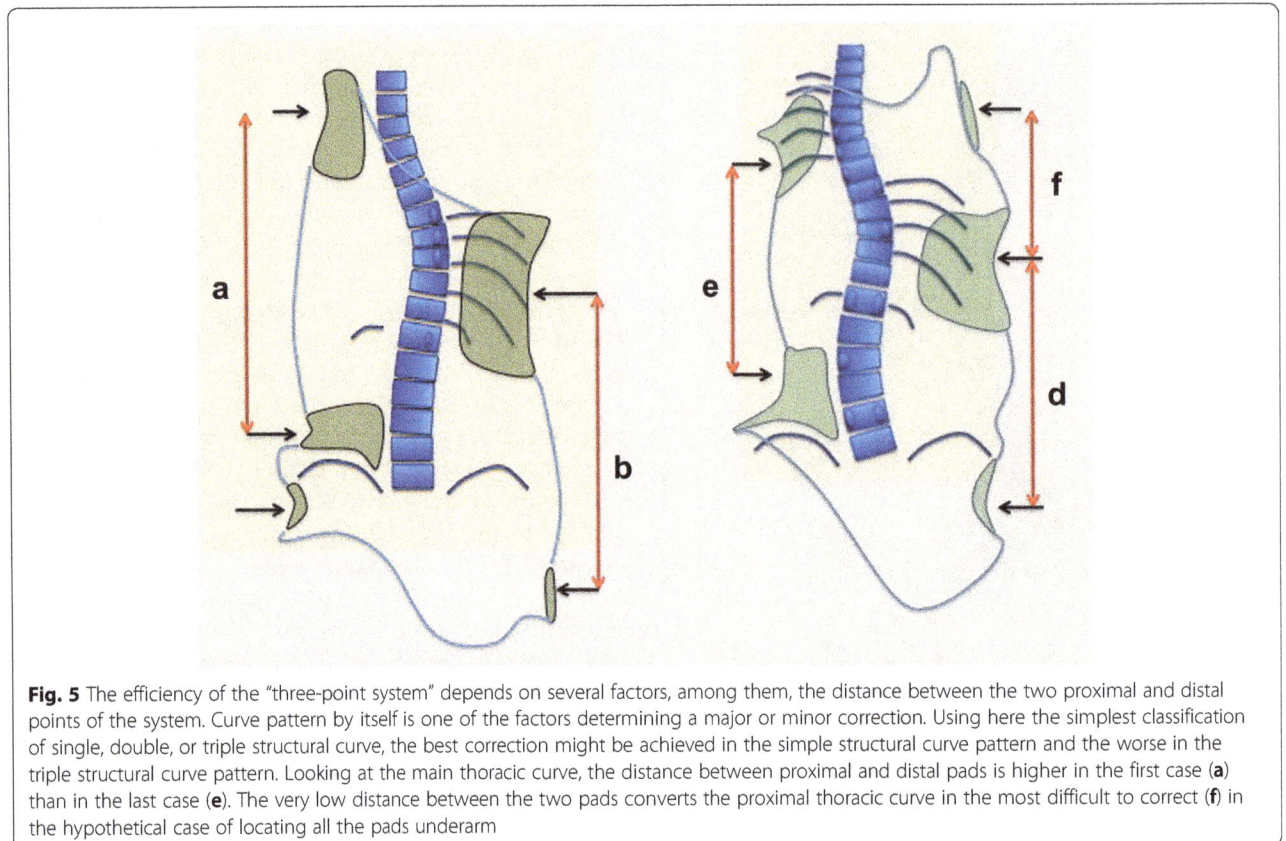

Fig. 5 The efficiency of the "three-point system" depends on several factors, among them, the distance between the two proximal and distal points of the system. Curve pattern by itself is one of the factors determining a major or minor correction. Using here the simplest classification of single, double, or triple structural curve, the best correction might be achieved in the simple structural curve pattern and the worse in the triple structural curve pattern. Looking at the main thoracic curve, the distance between proximal and distal pads is higher in the first case (**a**) than in the last case (**e**). The very low distance between the two pads converts the proximal thoracic curve in the most difficult to correct (**f**) in the hypothetical case of locating all the pads underarm

matter the design of the brace, the morphological flat back cannot be avoided.

The proposed principle against the anatomical flat back is not only related to the passive correction but also to a dynamic effect from the breathing mechanics. Figure 7 shows a transversal section of the brace profile at the apical level for a right thoracic scoliosis. The whole section is more or less translated to the left in relationship to the two distal and proximal sections, depending on how translated to the right this region is in the pathological situation. The transversal section shows the two main pads acting at this apical level: the dorsal pad and the ventral pad. It also shows the two main expansion spaces: the ventral expansion space on the right side and the dorso-lateral expansion space on the left side. The shape of this section remains a distorted ellipse rotated to the left (over-correcting the pathological right rotation). The two pads offer two main forces with an oblique direction. The orientation of the pads is always oblique and defines the direction of the forces: (1) the direction of the force coming from the dorsal thoracic pad is from dorso-lateral to ventro-medial and (2) the direction of the force coming from the ventral thoracic pad is from ventro-lateral to dorso-medial. However, the two forces are not in the same

direction because the pads are not parallel to each other but are mildly divergent in a dorsal direction. In other words, the ventral pad's orientation is slightly more frontally oriented than the dorsal pad. The shape of the pads is also an essential point. Both pads are round with a radius that is significantly larger than the radius of the contacted rib humps. Looking at the orientation and shape of the pads it can be noted that the dorsal pad maintains body contact until reaching the middle frontal plane (middle axillar line). On the left side, however, the ventral pad loses contact before reaching this line from the ventral. The main force produced by each pad can be decomposed in two vectors at each contact point and the direction of the vectors is (1) to ventral and to lateral from the dorsal pad and (2) to dorsal and to medial from the ventral pad. Consequently, two vector forces, to ventral and to dorsal, establish the pair-of-force system for derotation, where the vector to dorsal offered by the ventral pad is the major one. On the other hand, the vector force to medial produced by the dorsal pad is more significant than the vector force to medial produced by the ventral pad. Also addressed by the two pads, the whole rib cage section translates to the left, which cancels the vector force to medial created by the ventral pad. The humps adapt to the pads becoming less

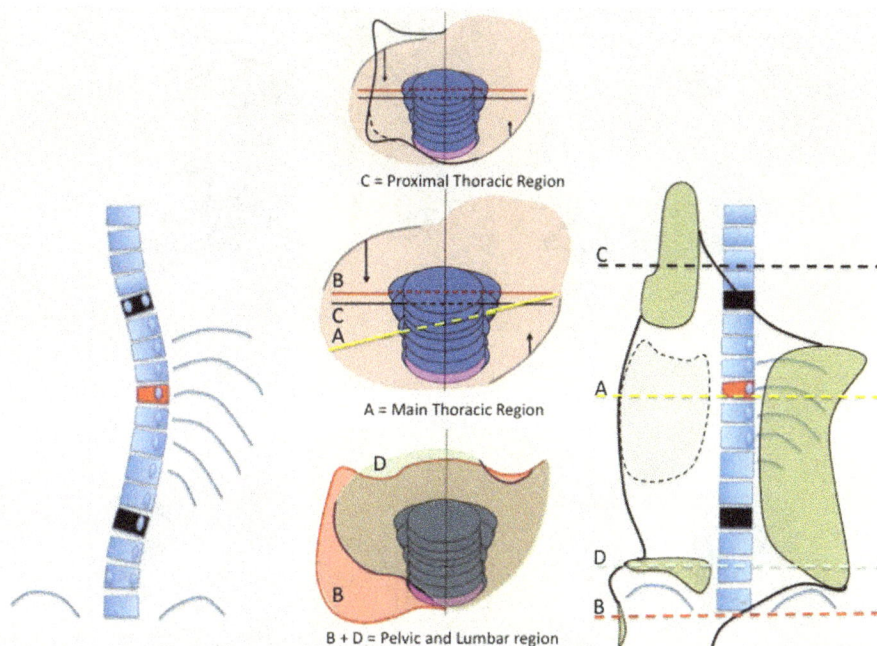

Fig. 6 This figure shows the corrective principles for a single long-low thoracic curve with the apical vertebra still in the main-low thoracic region (described later as A1 type in Rigo classification): "regional derotation" and "three-point system." The region of the trunk affected by the single structural curve is over-derotated to the left (yellow line A) throughout a dorsal-lateral pad and a ventral pad, against the two caudal and cranial regions. Pelvis and lower lumbar regions (B + D) are fixed in the frontal plane of reference (0° of rotation). The pelvis section of the brace is asymmetric, with the lateral-dorsal part opened in the right side and supported by left lumbar contact as well as anterior abdominal contact. The proximal thoracic region (C) is also fixed in the frontal plane of reference with a dorsal left counter-rotation pad. A left lateral to medial pad acts in the proximal thoracic region as the third proximal point of the "three-point system." The lateral component of the dorsal-lateral pad is the second point, on the right side. The left pelvis section together with the lateral component of the left lumbar support acts as the first caudal point of the system. The brace provides a left lateral-dorsal and a ventral right expansion rooms to facilitate breathing expansion and growth. The dorsal-lateral and anterior pads forming the pair of forces for derotation work both at the same level (maximum force at the apical level). This original design—A1 type—has shown to produce the highest percentage of in-brace correction [64]

angular, taking the shape of the pads. This reshaping effect is empowered by breathing mechanics, in inspiration. The ventral flat zone on the right side expands as well as the dorso-lateral concave area on the left. Thorax expansion also creates a dynamic pair-of-force system for derotation. As far as the major vector of force for derotation offered by the ventral pad in a dorsal direction, the apical vertebra, coupled to this force, comes backwards and the sagittal diameter of the thorax increases, with the consequent reduction of the anatomical lordosis or flat back. Each breathing cycle produces a gentle mobilization of the anatomical flat back in the corrective direction. This happens automatically, although the patient can increase this effect by forcing inspiration and trying to keep the two regions expanded during exhalation. Also, maintaining the distance between the sternum and the spine will increase the sagittal diameter of the thorax.

Pelvis section has to be fixed in the frontal plane of reference, with 0° of rotation, or can be mildly over-derotated when it is rotated in the pathological situation. This can be done using a fully closed pelvis section or a partially open pelvis section (i.e., plastic covering one hemi-pelvis). Indications are discussed later in this section (brace design according to curve pattern).

The proximal thoracic region is treated differently depending on the presence of a proximal structural curve or not. If there is no proximal structural curve, the design piece is called "classical." The classical proximal piece is not a real pad but a combination of two different counter pads. It works at the concave thoracic side and is composed first in a counter pad working oriented more or less on the sagittal plane as a third or proximal point of the three-point system correcting the main thoracic curve in the frontal plane (Fig. 8 explains this in more detail). The second component is a counter-derotation pad, from dorsal to ventral, fixing the proximal thoracic region and shoulder girdle region in the frontal plane of reference (also in Fig. 8). This counter-derotation force is necessary to prevent this region from coming back as a consequence of the over-

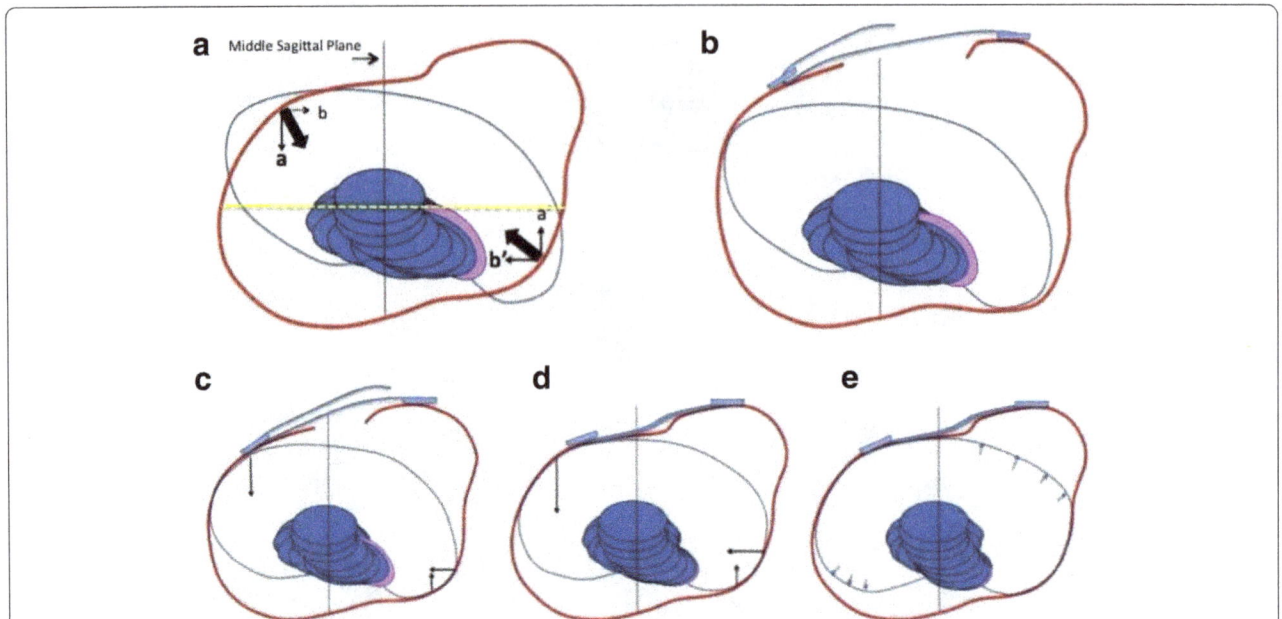

Fig. 7 The transversal section of the brace at the main thoracic region is shown in this figure **a**. The sequence **b, c, d**, and **e** shows the correction induced by the brace, while fitted, at the apical level of the main thoracic region for a right convex scoliosis. The orientation and shape of the pads facilitate local derotation, as shown in figure **a**. The right dorsal pad produces a main vector oriented from dorsal-lateral to ventral-medial direction. This main dorsal vector can be decomposed in two forces, one to medial (*b*) and the other one to ventral (*a*). The dorsal pad is closed enough to ventral in its anterior part to reach and still contact the middle axial line, providing lateral support enough. The ventral pad is oriented closest to the frontal plane and produces also a vector, which can be decomposed in two forces, one to dorsal (*a*) and a second to medial (*b*). The section of the brace at the frontal plane passing throughout the "middle axillar line" (*yellow line*) shows how the pad is still contacting the body on the right side but leaving room on the left side. The brace action (biomechanics) is explained by the final forces *a–a'*, forming a pair of forces for derotation, where *a* is a major force than *a'*, and *b'*, which produce the necessary right to left force for translation. While derotating to the left, the apical region will also translate to the left and at the same to the back coupled to the ribs (force *b* will be cancelled by this translation). Breathing mechanics will produce some dynamic reactive forces, increasing the three components *a, a'*, and *b'*, with the consequent expansion of non-contact areas. This expansion supposes an additional dynamic effect of derotation, reshaping the thorax, and fighting well against the morphological lordotization of the main thoracic region by increasing the sagittal diameter of the thorax

derotation force applied distally at the main thoracic region. As a counter-derotation pad, this sort of "stopping plate" is oriented on the frontal plane and has to be strictly perpendicular when observed from the lateral view (see next point about sagittal alignment and physiological profile). A second design is used when there is a primary or secondary (from previous brace usage) proximal thoracic structural curve. This second design is called "D modifier" (in accordance with the specific terminology used in the classification), and it is defined as a real proximal thoracic pad, which, like the main thoracic pad, is oriented to ventral and medial, and round shaped with a radius lightly bigger than the one of the ribs forming the proximal dorsal rib hump (Fig. 9 explains this in more detail). Most of the time, the "D modifier" pad needs to work in combination with a removable compression traction or just compression superstructure (Figs. 10 and 11). Please see further explanations in the text (cervico-thoracic region).

Correct balance and physiological alignment in the sagittal plane

A necessary base for correct trunk balance in the sagittal plane is a neutral pelvis inclination. Pelvis inclination must be in accordance with the individual "pelvic incidence." A correct sagittal balance depends basically on the relationship between pelvic indexes and the values of the maximum lumbar lordosis and maximum thoracic kyphosis, in absence of any sagittal morphological deformity. Thus, the possibility to achieve a correct sagittal balance and a more or less individualized correct sagittal alignment depends on the amount of morphological lordotization observed in the main thoracic region in relationship with the pelvic incidence. Reaching a correct sagittal balance and alignment is more difficult in cases with higher component of morphological lordotization in any region of the spine.

Therefore, this brace is not constructed to bring the pelvis into retroversion but supports its normal inclination to provide proximal continuity to the standard

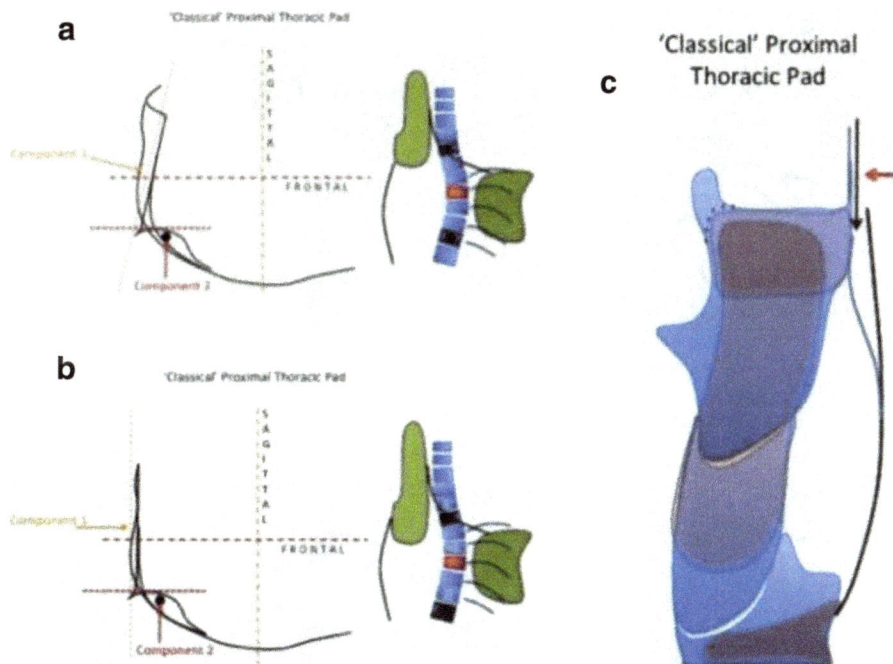

Fig. 8 This figure shows the classical proximal pad. It has two differentiated components: component 1 and component 2. Component 1 is the lateral component forming part of the "three-point system" correcting the main thoracic curve. This pad pushes the proximal thoracic region left to right, acting as the proximal point of the "three-point system." Its orientation depends basically on the observed plane of maximum deformity of the main thoracic curve. It is not so accurate like measuring the angle of the plane of maximum deformity. Scoliosis where the main thoracic curve is more oriented in the frontal plane, component 1 is oriented more in the pure sagittal plane (**b**). Scoliosis where the main thoracic curve is oriented in a more oblique plane to dorsal, component 1 is a little bit closed to ventral (**a**). Component 2 is a counter-rotation pad. Proximal region will tend to rotate to the left when the main thoracic region is over-derotated to the left. This pad stops rotation in the proximal region and help to produce a detorsional effect between the main thoracic curve and the proximal thoracic region. The orientation of this counter-rotation component when observed from the left side is perpendicular to the transversal plane of reference (**c**). The reason for is explained later in the text and Fig. 18. The proximal section is complemented by a ventral pad, which acts preventing the scapular anterior rotation

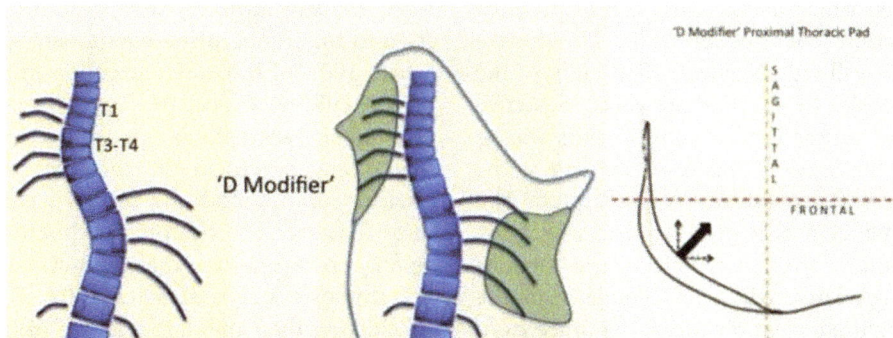

Fig. 9 The so-called D modifier is necessary when there is a structural curve in the proximal thoracic region. In such a case, the classical approach has to be modified to this "D modifier" design. The proximal pad has a unique component, like the main pad acting dorsally at the main thoracic region, but its radius is smaller. It does not work so high like the classical proximal pad but still high enough to produce correction of the main thoracic curve as the third proximal point of the "three-point system." The classical approach is not the best for this case because it will tend to increase the proximal structural curve, if this is already present in a clear way or hidden. The "D modifier" can be complemented by a compressing-traction principle (Fig. 12a)

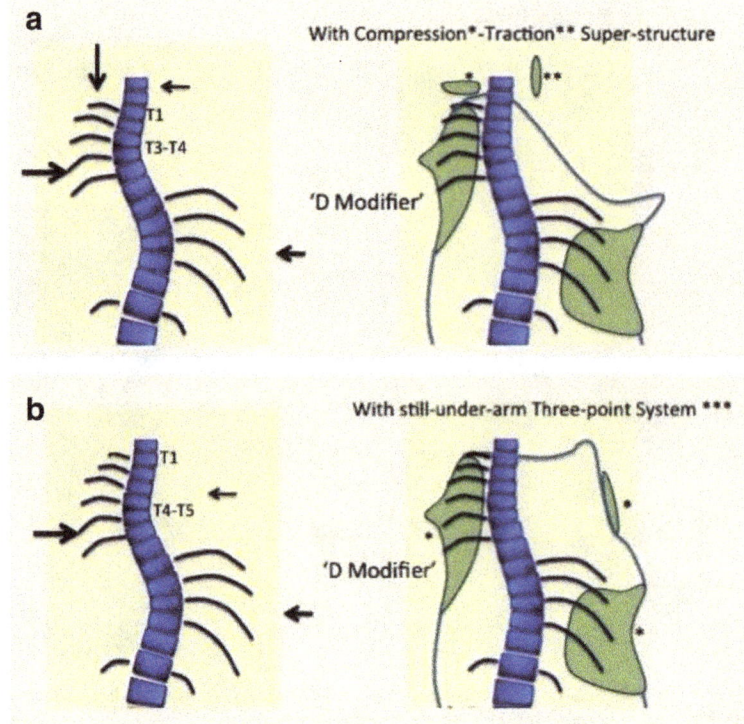

Fig. 10 The "D modifier" can be complemented by a compression-traction superstructure, when the apical region of the proximal curve is around T3–4 (**a**). The traction principle, applied from the left side, to pull the neck right to left, is the equivalent to the proximal point of the secondary "three-point system" working to correct the proximal curve, and it is complemented by a compressive force applied on the left trapezium prominent line, classically associated to the structural proximal curve. This proximal point of the "three-point system" can also be provided by an extra-high, but still underarm, right proximal pad, but only when the apical vertebra of the proximal curve is around T4–5 (**b**). Figure 13 shows the prototype of these two approaches

lumbar lordosis, all according to three basic sagittal types: (a) normal pelvic incidence, (b) high pelvic incidence, and (c) low pelvic incidence. Neither pelvis retroversion nor lumbar flattening is necessary to achieve good scoliosis correction when the above-explained principles are properly applied. Ventrally, the brace is constructed with expansion enough to produce abdominal contention but not pressure. Unselective abdominal pressure will only produce a flattening of the lumbar spine, opposite to the desired effect. Selective abdominal pressure, on the lumbar concave side, will be used to fix better the brace at this level, helping at the same time to derotate the lumbar scoliotic spine. The physiological sagittal alignment must be observed at the middle sagittal plane of the brace. Since some sections of the trunk are over-derotated, the physiological profile will be hardly recognized when observing the brace from one side or the other. In the classical design of a true double right thoracic/left lumbar curve, the brace will appear hypo-lordotic/hypo-kyphotic (lumbar and thoracic regions, respectively) when observed from the right convex thoracic side, while it will appear hyper-

lordotic/hyper-kyphotic when observed from the left concave thoracic side (Fig. 12).

No matter how physiological the brace shape, the sagittal alignment of the spine can hardly be reconstructed as 100% normal unless it is accepted that the correction of the anatomical lordosis in the thoracic region can reach 100% of in-brace correction. Bringing this expectation to the frontal plane component, is it reasonable to expect 100% of in-brace correction in the frontal plane? Why should we expect this in the sagittal plane? In any case, some very flexible spines, particularly those with single, long curves in the thoracic region can achieve total, or almost total, 3D in-brace correction. In most cases, however, the anatomical thoracic lordosis cannot be fully corrected such that the normal anatomical thoracic kyphosis is reconstructed 100%. For example, when considering the Cobb angle in the frontal plane, 50% of in-brace correction would be considered an excellent correction. Thus, a certain flattening of the spine will remain such that the geometry will usually be hypo-kyphotic in the thoracic region and, if well balanced, relatively hypo-lordotic in the lumbar region (Fig. 13).

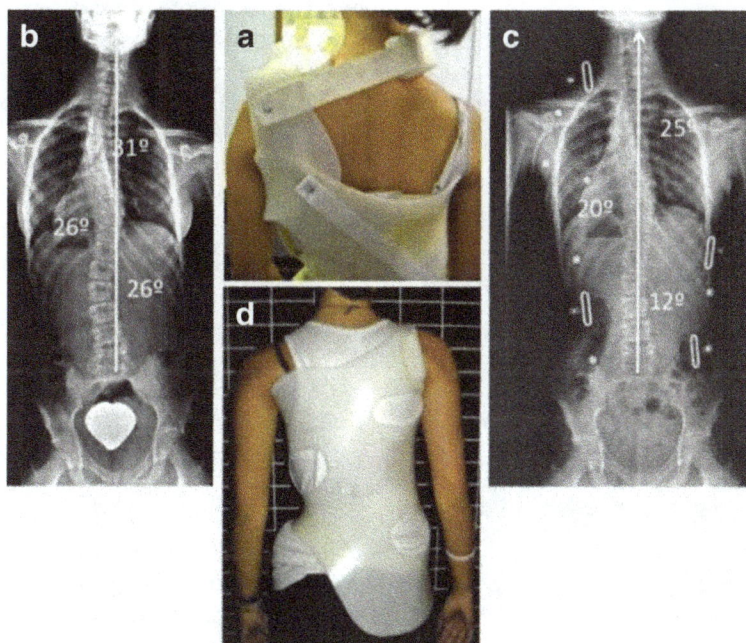

Fig. 11 A girl with a primary triple structural curve (left proximal 31°, right main thoracic 26°, and left lumbar 26°) (**b**), was fitted with a first prototype including "D modifier" proximal pad in combination with a removable compression-traction superstructure (**a**). The in-brace X-ray showed a mild correction of all the curves (**c**). Spinal balance was significantly improved with this brace, and proximal curve did not increased but decreased also significantly. After observing that the apical region of the proximal curve was relatively low (disc T4–5), it was decided to design a complex brace, which included a third "three-point system" still working underarm (**d**) (no X-ray available). This exclusive design formed by three underarm "three-point systems" had not been used ever before, to our knowledge, and helped to stabilize this scoliosis. The risk of failure is the highest for this curve pattern, especially in this particular case where the proximal curve is the major and most rigid one

The sagittal geometry of the spine is highly variable [27, 28]. To be pragmatic, scoliosis geometry in the sagittal plane can be described by using general terms: normo-kyphosis and normo-lordosis, hyper-kyphosis and hypo-lordosis, and hypo-kyphosis and hypo-lordosis. Additionally, the point where kyphosis becomes lordosis can be called geometrical transition, and should be located around the anatomical thoracolumbar anatomical region. In scoliotic spines, the geometrical transition can be located more proximally or distally to this region, such that the lumbar lordosis appears to be cranially extended or the thoracic

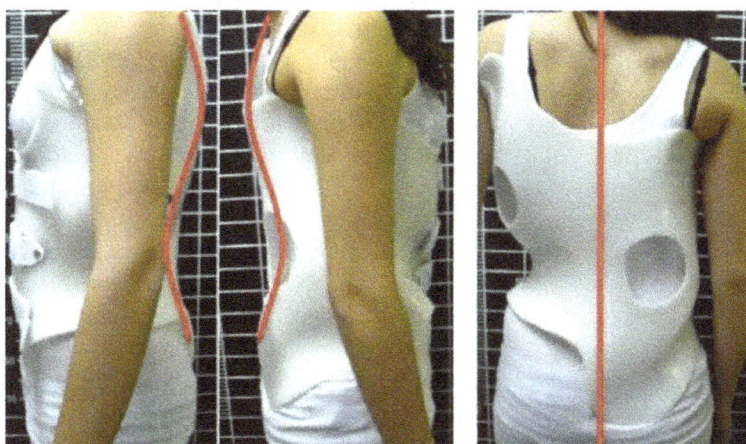

Fig. 12 The brace is always built with a more or less physiological profile. However, this cannot be observed from any side because it affects the middle sagittal plane. We currently suggest doing it more physiologic when the subject has a high "pelvic incidence" angle and less (hypo-lordotic/ hypo-kyphotic) when the subject has a lower "pelvic incidence" angle. In any case, sagittal postural balance will be the main sign confirming that the designed sagittal profile is accepted or not by any particular patient

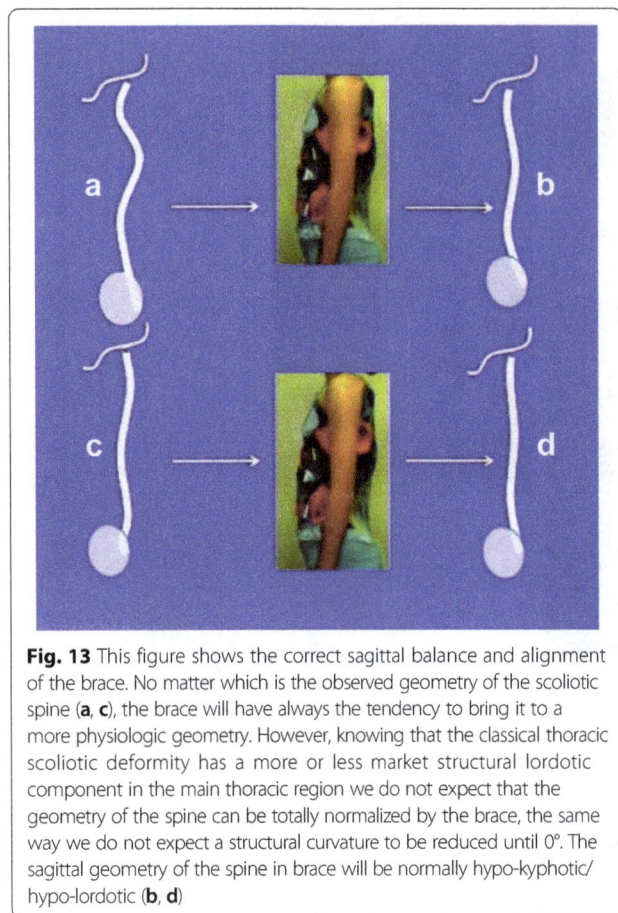

Fig. 13 This figure shows the correct sagittal balance and alignment of the brace. No matter which is the observed geometry of the scoliotic spine (**a**, **c**), the brace will have always the tendency to bring it to a more physiologic geometry. However, knowing that the classical thoracic scoliotic deformity has a more or less market structural lordotic component in the main thoracic region we do not expect that the geometry of the spine can be totally normalized by the brace, the same way we do not expect a structural curvature to be reduced until 0°. The sagittal geometry of the spine in brace will be normally hypo-kyphotic/hypo-lordotic (**b**, **d**)

kyphosis appears to be caudally extended. More so, the scoliotic spine can display better or worse harmony in its sagittal geometry; therefore, the regional thoracic and lumbar angles are not enough to describe the sagittal configuration of the scoliotic spine and should not be used to evaluate a brace's 3D correction. According to Bernhard and Bridwell [29], the anatomical thoracolumbar region (T10 to L2) should also act as the geometrical transition from thoracic kyphosis to lumbar lordosis; it should be neither fully kyphotic nor fully lordotic. This "normal" transitional geometry is observed in many scoliotic spines, while others present "abnormal" fully kyphotic or fully lordotic geometries. Figure 14 describes some examples that support this aforementioned variability in relationship with the curve pattern in the frontal plane.

During treatment, regardless of the curve pattern, a logical objective is to maintain the anatomical thoracolumbar region with its normal transitional kypho-lordotic geometry. As far as the brace using pads on both sides of the spine but not on the spine itself, the best possible restoration of the physiological spinal sagittal profile, including the anatomical thoracolumbar region with its transitional geometry, depends on how the pads from one side or the other are designed from the sagittal view. This method of pad placement is technically complex, as explained in Fig. 15.

The proximal thoracic region and the cervicothoracic transition are also considered from the sagittal perspective. The first thoracic vertebrae are still slightly lordotic. The designs of the Chêneau brace concept and some other TLSO concepts, but not all TLSOs, include an extension to the proximal thoracic region. For a classical right thoracic scoliosis, the Chêneau brace is extended cranially, reaching the proximal thoracic region on the left side (i.e., the concave thoracic side in opposition to the convex thoracic side on the right in this example). From one side, this upper extension provides a pure lateral-to-medial force and forms part of the three-point system designed to correct the frontal component of the main thoracic curve (also in Fig. 8). Alternatively, the upper extension also provides a counter-rotation force in a dorsal-to-ventral sense. In the classical Chêneau design, the counter-rotation support is applied on the dorsal aspect of the scapula on the concave thoracic side. From the lateral view, to provide the best counter-rotation force, the orientation of the support must be perpendicular (or parallel to the axial axis). Some orthotists, who were following Chêneau's principles but were most likely influenced by other concepts, designed this support to be ventrally tilted with the purpose of increasing the thoracic kyphosis (Fig. 16). However, this tilted support, combined with the anterior pad, forces the trunk into a flexion position, which produces an undesirable effect: the support brings the scapula in ventral rotation and does not effectively halt the dorsal rotation of the proximal ribs. This represents a failure of the counter-rotation effect, with the proximal vertebrae rotating in response to the correction exerted on the main thoracic region. Overall, this improper design, rather than creating kyphosis in the main thoracic region, facilitates the creation of a secondary proximal structural curve, which also develops with kyphosis.

The classical upper extension on the concave thoracic side can be generally used unless there is a structural proximal curve, primary or secondary to a previous brace treatment. In that case, we recommend applying a specific design called a "D modifier," where the upper extension works like a derotational pad rather than a counter-rotational pad. The D modifier is similar to the dorsal pad design for the main thoracic curve. The main limitation to treat a structural proximal curve is the theoretical need of a decollapsing effect on the proximal concavity. This can only be achieved by creating a three-point system with the use of a superstructure. The purpose of the superstructure is to provide a proximal

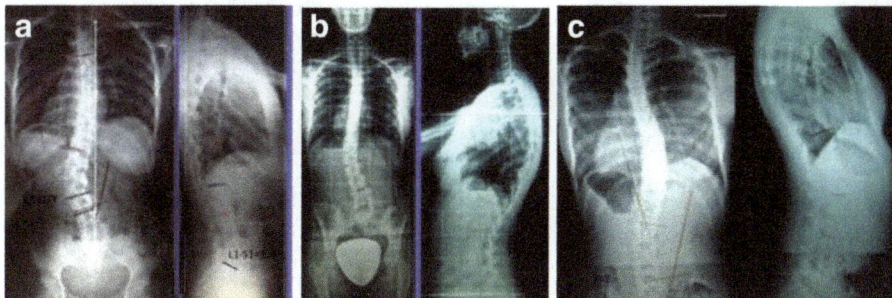

Fig. 14 The sagittal configuration of the scoliotic spine is too variable to be simplified with simplistic "dogmas" and solutions, like "scoliosis is a flat back deformity" or "scoliosis comes from **a** kyphotization of the thoracolumbar spine." The low thoracolumbar curve observed in **a** (apical vertebra L1) presents indeed a thoracolumbar kyphosis in the lateral projection, but the second one (**b**), with much less torsion, shows a still full lordotic configuration in the lateral projection. The very low thoracic curve observed in (**c**) is associated with a proximal thoracic curve and a distal short lumbar curve. The projection of this last scoliotic spine is clearly lordotic at the thoracolumbar region. Junctional thoracolumbar kyphosis is most commonly observed in true double major thoracic/lumbar curves. A torsional phenomenon rather than a single uniplanar failure can explain the high variability of sagittal configurations observed in relationship with the frontal curve pattern

counter-pressure applied on the lateral aspect of the neck on the convex thoracic side (main thoracic curve) while applying a compression mechanism for the proximal convexity on the trapezium prominence. Figure 13 has shown the D modifier working with a type of suggested superstructure, but any other design with similar effect could be used. In any case, the use of the superstructure makes the brace more visible and, thus, increases brace-related stress. We recently introduced a technical variation, which consists of an additional full three-point system, still working under-arm, but only in case the apex of the proximal curve is T4–5, not T3. Since adolescents do not readily accept the first technical solution, we previously recommended a removable superstructure to be used only at home, enabling patients to experience a social life without the more visible superstructure. The second technical solution is theoretically more acceptable

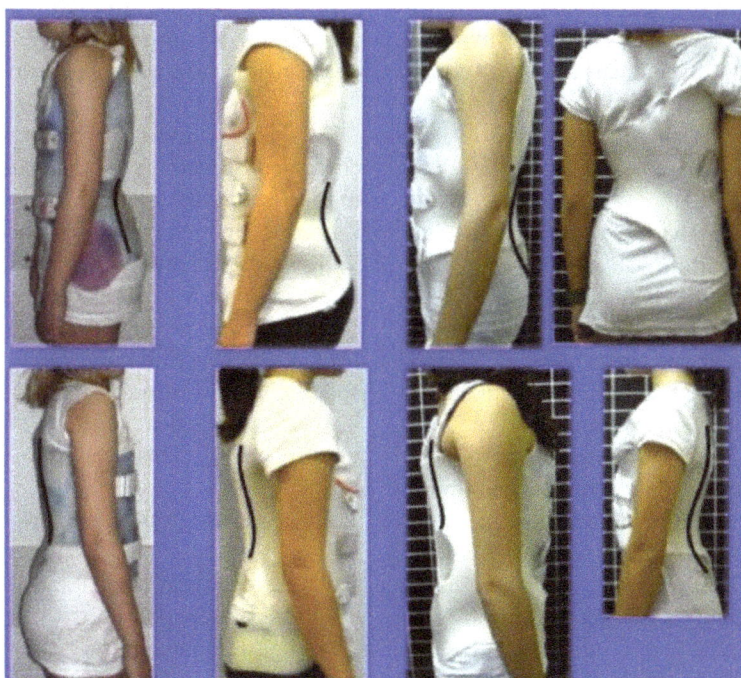

Fig. 15 This figure shows four different brace designs. All of them are physiological at the middle sagittal plane but their very market asymmetric design makes them appear very different when observed from one side or the other. First one is an A1 type, second is A2, third is B1, and last E1 (names according to the Rigo classification and brace design)

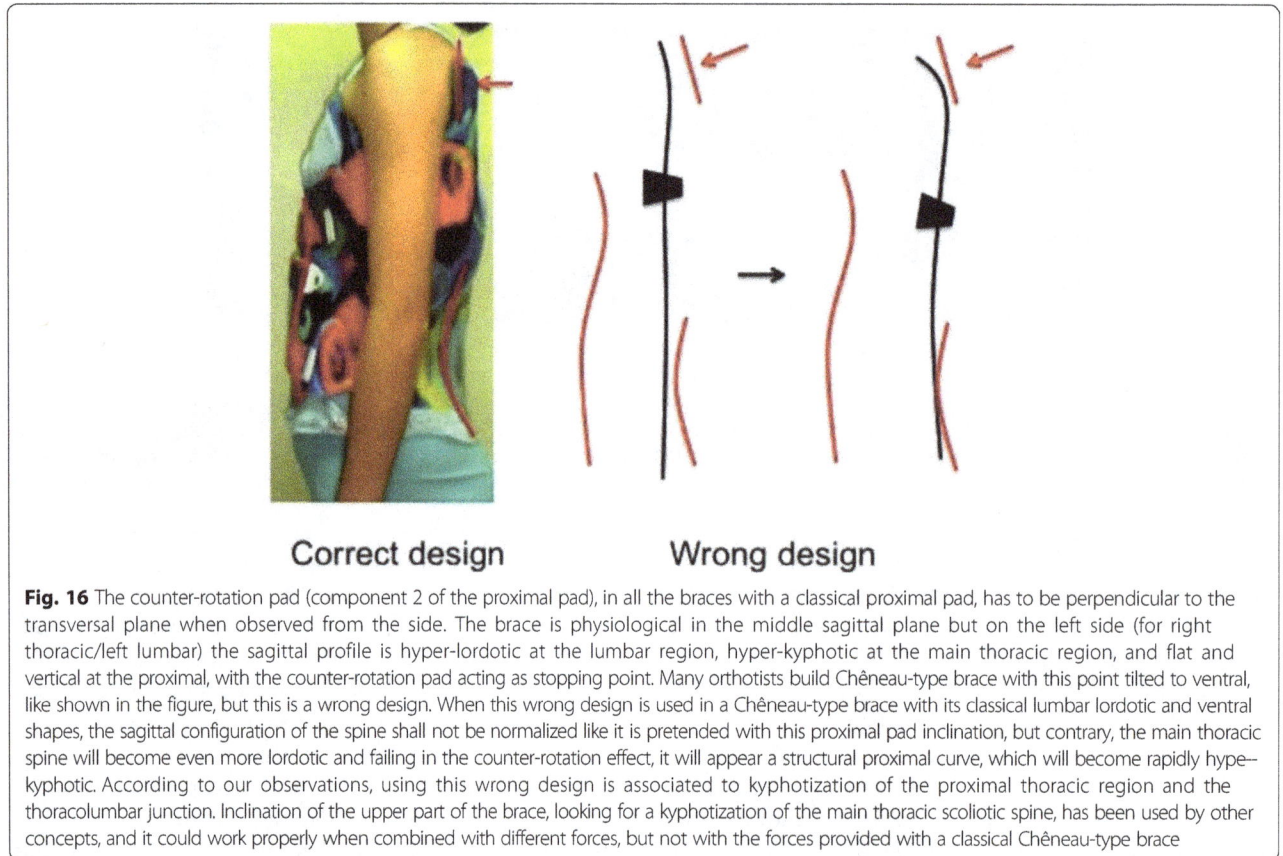

Fig. 16 The counter-rotation pad (component 2 of the proximal pad), in all the braces with a classical proximal pad, has to be perpendicular to the transversal plane when observed from the side. The brace is physiological in the middle sagittal plane but on the left side (for right thoracic/left lumbar) the sagittal profile is hyper-lordotic at the lumbar region, hyper-kyphotic at the main thoracic region, and flat and vertical at the proximal, with the counter-rotation pad acting as stopping point. Many orthotists build Chêneau-type brace with this point tilted to ventral, like shown in the figure, but this is a wrong design. When this wrong design is used in a Chêneau-type brace with its classical lumbar lordotic and ventral shapes, the sagittal configuration of the spine shall not be normalized like it is pretended with this proximal pad inclination, but contrary, the main thoracic spine will become even more lordotic and failing in the counter-rotation effect, it will appear a structural proximal curve, which will become rapidly hype–kyphotic. According to our observations, using this wrong design is associated to kyphotization of the proximal thoracic region and the thoracolumbar junction. Inclination of the upper part of the brace, looking for a kyphotization of the main thoracic scoliotic spine, has been used by other concepts, and it could work properly when combined with different forces, but not with the forces provided with a classical Chêneau-type brace

but, in practice, causes more discomfort due to the relatively short distance between points. Obviously, this curve pattern shows an increased risk of brace failure so clinical control should be very careful in these cases and expectations should be realistic.

Results

We describe in this section the brace design and blueprints according to curve pattern.

The brace design is based on the application of the aforementioned principles of correction, according to the different curve patterns. A curve pattern-specific classification was developed based on clinical and radiological criteria. The classification contains most of the curve types that require treatment and has been shown to be reliable [10]. In this paper, the classification has been revisited and, after years of use in a clinical setting, some minor changes have been introduced to facilitate its use.

To use the classification properly, we recommend first examining the patient and then reviewing the radiograph.

The first step is to identify one of the following four basic clinical types:

1) Three-curve pattern or A type

2) Four-curve pattern or B type
3) Non-3, non-4 or C type
4) Single lumbar/thoracolumbar or E type

This first clinical diagnosis is based exclusively on clinical observations of the patient, without any information from the radiograph. Christa Lehnert-Schroth was the first to describe these basic clinical types [30], whose descriptions herein are slightly different than Lehnert-Schroth's descriptions. The four basic types, showed in Figs. 17, 18, 19, and 20, have been previously described in the original paper about the specific classification [10].

Also radiological criteria have been previously described [10]. This is a short review, introducing few little changes.

Three radiological criteria are used:

1) Curve pattern compatibility
2) Transitional point offset
3) L4–L5 counter-tilting

1) First radiological criterion: curve pattern compatibility

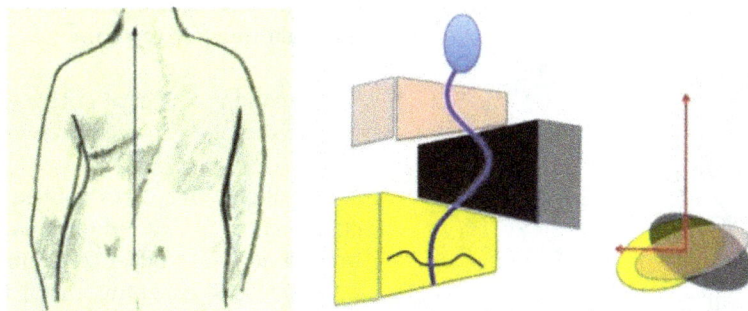

Fig. 17 This figure shows the clinical picture and the modified Schroth's schema of blocks for the functional three-curve pattern (3C). This functional pattern is called in Rigo classification A type. From observation of the clinical picture, the trunk can be here divided into three blocks or regions, with the main thoracic region affected by the main structural thoracic curve and the lower and upper trunk affected by both upper and lower compensations. The three consequent blocks are translated and rotated one against the other, collapsed on the concavities and expanded on the convexities. The main thoracic and proximal thoracic blocks are imbalanced to the right side according to the lower lumbo-pelvic block (including this last the central sacral line). The lumbo-pelvic block is translated to the left according to the polygon of sustentation, with the left hip joint in a relative adduction in comparison with the right hip joint. In case there is a lumbar structural curve, this is still coupled to the pelvis. The schema of blocks offers to the clinicians, physiotherapists, and orthotists a clear composition of the scoliotic phenomenon in 3D and can be taken as a guide for the 3D correction. When the main thoracic curve is convex to the right, the used term is "right 3D or right A type." The mirror case exists and it is called "left 3C or A type"

The curve pattern is defined according to a modified Moe and Kettleson classification [31]. Following is the SRS terminology that is used to define the name of the curve [32].

Figure 21 summarizes the initial radiological criteria, which is used as a first step in the confirmation protocol once a clinical diagnosis of first suspicion is made. Curve pattern compatibility means that not all curve patterns fit in a particular basic type. As described below, every basic type finds some curve patterns that fit with it and, at the same time, defines a subtype: A1, A2, A3, B1, B2, C1, C2, E1, E2.

Two relevant changes from the original description:

Subtype A1 is characterized by a long-low single thoracic curve. Low means that apical vertebra use to be in the low thoracic region (T9, T10, T11). Long means that the curve goes down into the lumbar region, being L4 the first horizontal vertebra (sometimes L5). If L3 is horizontal, we classify then A2, no matter whether the curve is long and low. In B type, there are always two structural curves, one in the main thoracic region and another in the lumbar or thoracolumbar region. B type is typically a double major curve or a double major/minor, with the lumbar or thoracolumbar curve being

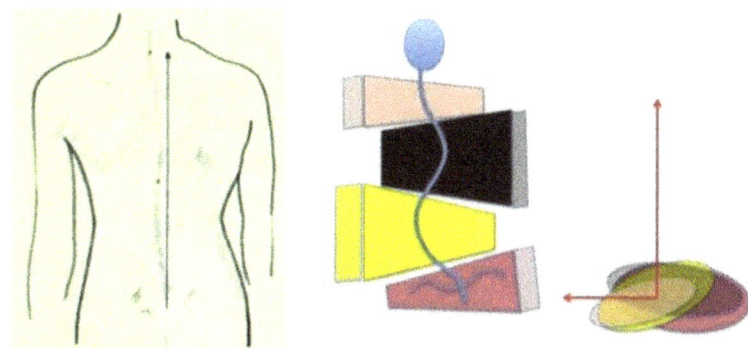

Fig. 18 This figure shows the clinical picture and schema of blocks or regions for a four-curve pattern. This is called B type in Rigo classification. This type is characterized by a lumbosacral compensatory curve. The trunk is consequently divided into four blocks or regions, translated and rotated one against the other, collapsed on the concavities and expanded on the convexities. The three upper blocks, lumbar or thoracolumbar, main thoracic and proximal thoracic are imbalanced to the left according to the most caudal pelvic block (including this last the central sacral line). Pelvis is translated to the right according to the polygon of sustentation, so right hip joint is in relative adduction in comparison with left hip joint. This description corresponds to a "right 4C or B type." The mirror case exists for a left convex thoracic curve combined with right lumbar or thoracolumbar and it is called "left 4C or B type"

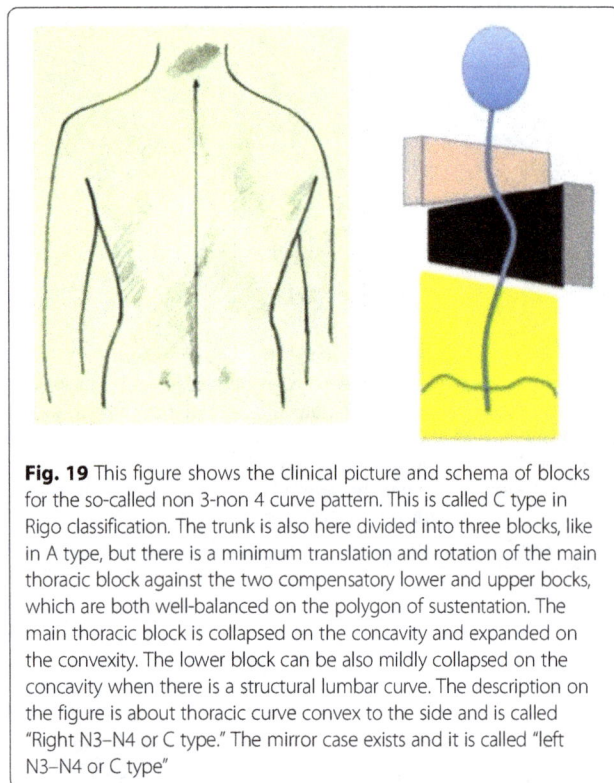

Fig. 19 This figure shows the clinical picture and schema of blocks for the so-called non 3-non 4 curve pattern. This is called C type in Rigo classification. The trunk is also here divided into three blocks, like in A type, but there is a minimum translation and rotation of the main thoracic block against the two compensatory lower and upper bocks, which are both well-balanced on the polygon of sustentation. The main thoracic block is collapsed on the concavity and expanded on the convexity. The lower block can be also mildly collapsed on the concavity when there is a structural lumbar curve. The description on the figure is about thoracic curve convex to the side and is called "Right N3–N4 or C type." The mirror case exists and it is called "left N3–N4 or C type"

thoracic region. E2 is like B2 lacking structural curve at the main thoracic region.

2) Second radiological criterion: transitional point (TP) according to the central sacral line (CSL)

Transitional point was defined in the original paper on classification [10]. We do not use more T1 offset but just transitional point offset to confirm A, B, or C type. The reference is the central sacral line (CSL). Transitional point offset is to the convex thoracic side in A types and to the concave thoracic side in B types. In C type, transitional point is more or less balanced on the CSL. We have not been able to establish a threshold offset value to confirm A or B type at this present time, but we are working on this. It is not easy to differentiate between A and C types in some cases, when TP is not perfectly balanced on the CSL but the offset is not enough to produce a clinical picture where thorax-pelvis imbalance is so clear.

3) Third radiological criterion: L4–L5 counter-tilting

This criterion was also described in the original paper on classification [10]. It is positive when L4 is more tilted than L5 and negative when L4 and L5 are parallel. This criterion is only necessary to confirm B type and, when necessary, to differentiate between B type and C type. B types are associated with a positive L4–L5 counter-tilting. C types are associated with a negative L4–L5 counter-tilting.

E types are like B when describing the lumbosacral region, so it will always show a positive L4–L5 counter-tilting (at least in idiopathic scoliosis).

the major one. However, it can be also major thoracic and minor lumbar or thoracolumbar. The subtype B1 is defined by the apical vertebra of the lower structural curve at L2 or L1. The subtype B2 is defined by the apical vertebra at T12, the same for subtypes E1 and E2. E1 is like B1 without structural curve at the main

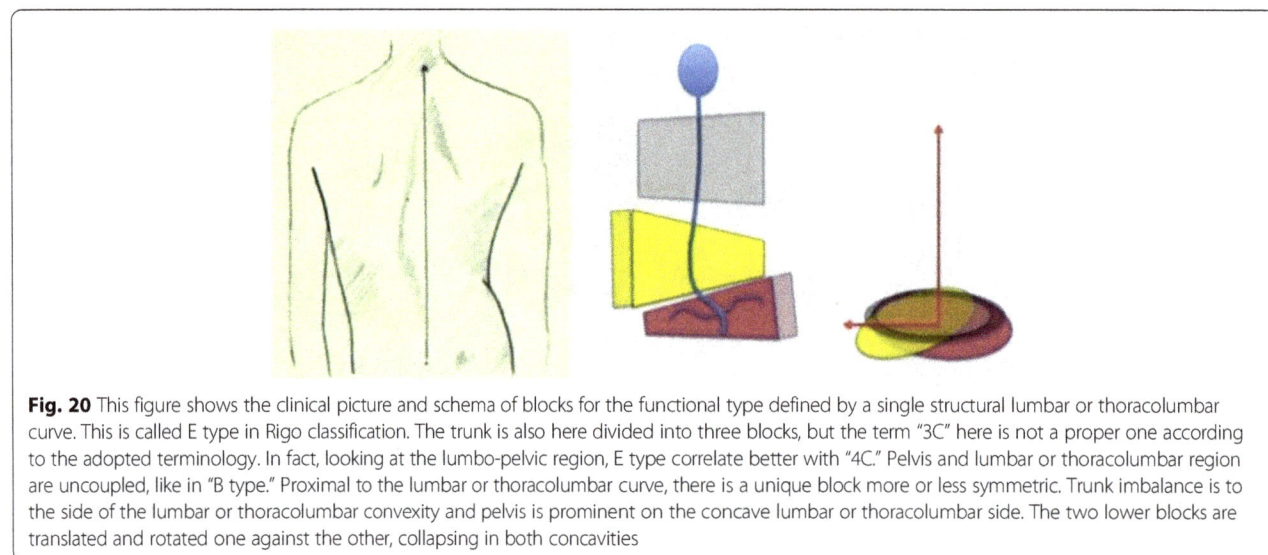

Fig. 20 This figure shows the clinical picture and schema of blocks for the functional type defined by a single structural lumbar or thoracolumbar curve. This is called E type in Rigo classification. The trunk is also here divided into three blocks, but the term "3C" here is not a proper one according to the adopted terminology. In fact, looking at the lumbo-pelvic region, E type correlate better with "4C". Pelvis and lumbar or thoracolumbar region are uncoupled, like in "B type." Proximal to the lumbar or thoracolumbar curve, there is a unique block more or less symmetric. Trunk imbalance is to the side of the lumbar or thoracolumbar convexity and pelvis is prominent on the concave lumbar or thoracolumbar side. The two lower blocks are translated and rotated one against the other, collapsing in both concavities

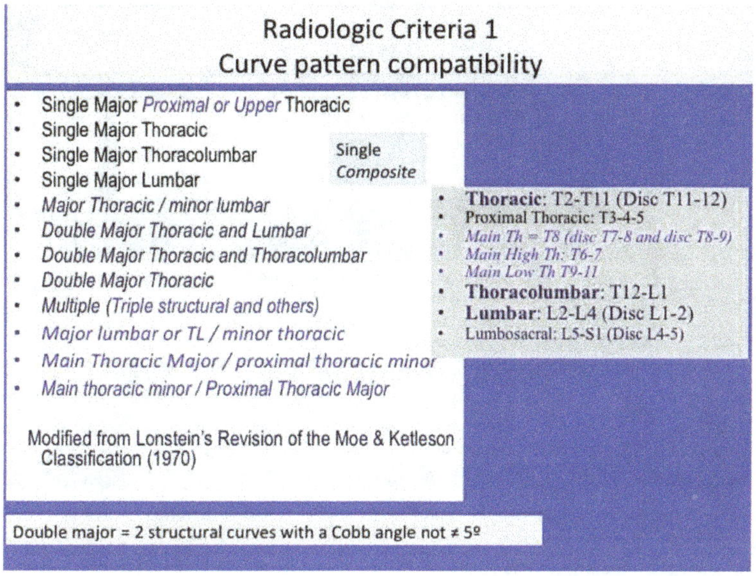

Fig. 21 The first radiological criterion is called "curve pattern compatibility." Any curve is defined according to the apical level following SRS terminology. Structural curve is not defined directly from the radiograph but from clinical observation and exploration. A clinically defined structural curve is used to be confirmed on the radiograph by certain amount of rotation or vertebral wedging (no matter the Cobb angle). Once the curve/s have been defined, we use a modified Lonstein's revision of the classical Moe and Kettleson classification. Double major is defined when two structural curves have a Cobb angle not different to 5°. Single curve is used just when there is one single structural curve. One pattern more is defined in the composite group, called "major lumbar or thoracolumbar with minor thoracic." This is here necessary because a real single lumbar or thoracolumbar is classified as E type and will get a short brace while "major lumbar or thoracolumbar with minor thoracic" is classified B type and will get a long brace. The term structural proximal curve is not only used for thoracic double major curve. A minor structural proximal curve can be observed, primary or secondary to bracing. Sometimes the proximal curve is clearly visible clinically but not easy to confirm radiologically (hidden proximal curve). Clinical signs for a proximal thoracic curve are elevation of the shoulder with a prominence of the trapezium line in combination with a deviation of the spinous processes line and costal prominence in forward bending. The proximal curve can be also a major, combined with a minor structural curve in the main thoracic region

The "D modifier."

Any of the above described A, B, or C type could be associated with a primary or secondary (from previous bracing) proximal structural curve.

A full description of all the radiological criteria confirming the different subtypes A1, A2, A3, B1, B2, C1, C2, E1, and E2 can be seen in Figs. 22, 23, 24, 25, 26, 27, 28, 29, 30, 31, 32, 33, 34, 35, 36, and 37.

The brace (blueprints)

Every basic type 3C (A type), 4C (B type), N3N4 (C type), or single lumbar/thoracolumbar (E type) is treated following specific principles that were described in the previous sections. Below is the more specific application of the three-point system principle according to the different types.

Specific designs and construction for "A" types

The A1 type is treated with a simple main three-point system, while A2 and A3 need a secondary three-point system to complement the main one. Figures 6 and 38 show the application of corrective principles for A1 and

A2/A3, respectively. Figures 39, 40, 41, and 42 show the blueprints and brace examples.

The function of the three-point system is to bring the trunk into the best possible correction in the frontal plane. For a classical right convex thoracic scoliosis, we need to translate the main thoracic region right to left in between the two caudal (lumbo-pelvic) and cranial (proximal thoracic) regions. A caudal pelvic pad with a strong dorso-lateral lumbar support on the left side, a more proximal main thoracic pad on the right side, and the most cranial pad for the proximal thoracic region on the left side form the main three-point system. When constructing these pads on the positive mould and to achieve the best possible correction, the technician should bring the left proximal pad as high and medial as possible. As described above, the orientation of the main thoracic pad allows it to work from one side and in its lateral component as a part of this main three-point system, while forming part of the dorsal component of the pair-of-force for derotation. The lumbo-pelvic as well as the proximal thoracic regions, including the shoulder girdle, have to be maintained in the best case

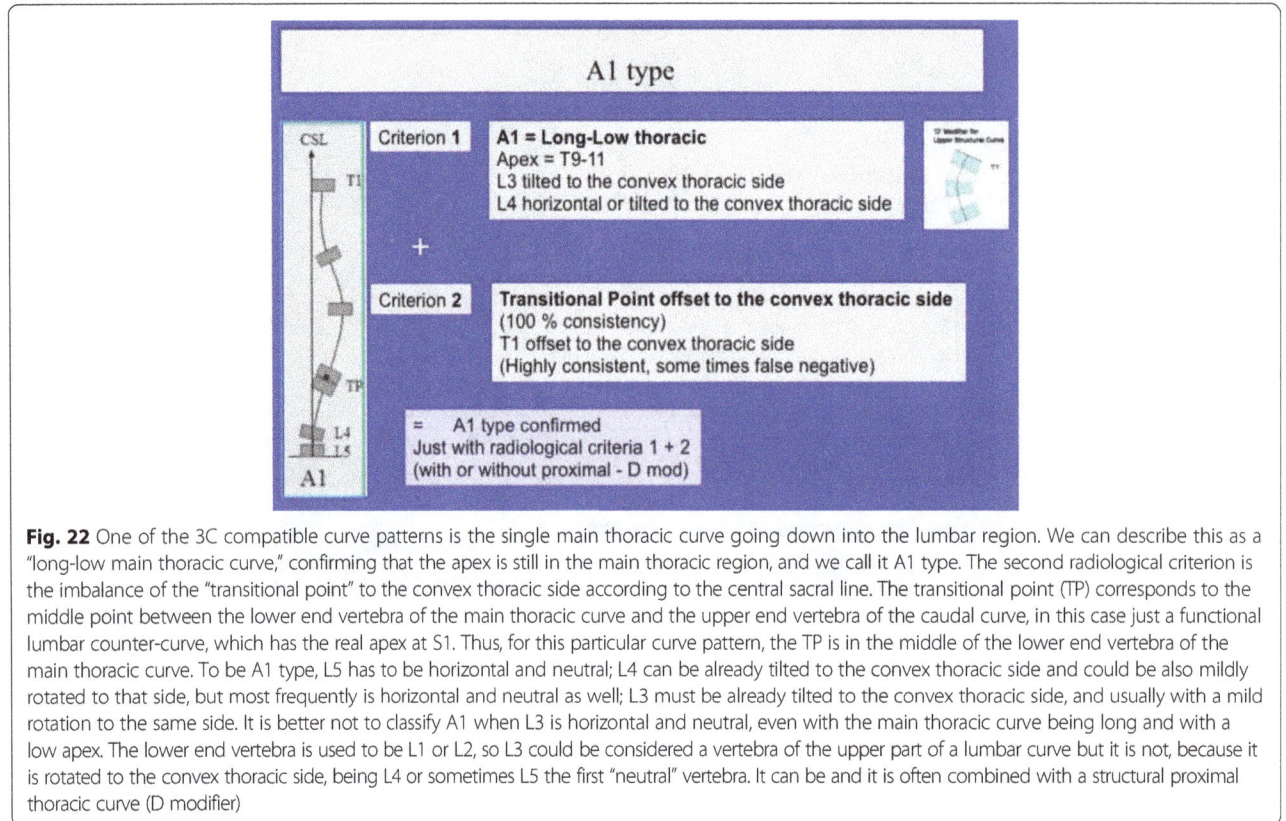

Fig. 22 One of the 3C compatible curve patterns is the single main thoracic curve going down into the lumbar region. We can describe this as a "long-low main thoracic curve," confirming that the apex is still in the main thoracic region, and we call it A1 type. The second radiological criterion is the imbalance of the "transitional point" to the convex thoracic side according to the central sacral line. The transitional point (TP) corresponds to the middle point between the lower end vertebra of the main thoracic curve and the upper end vertebra of the caudal curve, in this case just a functional lumbar counter-curve, which has the real apex at S1. Thus, for this particular curve pattern, the TP is in the middle of the lower end vertebra of the main thoracic curve. To be A1 type, L5 has to be horizontal and neutral; L4 can be already tilted to the convex thoracic side and could be also mildly rotated to that side, but most frequently is horizontal and neutral as well; L3 must be already tilted to the convex thoracic side, and usually with a mild rotation to the same side. It is better not to classify A1 when L3 is horizontal and neutral, even with the main thoracic curve being long and with a low apex. The lower end vertebra is used to be L1 or L2, so L3 could be considered a vertebra of the upper part of a lumbar curve but it is not, because it is rotated to the convex thoracic side, being L4 or sometimes L5 the first "neutral" vertebra. It can be and it is often combined with a structural proximal thoracic curve (D modifier)

with no rotation (i.e., the frontal plane of both regions should coincide with the frontal plane of reference). The proximal thoracic region will need a counter-rotation force integrated in the upper pad. In A2 and A3 types, a counter-trochanter pad is necessary on the right side to provide a secondary three-point system, facilitating a better postural balance in

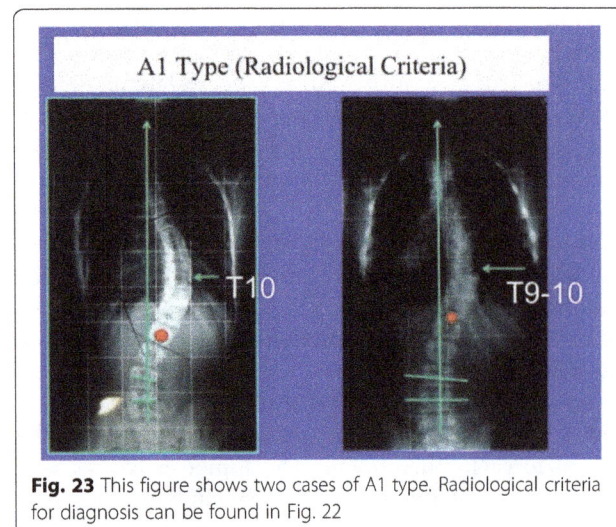

Fig. 23 This figure shows two cases of A1 type. Radiological criteria for diagnosis can be found in Fig. 22

the frontal plane. To keep the patient vertical, it is necessary to stretch the soft tissues from the lumbo-pelvic concavity, which are shortened in the axial direction; otherwise, the trunk would bend to the right side due to their tension. In A1 type, the main thoracic pad is larger in the cranio-caudal direction compared with A2 and A3 types and enables the shortened soft tissues from the lumbo-pelvic concavity to be stretched more efficiently with the frontal plane translation obtained from the action of the left lumbo-pelvic pad and the right large thoracic pad, including the upper lumbar, the thoracolumbar, and the main thoracic regions. In this way, the A1-type brace can be constructed without the right counter-trochanter pad and the pelvic area can be opened on the right side.

Specific designs and construction for "B" types

The B type is treated with two main three-point systems (the principle of correction can be seen in Fig. 43). The caudal system is designed to correct the lumbar or thoracolumbar structural curve and a more proximal system acts on the main thoracic curve. In B types, the pelvis and lumbar regions are not coupled, so they cannot be corrected together against the main thoracic region, but one against the other. Thus, for a classical left

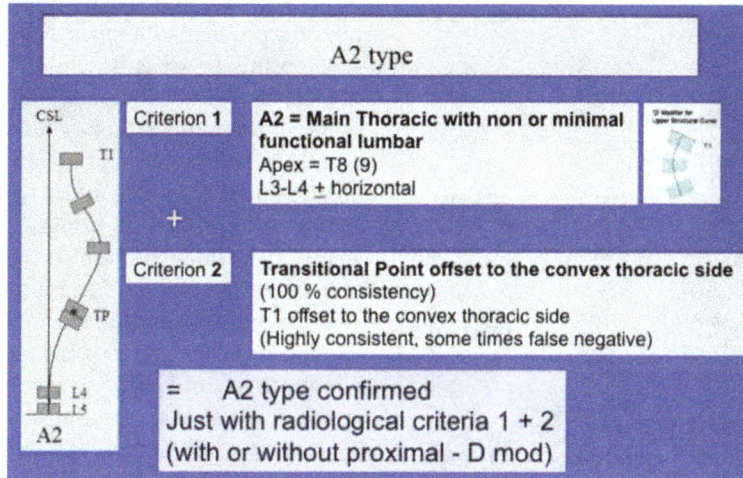

Fig. 24 The second 3C compatible curve pattern is the classical "single main thoracic curve" with no lumbar or just a mild totally functional lumbar curve. This is called A2 type. Second criterion for diagnose is the TP offset to the convex thoracic side. It can be combined with a structural proximal thoracic curve (D modifier)

lumbar/thoracolumbar combined with right thoracic, the most distal pad of the caudal system is located on the lateral aspect of the right pelvis, between the iliac crest and the trochanter; the medium pad pushes on the left lumbar or thoracolumbar prominence; and the most proximal pad puts pressure on the thoracic rib hump. When doing the modification of the positive mould, pelvis has to be translated to the concave thoracic side (right to left for a right thoracic/left lumbar) in about 10 cm or more, while lumbar pad is built gently to offer

a stopping point. For the proximal three-point system, the most distal pad presses on the lumbar or thoracolumbar prominence, the medium pad pushes on the thoracic rib hump, and the proximal pad puts pressure on the left proximal thoracic region. The construction of this proximal system in B type is similar to the A type, although it may be shorter in the cranio-caudal direction.

The B-type brace can be built with the pelvis open in most cases, but it may be necessary to use a counter-

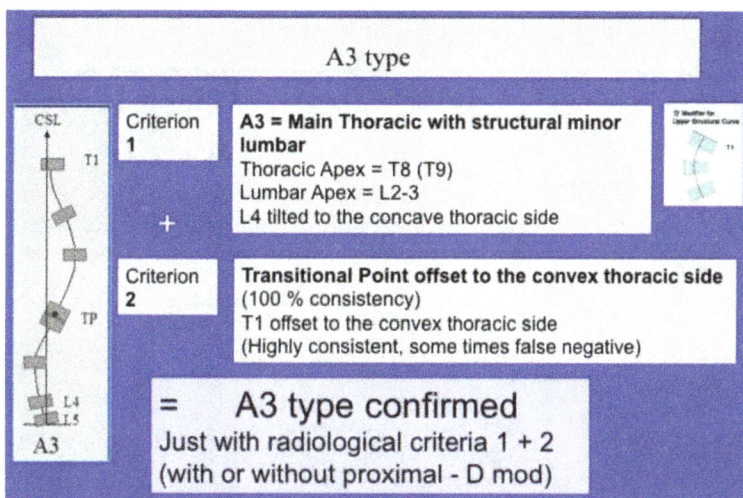

Fig. 25 The third 3C compatible curve pattern is the composite "major main thoracic"/"minor lumbar." Both curves are structural but lumbar is a more flexible, minor, probably secondary curve. This is called A3 type and the second radiological criteria to confirm 3C is the TP offset to the convex thoracic side, like in A1 and A2 types. Due to the lumbar structural curve, it is wrongly taken like 4C by many Chêneau followers, but a structural lumbar curve is not criterion enough to decide about using a 4C brace design. It can be combined, like most of types by a primary or secondary or iatrogenic proximal thoracic curve

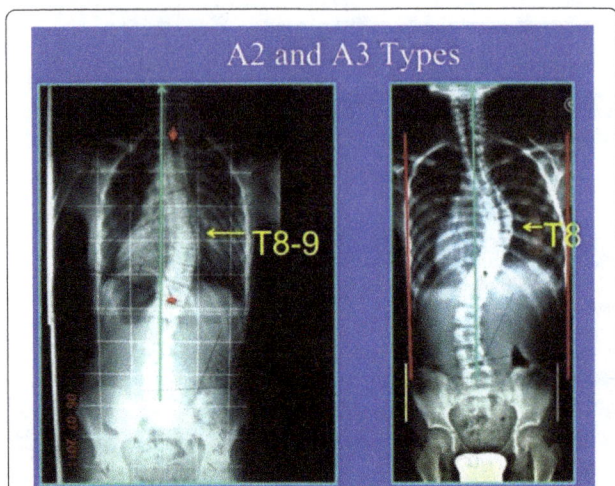

Fig. 26 This figure shows two cases of A2 type (*left*) and A3 type (*right*). Radiological criteria can be found in Figs. 24 and 25

trochanter pad on the left side (for the example used here of right thoracic/left lumbar or TL). However, the decision about when to use an open pelvis or when to close it to provide the counter-trochanter pad is not based here, as in A type, on the diagnosis of a particular subtype. Both B1 and B2 can be built with a complete pelvis or with an open pelvis. We cannot give an evidence-based explanation about the cause or causes of the frontal plane imbalance in B type scoliosis, so we cannot explain why some patients attain in-brace

balance of T1 and TP on the CSL, accepting with no relevant problems the open pelvis design.

Blueprints to treat B1 and B2 are the same (Figs. 44, 45, 46, and 47). The main difference is the size and shape of the lumbar/thoracolumbar pad. B1 is a more or less wide pad in the cranio-caudal direction, depending on the apical level, the most typical L2 and L1. We design a real pad, which brings, with a highly anatomical shape, the whole prominent region to a more ventral and medial position. Covering the lower ribs with the pad has historically not been a problem when allowing enough room ventrally at the same level and dorsally in a lower level, and allowing pelvis ante-version, especially at the gluteus region on the same side. The pad in B2 is a very large thoracolumbar pad, which has to provide the maximum derotational effect at the T12 level. The pad has a very accurate and difficult-to-achieve 3D shape and orientation, contributing in its lower part to create lumbar lordosis, in its upper part to allow thoracic kyphosis, and as a whole to maintain the thoracolumbar region as a geometrical transitional region.

Specific designs and construction for "C" types

C1–2 braces are built now most with the pelvis open, like 4C, at the concave thoracic side, but while modifying the positive mould, the pelvis section is considered the neutral caudal reference and consequently shall not be translated like in 4C. Pelvis can be fixed between a lumbar support and a counter supra-trochanter pad on the convex thoracic side. Although it looks like in B

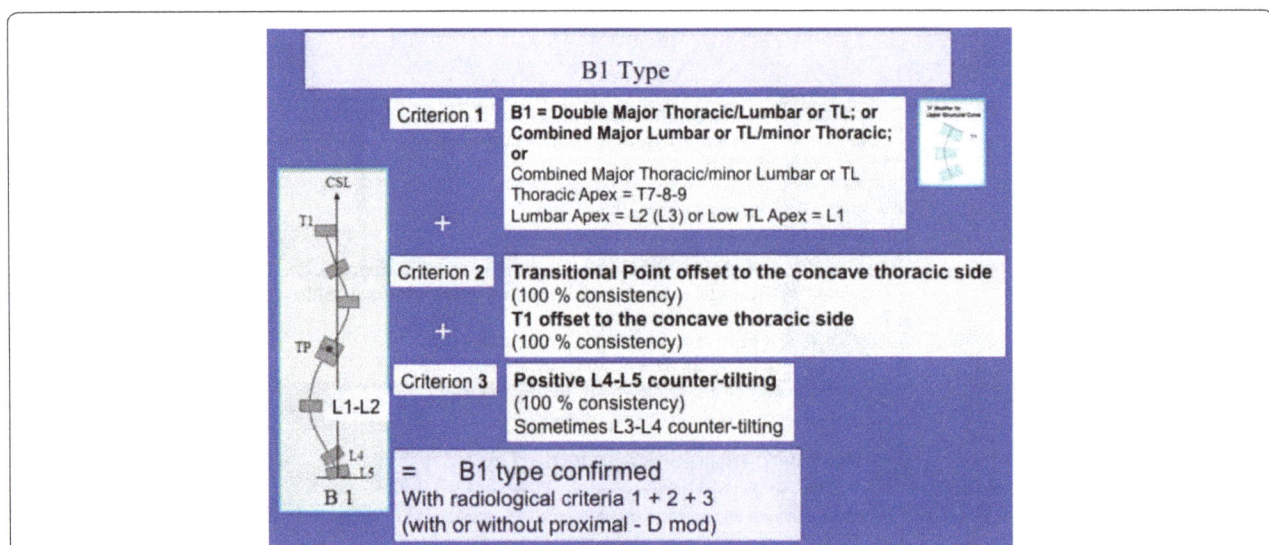

Fig. 27 Classical double structural scoliosis, main thoracic/lumbar (apex L2) or low thoracolumbar (apex L1) is the most common 4C compatible curve pattern. This is called B1 type. It can be double major, major lumbar-low thoracolumbar/minor thoracic, or rarely major thoracic/minor lumbar-low thoracolumbar. The second radiological criterion is the TP (and T1) offset to the concave thoracic side according the CSL. A third criterion is the L4–L5 positive counter-tilting. It can be combined with a structural proximal thoracic curve (triple structural scoliosis)

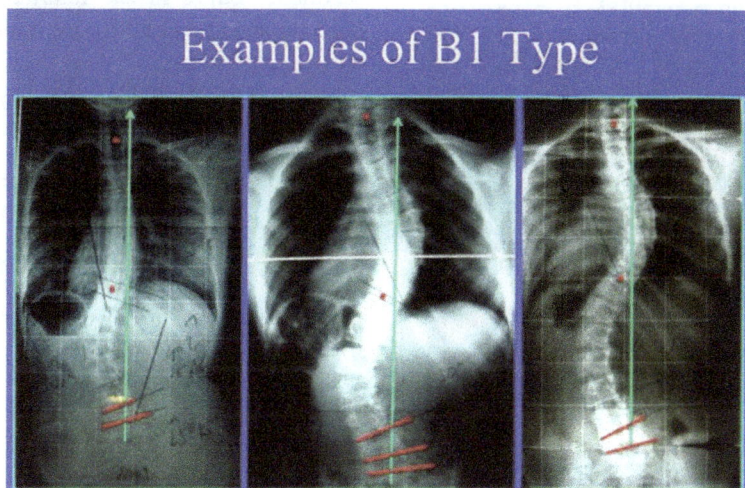

Fig. 28 This figure shows three different cases fulfilling all the criteria for B1 type

type, it is not. There is a significant difference in the design of the B lumbar pad and the C lumbar support as can be seen in Figs. 48 and 49. Lumbar support and counter-supra-trochanter pad form a system to block the pelvis in a stable position, balanced on the polygon of sustentation and well oriented in the frontal plane.

Specific designs and construction for "E" types

The brace design for E1 and E2 is a short one, with a single three-point system to correct the single lumbar/thoracolumbar curve. At lumbo-pelvic level, the brace has exactly the same design as B1 and B2, respectively, with or without the counter-trochanter pad. However, the short brace is not just a long brace where the proximal thoracic pad has been eliminated. Since there is no structural main thoracic curve, it is not necessary to design a "deflection-derotation system" acting on the main thoracic region. At the main thoracic region, simply a counter-thoracic lateral pad is necessary to prevent the secondary formation of a functional thoracic curve, which could become structural later. This counter-thoracic pad has to act from lateral to medial and just caudal to the virtual apex of the secondary curve

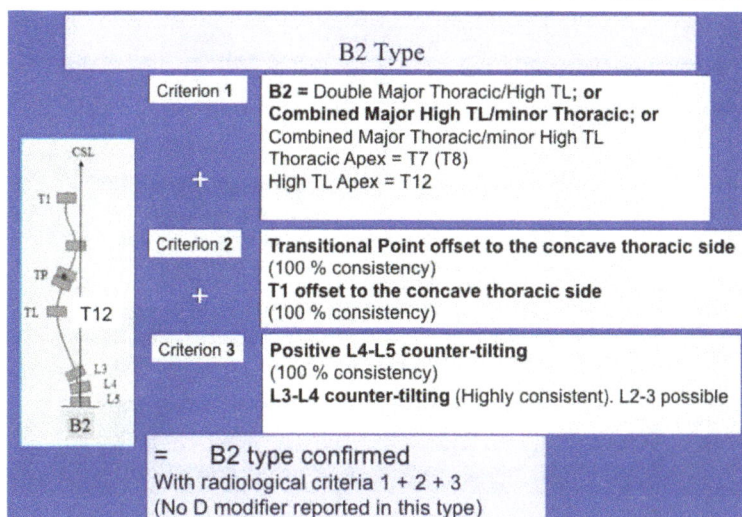

Fig. 29 The so-called B2 type is a 4C compatible curve pattern defined by a high main thoracic structural curve combined with a long-high thoracolumbar curve, with the apex at T12. The second and third radiological criteria for 4C are also accomplished (TP offset to the concave thoracic side and L4–L5 positive counter-tilting). Very rarely it can be also combined with a short structural proximal thoracic curve (mostly iatrogenic)

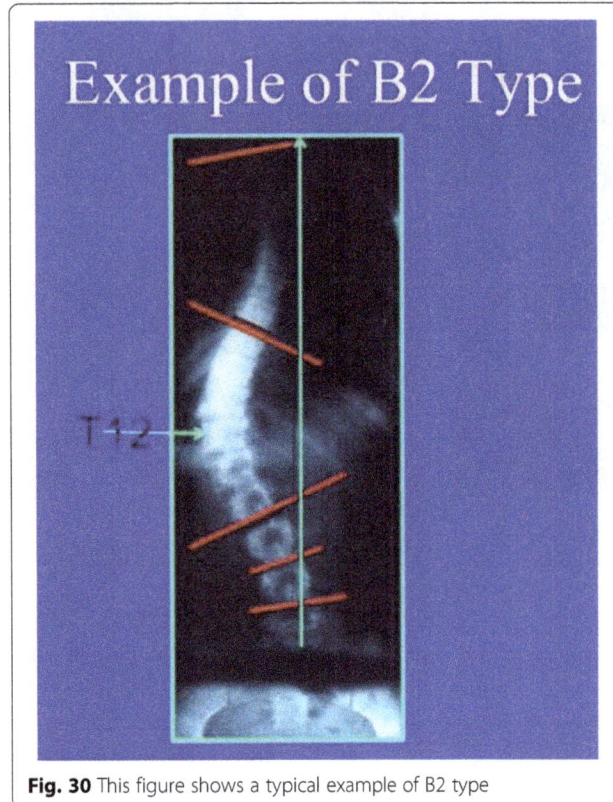

Fig. 30 This figure shows a typical example of B2 type

produced in the main thoracic region. Dorsally, the brace can extend from cranial to the virtual apex to produce a stopping counter-rotation effect, but laterally it has to be cut caudal to the level of the virtual thoracic apex; otherwise, it will facilitate the formation of a

secondary curve in the main thoracic region that can become structural and potentially progressive (Figs. 50 and 51).

How to prescribe the brace?

It is a more or less generalized rule in this field that different curve patterns require different brace concepts or orthopedic products, which can be prescribed according to the doctor's specific knowledge, experience, and preferences. However, although a prescription of "Chêneau brace" exists with its own reference code number in the list of orthopedic products covered by the public health system in many countries, this does not guaranty the minimum quality and standard required treating the patient effectively, efficiently, and safely. RSC® has a number, but only in Germany, and cannot be used by custom-made braces and other CAD CAM systems. Thus, the Rigo-Chêneau brace can and must be prescribed under the name "Chêneau brace" according to Rigo principles and classification. However, the so-called Chêneau brace is a "highly specific corrective device" that has to be built not only according to the principles for each curve pattern but also taking into consideration individual factors like the patient's morphology and correctibility. The whole concept was inspired in the plaster cast technique applied by the old masters, so it is not possible to build a good standard Chêneau brace with repeatability and consistency without specific and deep knowledge of the 3D nature of idiopathic scoliosis and extensive experience with scoliosis correction. A good Chêneau brace can only be constructed and fitted by an experienced medical doctor with specific

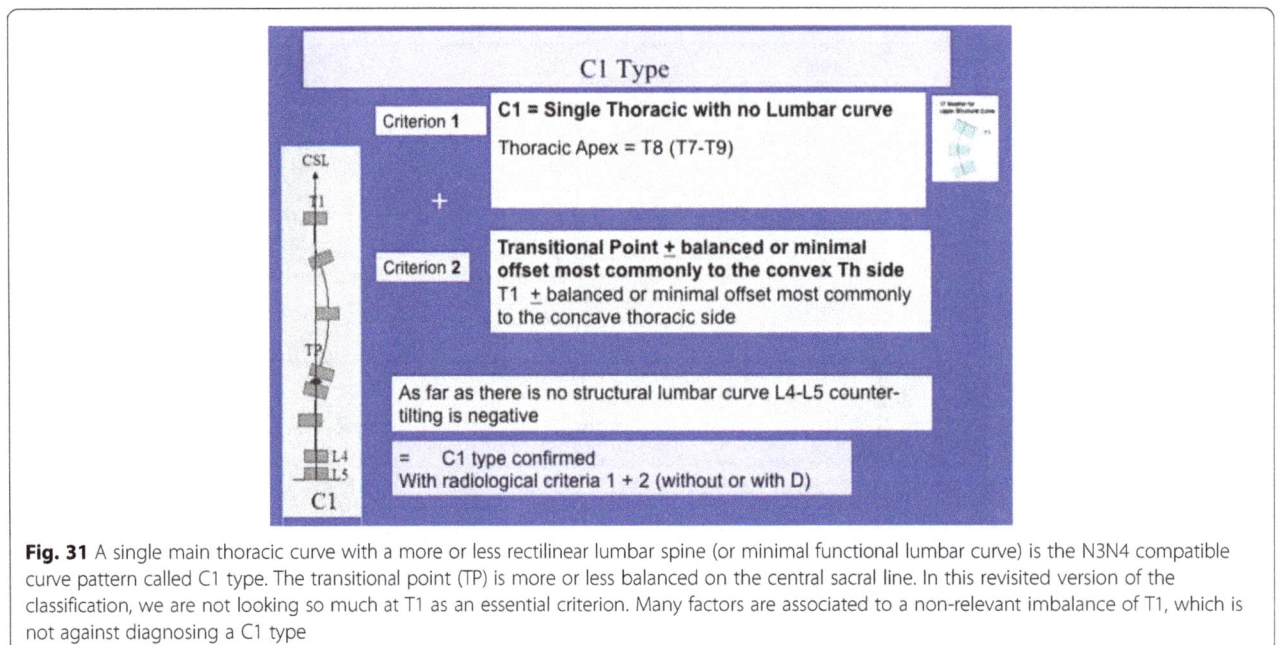

Fig. 31 A single main thoracic curve with a more or less rectilinear lumbar spine (or minimal functional lumbar curve) is the N3N4 compatible curve pattern called C1 type. The transitional point (TP) is more or less balanced on the central sacral line. In this revisited version of the classification, we are not looking so much at T1 as an essential criterion. Many factors are associated to a non-relevant imbalance of T1, which is not against diagnosing a C1 type

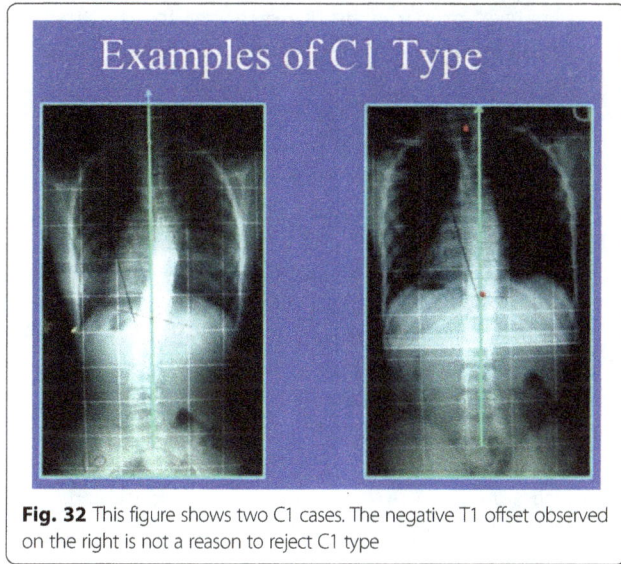

Fig. 32 This figure shows two C1 cases. The negative T1 offset observed on the right is not a reason to reject C1 type

knowledge of scoliosis correction, assisted by an orthotist, or by a highly educated and experienced orthotist working in full collaboration with a multidisciplinary team coordinated by a medical doctor, who is also highly educated in this technique, and a scoliosis physiotherapist, who provides his/her specific knowledge about the patient's correction throughout posture and movement.

Historically, the contamination by other brace concepts has produced unacceptable failures in the technique.

How to build the brace?

Following are the three different ways to construct the Rigo-Chêneau brace:

1) Classical hand-made technique, which is based on the modification or correction of a positive mould of the patient's trunk from a negative mould taken directly on the patient using plaster bands. Eventually, the positive mould can be reproduced by CAD CAM after a laser capture of the patient's trunk. The modification of the positive mould consists in shaping all pad areas and expansion spaces according to the desired curve pattern-specific design. It is generally assumed that pad areas are built by removing plaster from the positive, while adding plaster forms the expansion spaces. However, depending on the design, it is common for pad areas to be shaped by adding plaster and for spaces to be created by removing plaster. The brace itself is built by modeling a thermoplastic structure, which is commonly 4 mm of polypropylene-copolymer, on the modified positive mould. The knowledge about how to affix the plastic to the mould is part of the general knowledge

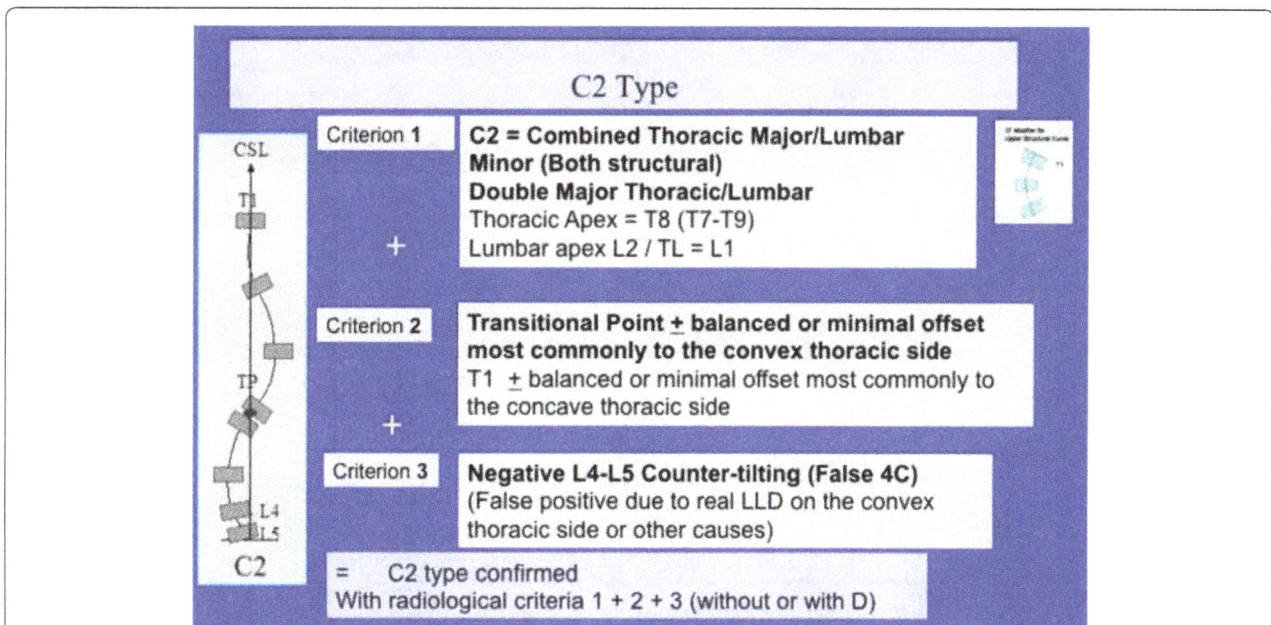

Fig. 33 A composite structural scoliosis, main thoracic and lumbar is compatible with N3N4 and it is called C2 type. It can be major thoracic/minor lumbar or double major but we have not seen any N3N4 with lumbar structural curve where the lumbar component was major and the thoracic minor. The second radiological criterion is the TP and T1 on the CSL. Minimal offset (±4 mm) is considered not a reason to reject diagnosis of C2. The third radiological criterion is a L4–L5 negative counter-tilting (it can be observed a mild false positive counter-tilting, for example due to leg length discrepancy or pelvis asymmetry)

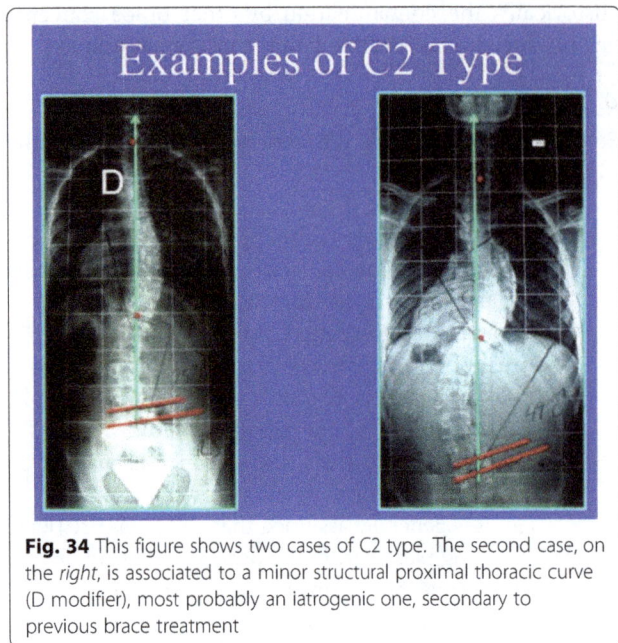

Fig. 34 This figure shows two cases of C2 type. The second case, on the *right*, is associated to a minor structural proximal thoracic curve (D modifier), most probably an iatrogenic one, secondary to previous brace treatment

of a certified orthotist and is not explained in this paper. The trim lines, however, are essential to the success of the brace and are determined during the fitting process. Improper trim lines can destroy a well-constructed brace. Generally speaking, the

plastic is prepared by the orthotist for the first fitting such that all trim lines are slightly higher (on the top) or lower (on the bottom) than necessary for the initial fitting.

2) Similar to the classical procedure, the CAD CAM system enables the orthotist to laser capture the patient's trunk and use a software program to modify the virtual mould. The program offers a partially predesigned mould according to the two basic types: 3C and 4C. The authors are not familiar with this procedure and, although many orthotists use this system to build Chêneau-type braces and derivatives, they know of no orthotist who uses it to specifically build a Rigo-Chêneau-type brace.

3) Using a CAD CAM system from a predesigned library, a fully predesigned mould is selected and modified according to the patient's specifications, including static as well as dynamic measurements. The library can be based on a somewhat complex and complete set of models and the selection can be based on a somewhat complex and complete classification.

This paper describes the principles that provide a better understanding of how to build a custom brace. CAD CAM procedures are not described herein.

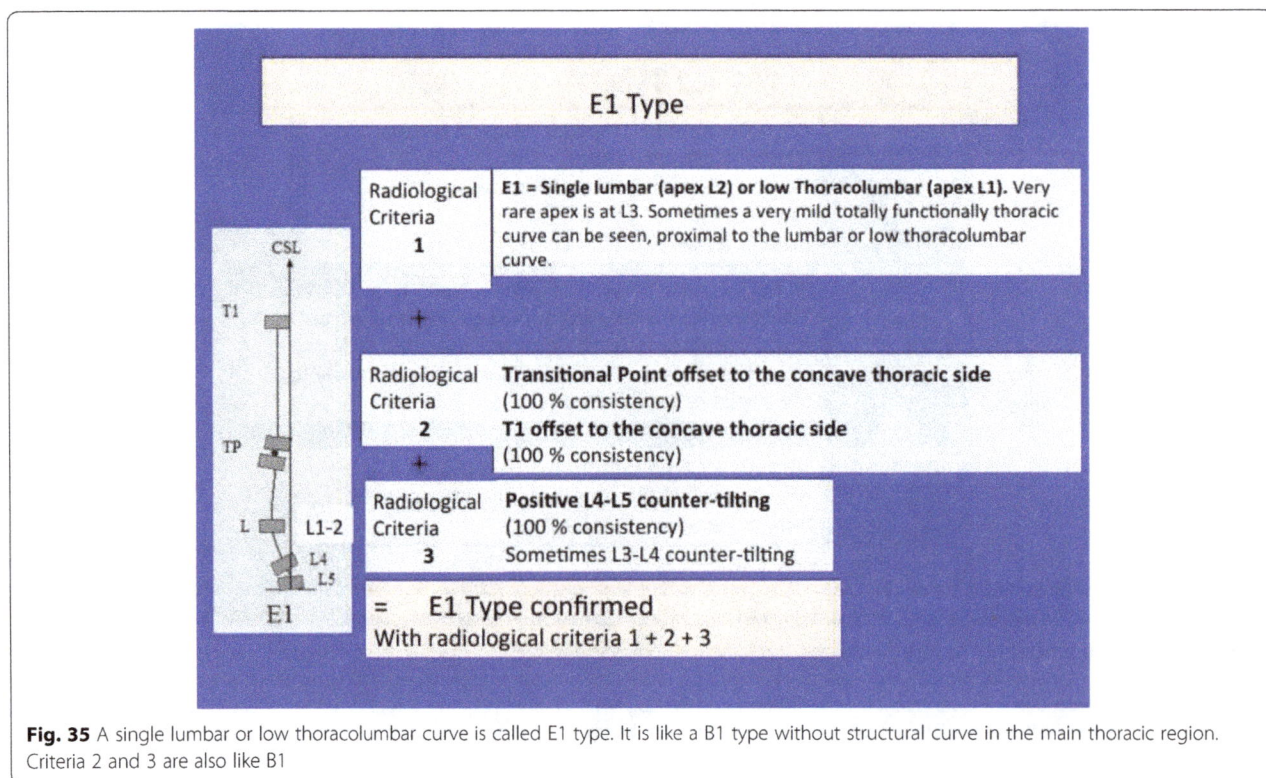

Fig. 35 A single lumbar or low thoracolumbar curve is called E1 type. It is like a B1 type without structural curve in the main thoracic region. Criteria 2 and 3 are also like B1

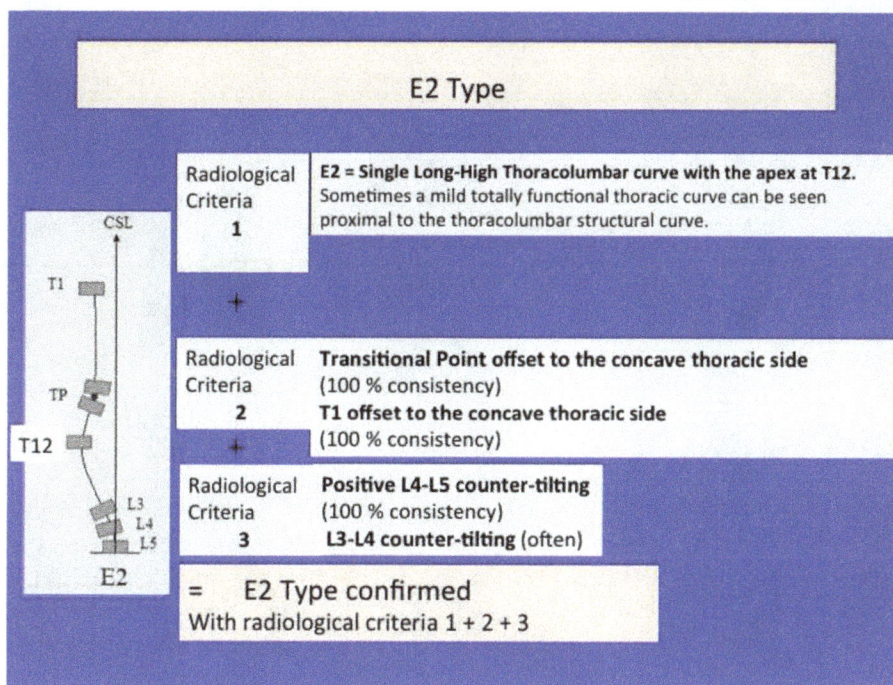

E2 Type

Radiological Criteria 1	E2 = Single Long-High Thoracolumbar curve with the apex at T12. Sometimes a mild totally functional thoracic curve can be seen proximal to the thoracolumbar structural curve.

+

Radiological Criteria 2	**Transitional Point offset to the concave thoracic side** (100 % consistency) **T1 offset to the concave thoracic side** (100 % consistency)

+

Radiological Criteria 3	**Positive L4-L5 counter-tilting** (100 % consistency) **L3-L4 counter-tilting** (often)

= **E2 Type confirmed**
With radiological criteria 1 + 2 + 3

Fig. 36 A single long-high thoracolumbar curve with the apex at T12 is called E2. It is like B2 type without structural curve in the main thoracic region. Criteria 2 and 3 are like B2

How to check the brace?

In our particular case, the orthotist and MD make the first fitting. First, in case the patient is fitted for the first time (no previous brace treatment), the doctor explains the brace objectives to the patient. Depending on curve flexibility, the patient feels more or less pressure from the pads. The more rigid the curve, the more pressure the patient will note, and the more marked the trunk posture will be changed. From one side, pressure produces physical discomfort and, depending on the patient's sensitivity, this first contact with the brace can be a determinant for brace acceptance. Alternatively, the change of trunk posture creates a neurological discomfort by changing suddenly, without adaptation, the body schema. As a result, the patient must be managed calmly and respectfully. For the first trials, the orthotist will help the patient put the brace on, but the brace will be closed only with the patient lying in the supine position. Typically, the brace is finished with three straps in the front, but for the fitting phase, two straps are adequate. The two straps are closed gradually until the right side of the plastic overlaps the left side (for a right thoracic curve). The brace has been built such that extra volume will guaranty the life of the brace for at least 10 to 12 months, even in the accelerated growth phase before and during the peak of growth. A well-constructed brace adapted after menarche should usually work until the end of treatment. The brace is fitted alternating the caudal and cranial strap, and once it is finally fixed in the lumbo-pelvic region, we ask the patient to breathe deeply while observing thorax expansion. At a certain point, the patient has to fight against the brace to make a full inspiration. When this happens, we use the exhalation phase to completely fasten the straps to their final position and mark the straps with the "maximum"

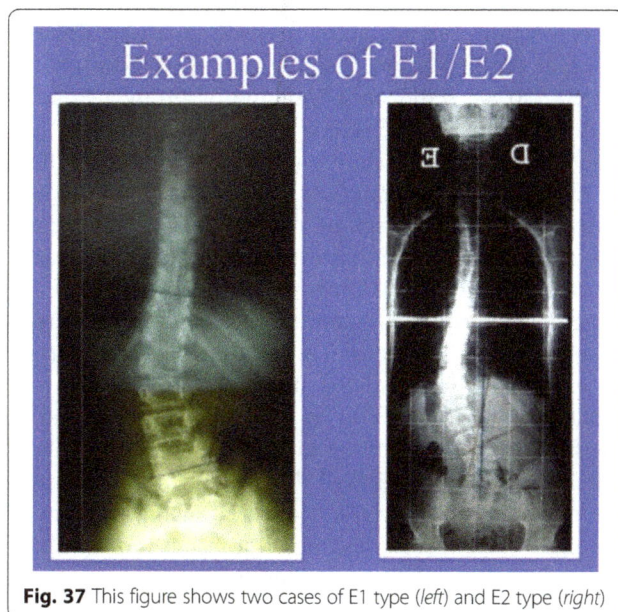

Fig. 37 This figure shows two cases of E1 type (left) and E2 type (right)

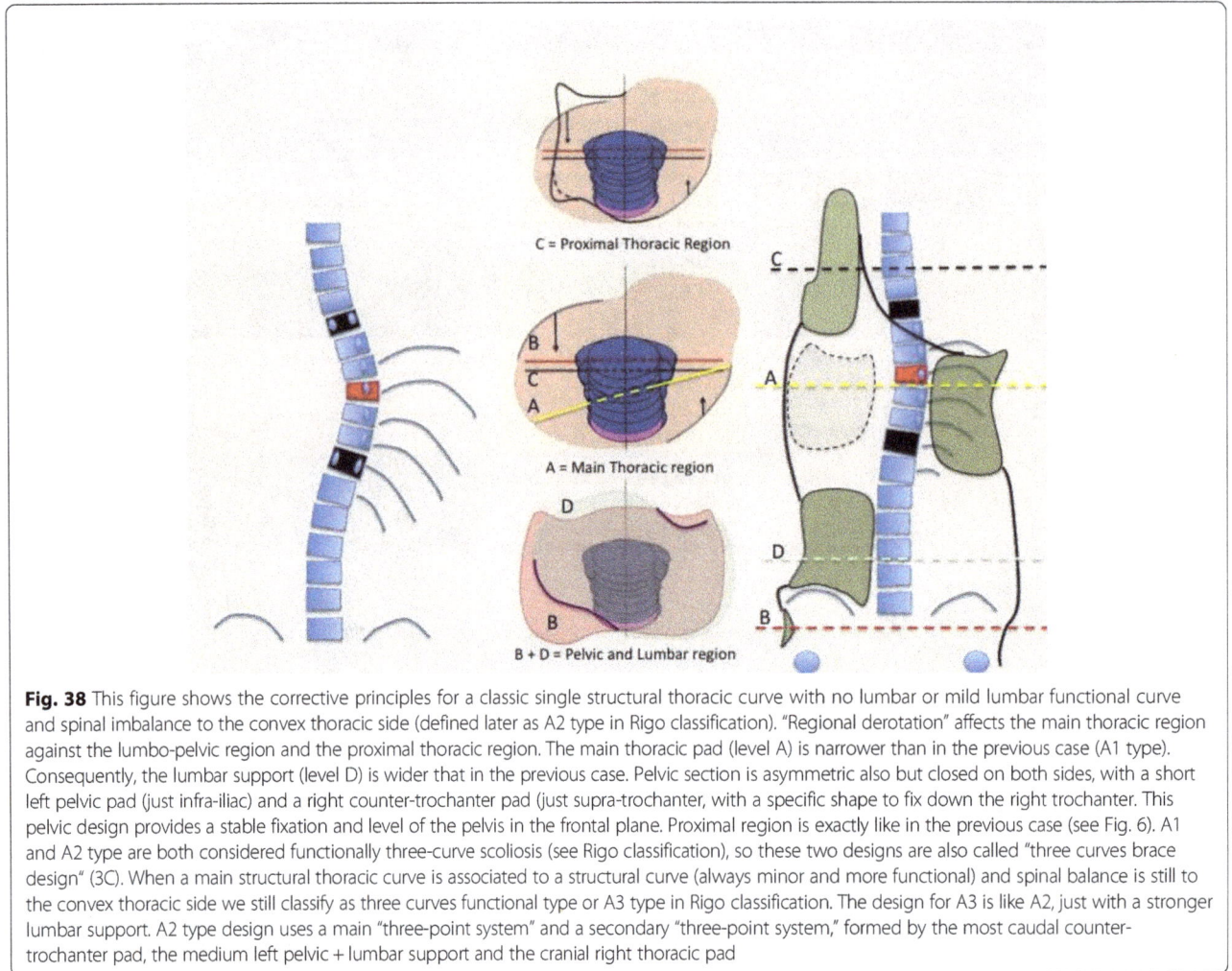

C = Proximal Thoracic Region

A = Main Thoracic region

B + D = Pelvic and Lumbar region

Fig. 38 This figure shows the corrective principles for a classic single structural thoracic curve with no lumbar or mild lumbar functional curve and spinal imbalance to the convex thoracic side (defined later as A2 type in Rigo classification). "Regional derotation" affects the main thoracic region against the lumbo-pelvic region and the proximal thoracic region. The main thoracic pad (level A) is narrower than in the previous case (A1 type). Consequently, the lumbar support (level D) is wider that in the previous case. Pelvic section is asymmetric also but closed on both sides, with a short left pelvic pad (just infra-iliac) and a right counter-trochanter pad (just supra-trochanter, with a specific shape to fix down the right trochanter). This pelvic design provides a stable fixation and level of the pelvis in the frontal plane. Proximal region is exactly like in the previous case (see Fig. 6). A1 and A2 type are both considered functionally three-curve scoliosis (see Rigo classification), so these two designs are also called "three curves brace design" (3C). When a main structural thoracic curve is associated to a structural curve (always minor and more functional) and spinal balance is still to the convex thoracic side we still classify as three curves functional type or A3 type in Rigo classification. The design for A3 is like A2, just with a stronger lumbar support. A2 type design uses a main "three-point system" and a secondary "three-point system," formed by the most caudal counter-trochanter pad, the medium left pelvic + lumbar support and the cranial right thoracic pad

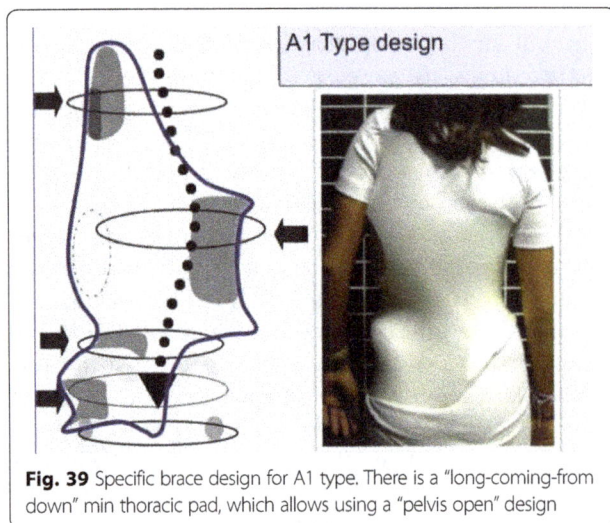

A1 Type design

Fig. 39 Specific brace design for A1 type. There is a "long-coming-from down" min thoracic pad, which allows using a "pelvis open" design

closing point. In flexible curves, this position is well accepted from the beginning. In rigid curves, fitting the brace at the maximum position can be stressful for the patient, so we settle on a "minimum" fitting point. To find this point, we unfasten the upper strap but keep the brace closed in its maximum position, asking the patient to fully inhale while carefully releasing the strap, finally fastening it in the minimum position, where the patient can achieve full inspiration with practically no resistance from the brace. At this time, we leave the patient in the lying position for a couple of minutes and move away to observe his/her reactions. Then, we help the patient get up and observe how she/he stands at the very first moment. The patient should be able to stand balanced in the frontal as well as in the sagittal plane for a couple of minutes if the brace is well designed. During this time, the orthotist can mark the trim lines, taking care not to cut more than necessary. It is better to cut too little than too much in this first trial. The brace is then prepared for a second trial and the procedure is repeated. In the

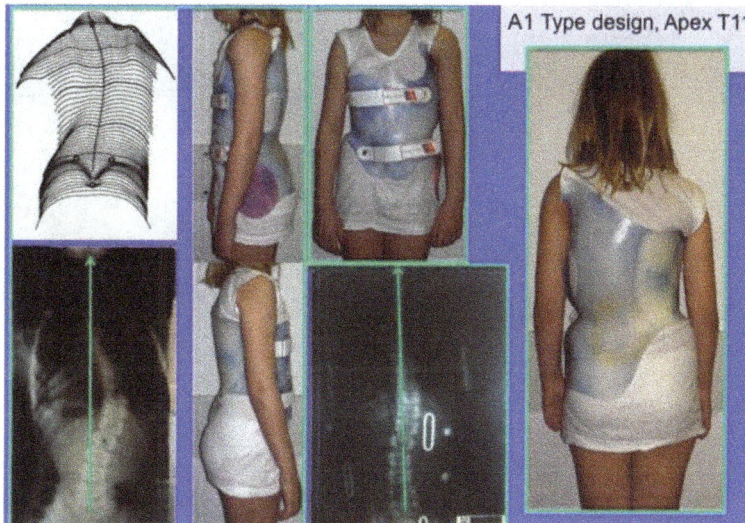

Fig. 40 The specific brace design for A1 type has been related to the best in-brace correction as shown in this figure. In-brace correction of the Cobb angle has been reported to be 76% with this specific brace design, the highest in comparison with other curve patterns and brace designs

second trial, the patient is usually able to stay in the upright position longer so the orthotist can spend more time deciding on the position of the final trim lines in both the upright and sitting positions. The orthotist and MD then consider whether the combined pressure points bring the patient into the maximum possible correction in all three planes. Pads should be touching the body at the right points and in the right direction

according to the aforementioned principles. One of the most controversial issues is how high the brace should be on the convex thoracic side. There is no clear rule but, generally speaking, in flexible scoliosis the brace can be cut lower, slightly cranial to the apical level of the thoracic curve (warming the plastic and releasing pressure up to the apex, but maintaining some plastic to prevent the brace from being too short when the patient

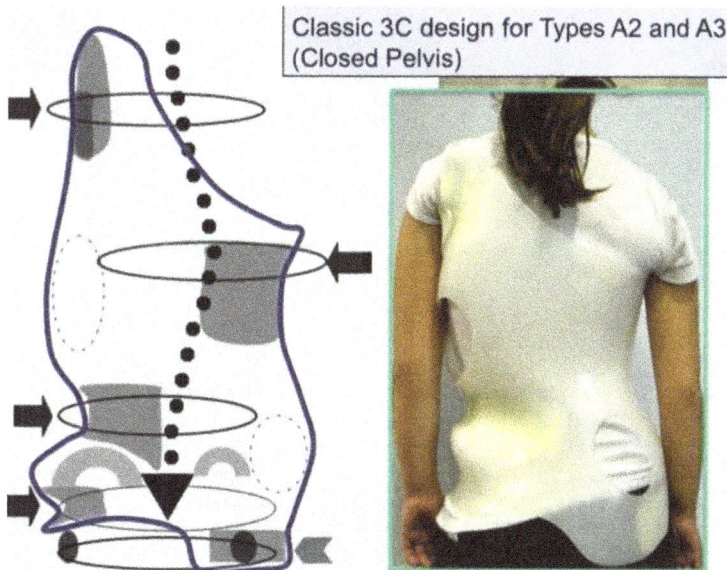

Fig. 41 Brace design for A2 and A3 types is the same. The main thoracic pad is not so large like in A1 type. There is some expansion room caudal to the main thoracic pad, for the lumbar concavity. Pelvis has to be fixed by closing the pelvis, in order to provide a counter-trochanter pad on the convex thoracic side

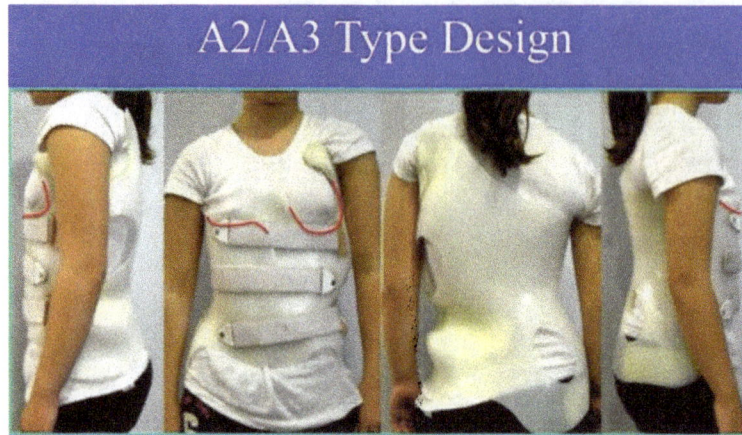

Fig. 42 Brace design for A2 and A3 observed from ventral, dorsal, and both sides. It is important to note the sagittal balance and profile. Both sides show a different profile due to the asymmetric design. From the left it looks like the thoracic kyphosis is extended to caudal. From the right it looks like the lumbar lordosis is extended to cranial. In the middle sagittal plane the profile is more or less physiologic

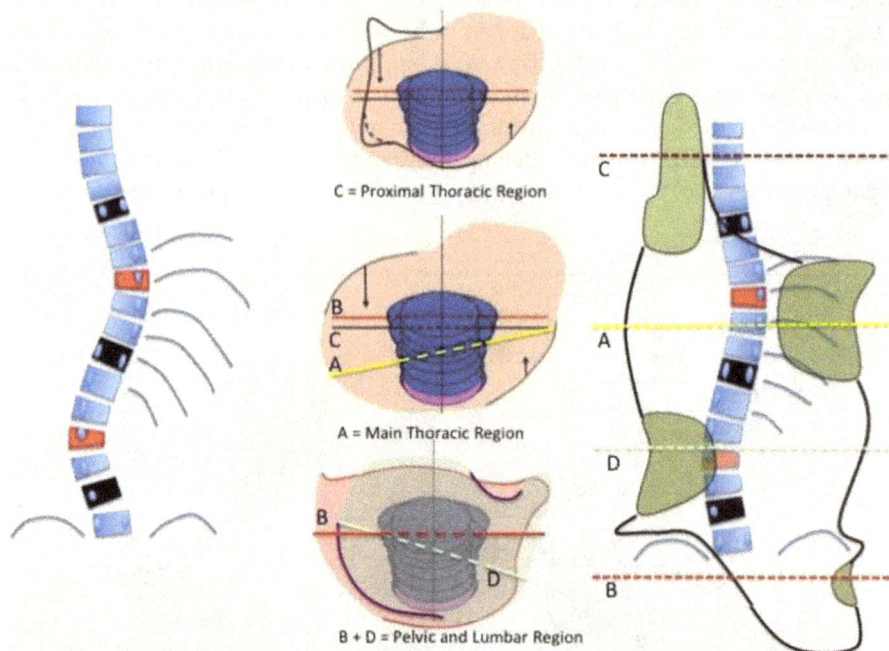

Fig. 43 This figure shows the principle of correction for a true double structural curve. Most but not all the double structural curves are classified as "four-curve pattern" (4C) or "B type" (B1 and B2). The objective criteria to classify 4C (or B types) can be seen later in the main text and some more figures. This current figure is about a classical B1 type, with the apical vertebrae of the right main thoracic curve at T8 and the left lumbar curve at L2. "Regional derotation" is applied here at these two regions. The main thoracic region is over-derotated to the left (*yellow line A*) like in previous cases. The lumbar region is over-derotated to the right with the combination of a couple of forces formed by a real left lumbar pad and a right low abdominal pad (*green line D*). The lumbar pad is dissociated or uncoupled from the pelvic region (it is not just a lumbar support coupled to the pelvis section) and approaches the lumbar convexity, reaching the maximum pressure at the apical level, leaving room down. Pelvis region has to be translated to the left, bringing also the lower lumbar vertebrae to the left, to the provided room caudal to the lumbar pad. Pelvis is not only translated but also derotated to the left (not over-derotated but just derotated to 0°, fixing the pelvis region in the frontal plane of reference—*red line B*). Two main "three-point systems" are formed with the lateral component of all the pads. The right pelvic pad, the left lumbar pad, and the right thoracic pad form the lower "three-point system"

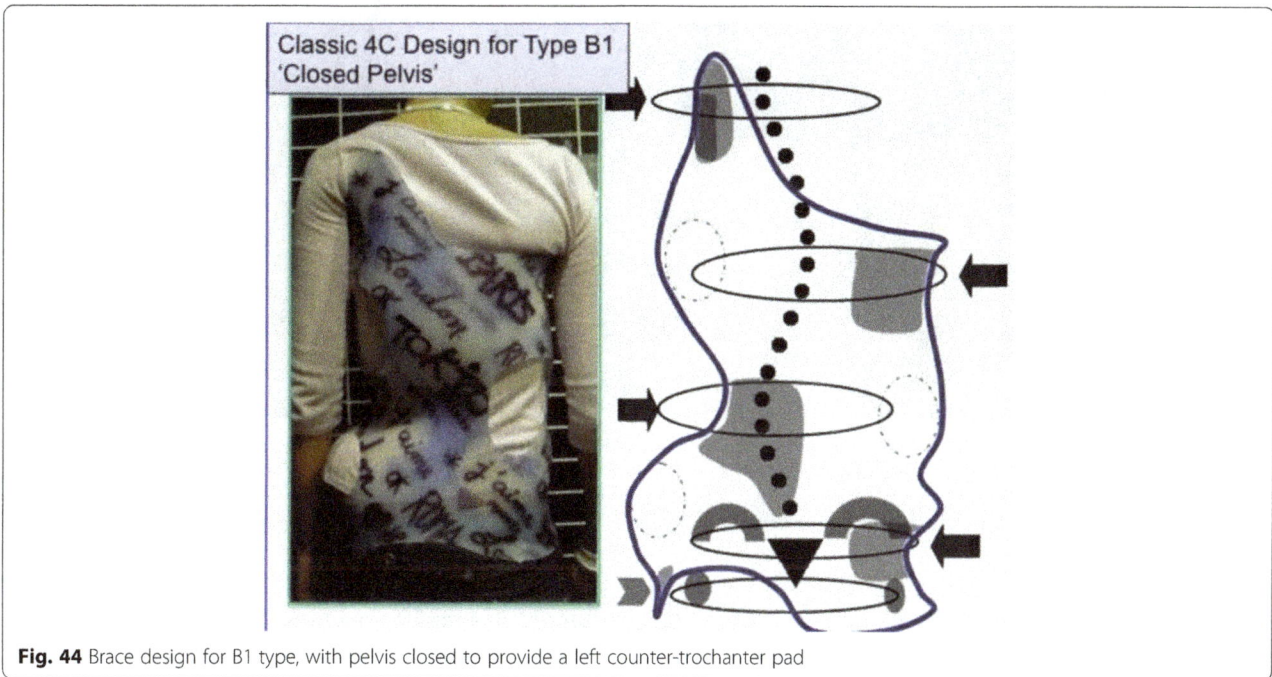

Fig. 44 Brace design for B1 type, with pelvis closed to provide a left counter-trochanter pad

grows). In rigid curves, it is better to leave more plastic cranially. In this case, the maximum pressure goes to the more prominent part of the rib hump and, as long as the curve is not immediately corrected, the upper plastic will not push the ribs, so there is no need to warm and release pressure there. Do not cut the plastic because the plastic will not be visible, and it is always better to

have additional plastic cranially to the apex to continue reaching the apex after the patient grows. The counter-pressure point working at the proximal thoracic region has to be totally adapted to the upper ribs, pushing to medial but with a very light dorsal direction to form a pair-of-force for deflection with the main thoracic pad. It should not be possible to bring the patient passively

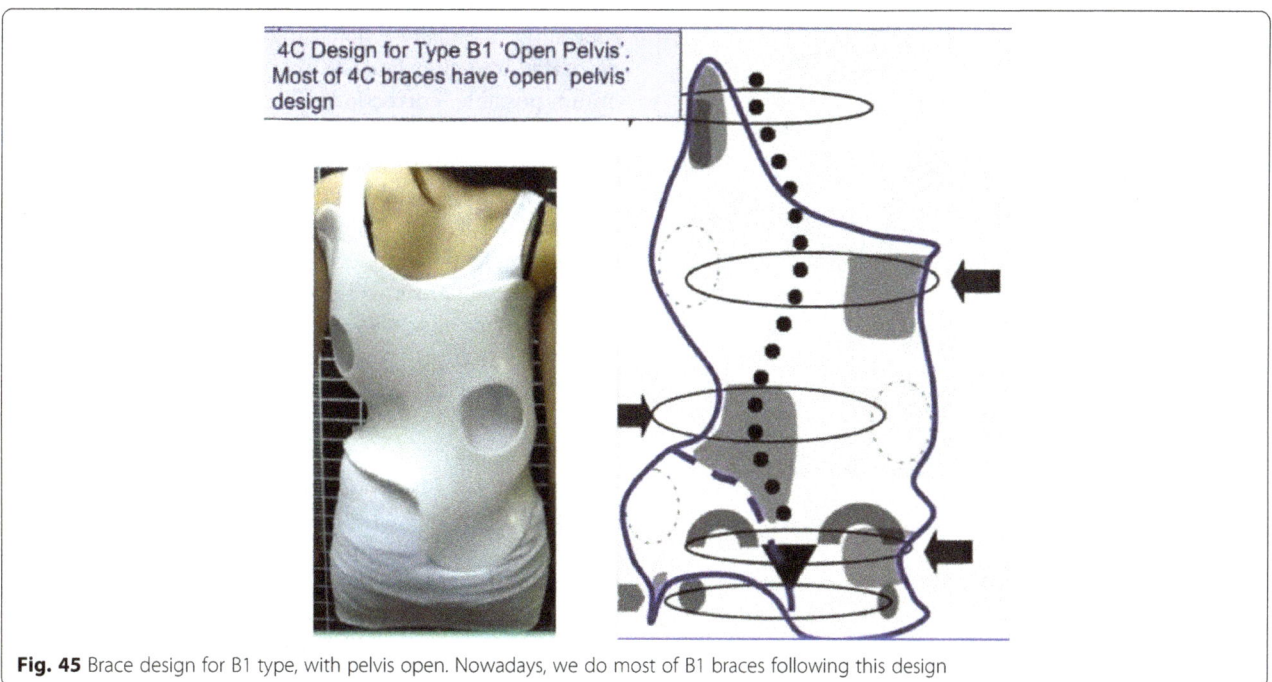

Fig. 45 Brace design for B1 type, with pelvis open. Nowadays, we do most of B1 braces following this design

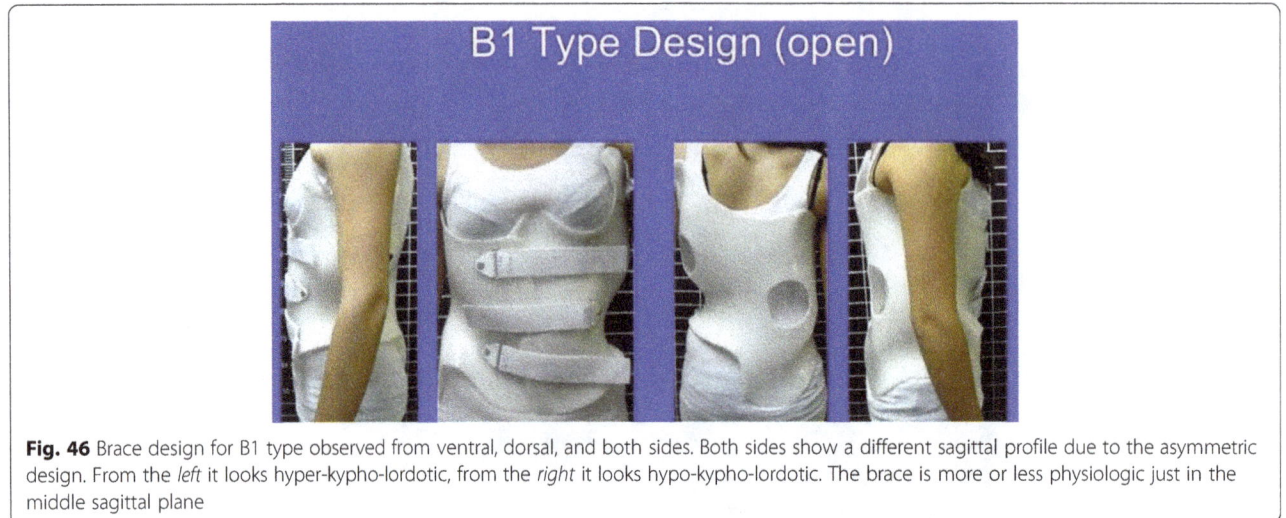

Fig. 46 Brace design for B1 type observed from ventral, dorsal, and both sides. Both sides show a different sagittal profile due to the asymmetric design. From the *left* it looks hyper-kypho-lordotic, from the *right* it looks hypo-kypho-lordotic. The brace is more or less physiologic just in the middle sagittal plane

with our hands or actively by asking him/her to bend to the convex thoracic side to a bigger correction. The patient has to be blocked in the maximum possible correction in the frontal plane through these two forces provided by the main thoracic pad and the upper thoracic counter pad. If this correction is not achieved, consideration should be given to increasing the pressure by adding internal pads or cutting the upper counter pad to bring it to a more medial position by using metal

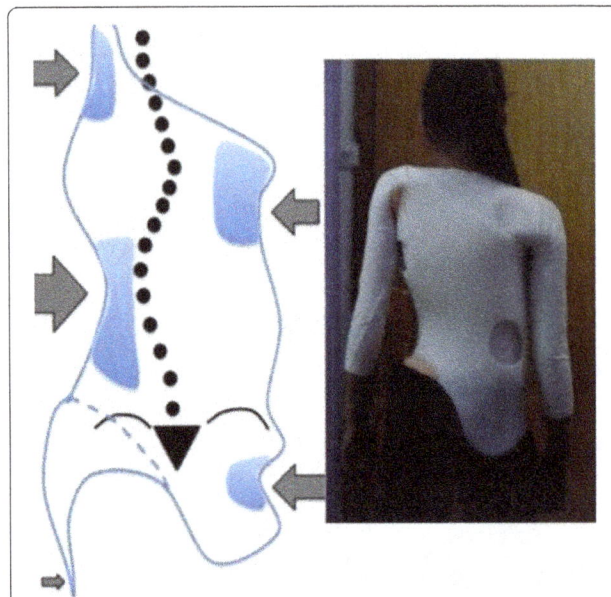

Fig. 47 Brace design for B2 type. There is a large 3D-shaped thoracolumbar pad, very difficult to perform when correcting the positive mould by hand. On the *right*, a B2-type brace made by the junior author MJ (left thoracic/right TL curve, mirrored)

extensors (Fig. 58). Sometimes, especially in very flexible curves, the correction is poor enough to consider remaking the brace as the best and most practical option.

The brace action also must be checked at the lumbopelvic region. Lumbar support in A and C types has to push on the lumbar convexity from below the apex and just reaching the apex, with no need to go over the apex. This support is, in a way, integrated into the pelvis section. The difference between the lumbar support and the real lumbar pad from B types has been explained above. In B types, it is necessary to check that the pelvis is brought fully to the left (in the example of a right thoracic/left lumbar scoliosis) and maintained by the brace in the frontal plane of reference (with 0° of axial rotation). Cranially, the lumbar region has to be derotated and translated to the right, reaching the maximum possible correction. The anterior design of the brace is essential to achieve this effect. The lumbar pad, which pushes from dorso-lateral to ventro-medial, needs an "escaping" space exactly at the same level in the anterior-lateral part. The body will totally fill this space in the upright position, and abdominal expansion during breathing mechanics will occur mostly laterally and back on the lumbar concavity. The anterior abdominal pad on the right side pushes from ventro-lateral to dorso-medial, exactly in the opposite direction of the lumbar pad, but at a lower level, to prevent any compression or "sandwich effect." Otherwise, the best correction cannot be reached because the translation between the pelvis and lumbar regions is blocked. The anterior abdominal pad, which works in combination with the lateral pelvic pad, should help to stabilize the pelvis into the best possible 3D correction.

The brace is then finished by the orthotist and MD, who indicate a schedule for adaptation after training the

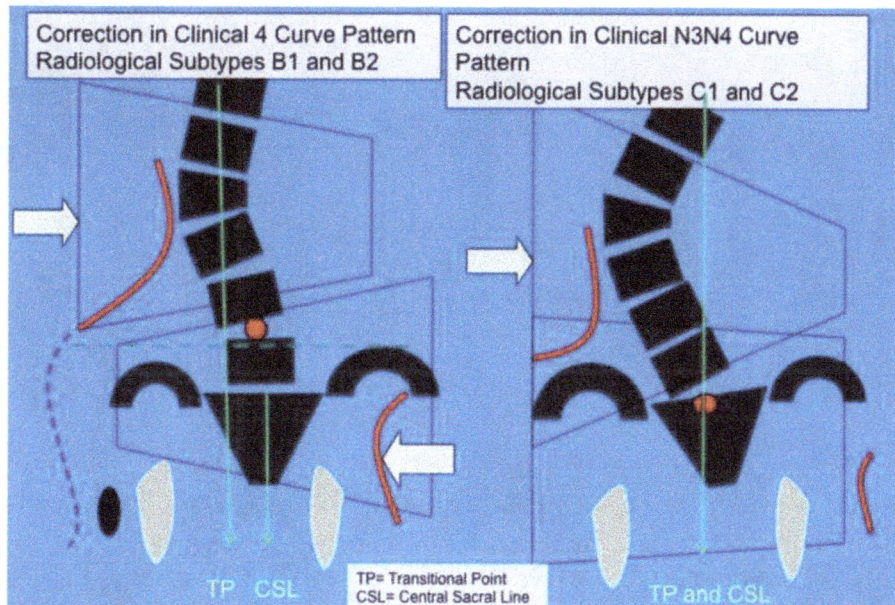

Fig. 48 This figure shows the main difference in designing B and C types. In B type, the pelvis region is first translated around 8 cm, taking off plaster from the pelvis region at the convex thoracic side. This is not necessary in C type. Later, the pads are designed. In both types, pelvic pad is very similar, if perhaps it works lightly more caudal, just supra trochanteric, in C type. This pad braces the whole hemi-pelvis on the convex thoracic side, as it is extended to dorsal. On the concave thoracic side, B type presents a real lumbar pad reaching its maximum pressure at the apical level of the lumbar curve and approaching this level coming inclined from caudal to cranial and from lateral to medial. This pad works as a counter-stop point at the apical level against the pelvis a low lumbar region translation. The room caudal to the apex is necessary allowing translation. In C type, pelvis cannot be translated because it is a coupled lumbar region, so correction can be only achieved by keeping the pelvis stable and pushing the lumbar curve from caudal to cranial. The lumbar support goes practically horizontal from lateral to medial and reached the maximum pressure in the lower lumbar hemi-convexity

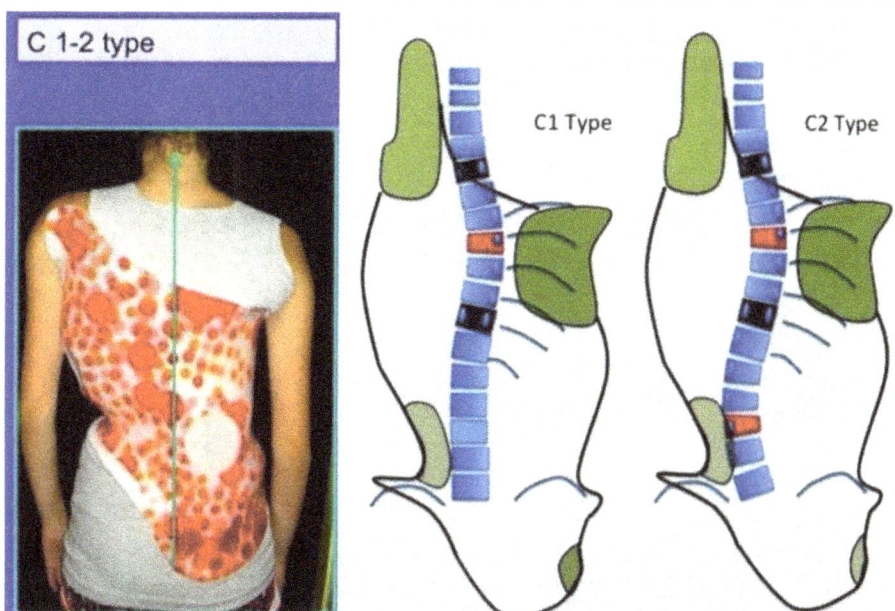

Fig. 49 An example of C-type brace can be seen on the *left side* of this figure. No significant difference exists between the C1 and C2 brace design, as showed on the *right side* of the figure

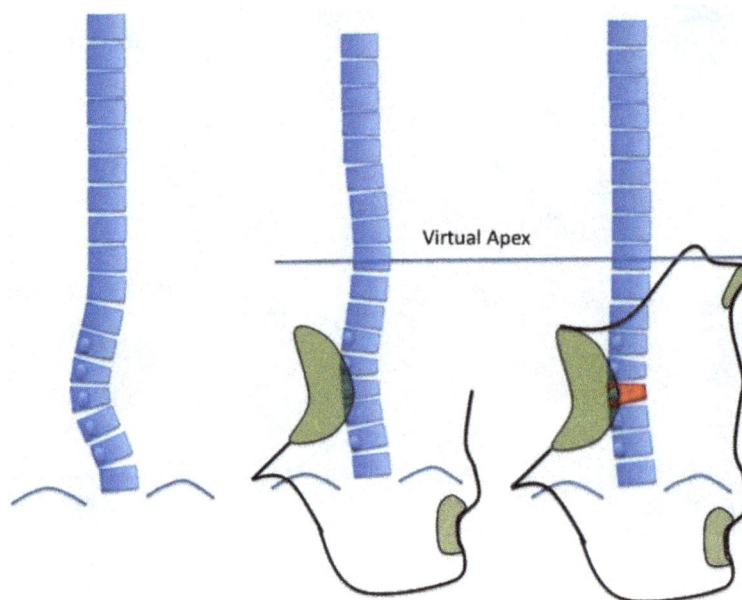

Fig. 50 Brace design for E type. The difference between E1 and E2 is the same difference in the size of the main pad. A long-high thoracolumbar with apex at T12—E2 type—needs a larger pad in comparison with E1. The main thoracic pad works mainly as a counter-rotation force and a counter lateral to medial force worn the virtual apex of the compensatory functional thoracic curve. Although this curve does not exist originally it tends to appear when the structural lumbar or thoracolumbar curve are corrected

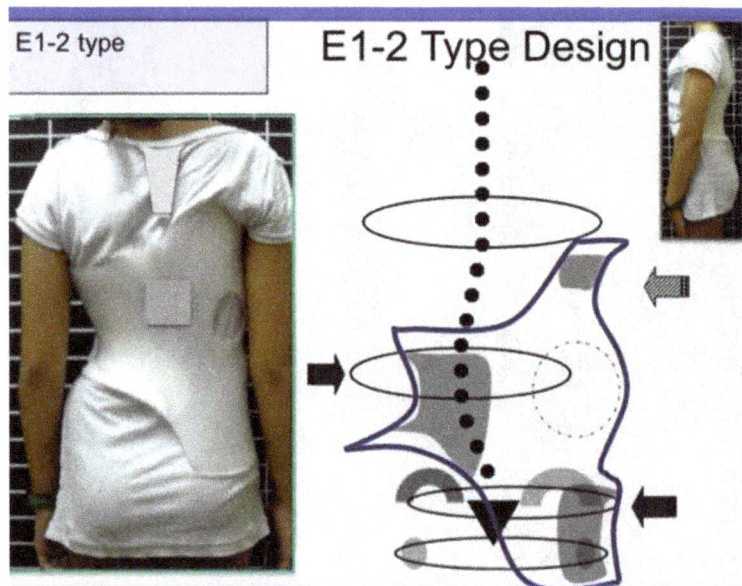

Fig. 51 This figure shows an example of E1-type brace

patient/parents to put the brace on and take it off by herself/himself.

Protocols and everyday usage

We currently recommend the following three schedule alternatives:

1) Full-time: the patient must wear the brace 20–23 h per day
2) Part-time: the patient must wear the brace 14–16 h per day
3) Nighttime: the patient wears the brace only at night

Full-time is the most common recommendation for patients with a scoliotic curve over 25° and in the rapid period of growth at Tanner 2–3, Risser 0–2, pre-menarche, or 1 year after menarche (in girls).

Two different schedules for adaptation are indicated to reach full-time, but this aspect is flexible and many variations are made according to individual characteristics. In general, we recommend that the patient first sleep in the brace, then adapt to daytime wearing at home, and finally wearing the brace outside the home.

Historically, one to five trials has been necessary to sleep a full night in the brace. When the patient can wear the brace the entire first night, we recommend a rushed adaptation schedule. When the patient needs more than one night, we recommend a slower adaptation schedule. In the rushed schedule, after the first night, the patient wears the brace at home for 1 h the first day, then doubling the time each day until fully filling all the hours at home. Then she/he can go to the school wearing the brace, reaching full-time in a few days. In the slower schedule, the patient repeats each step one or two times (e.g., wearing the brace for 2 days only at night, then wearing the brace 1 h for 2 days at home, then 2 h for 2 days, 4 h for 2 days, and so on). It can be even slower, repeating daytime during 3 or 4 days. Basically, the schedule depends on the scoliosis rigidity.

One month after reaching full-time, the in-brace correction is checked in a radiograph. To reduce the number of radiographs as much as possible, we check in-brace correction in the AP/PA radiograph, while the sagittal plane alignment is followed out of brace by surface topography.

The brace progress is checked every 3 months during the period of rapid growth, especially before menarche. Clinical control is made every 6 months by measuring anthropometrics, ATI, breathing function, surface topography, clinical photos, self-perception, and HRQL (in our protocol TAPS and SRS-22). We do not repeat a new radiograph every 6 months when patients/parents report good compliance and the clinical picture has improved. No clinical changes or worsening or suspicion of a change in the curve pattern is considered a reason to repeat a radiograph out of brace. At this point, it is not necessary for the patient to remove the brace many hours before the radiograph is taken; 2–4 h is enough. Failure of bracing or a change in the curve pattern necessitates the development of a new strategy.

The life of the brace, on average, is around 1 year during the period between 1 year pre-menarche and half a year post-menarche. One year and a half/2 years before this period, and even longer when the brace is made 6 months after menarche.

When the brace becomes too small due to growth and development, a new brace is indicated when necessary and a new in-brace radiograph is prescribed to check correction. It is not rare to find a loss of correction into the second or third brace, but in our experience the out-of-brace value of the Cobb angle is not far from the in-brace value in those cases. Good responders use to show continued improvement of correction.

The full-time regime is followed by most patients until 2 years after menarche and Risser sign 3 (European)/4 (American). The patient is then recommended to wear the brace part-time. An out-of-brace radiograph is prescribed after 1 month of part-time wear (8 h out of the brace before the radiograph). When values are acceptable, part-time is maintained for 3 to 6 months and the patient then wears the brace only at night for 1 year. Out-of-brace radiographs are repeated 1 month after wearing the brace only at night, as well as 1 month and 1 year after weaning.

Outside of the weaning period, part-time wear is indicated for patients who will not wear the brace outside of the home. These patients are informed about the dose-effect response of bracing and are made aware of the risks for failure.

Nighttime use was formerly recommended in pre-puberal cases with good-to-excellent in-brace correction and rapid improvement of the clinical values. Nighttime bracing often allows us to increase the brace correction, but we follow the same basic principles.

A radiograph every 6 months is recommended when the patient is under the partial or nighttime regime or for full-time non-compliant patients, unless clinical values improve in a relevant way.

Exercises

Most patients combine bracing with a regular regime of exercises according to the Barcelona Scoliosis Physical Therapy School (BSPTS), which basically follows Schroth's principles [30, 33]. The patient removes the brace to perform her/his Schroth exercises. In fact, the principles of correction used by the Rigo-Chêneau-type brace come from the evolution of the Schroth principles established by the BSPTS. We do not use to prescribe specific exercises in-brace, but patients can practice physical activities with the brace. It is recommended to remove the brace to participate in-group sports to avoid injuring others (in case of competition).

Discussion

In spite of its growing popularity, literature about the Chêneau-type brace is limited in comparison with other popular brace concepts. With the exception of some well-designed prospective studies, the methodology of most of the published series is low in quality. It is first necessary to provide some background on the efficacy of brace treatment, in general terms, and related to the initial in-brace correction as a predictive factor of the end result.

Weinstein et al. recently published the results of a multicenter study on the effects of TLSO bracing in adolescents with idiopathic scoliosis, enrolling both a randomized cohort and a preference cohort, concluding that bracing significantly decreased the progression of high-risk curves to the threshold for surgery [3]. The external evidence for bracing, when a TLSO brace is used, strongly supports its effectiveness. Thus, the question is not whether bracing works or not but how to achieve the best possible result in terms of preventing surgery as a main goal, preventing progression as a primary goal, and permanently decreasing the pretreatment angle as a secondary goal, all while improving the trunk shape and back asymmetry with no significant deterioration of function and, generally speaking, health-related quality of life (HRQL). The Weinstein paper also corroborated, in this case, the highest methodological quality, the previously suspected strong brace dose-response relationship. Previous prospective studies had shown the relationship between the short-term in-brace correction and end result. For whatever reason, in-brace correction is not reported in the Weinstein paper so, unfortunately, this relationship has not been confirmed in this paper. Nevertheless, even admitting its low quality, the existing evidence cannot be ignored.

In one of the classical references on brace treatment published in 1980, Carr et al. suggested that an initial in-brace correction of more than 50% was a predictive factor for a significant and permanent final correction [34]. In this study, however, 133 patients were treated with a Milwaukee brace, and by 1980, it was already known that the Milwaukee brace rarely achieved such a high in-brace correction on a regular basis. In a short series of 62 patients treated with the Milwaukee brace, Heine and Gotze [35] showed a very poor in-brace correction of less than 10%. In-brace correction as a predictor of the end result was also supported in the study from Noonan et al. [36], where patients treated

with a Milwaukee brace and a progressing curve that required surgery showed a very poor in-brace correction of 8%, while those not needing surgery were initially corrected by the brace with a mean percentage of 20. Surprisingly, in this last series, a good result could still be expected with a poor in-brace correction based on today's standards.

Later, three papers have stressed the relationship between initial in-brace correction and final outcome. Katz et al. [37] investigated the factors that could be predictive of the final outcome in patients with large curves treated with the Boston brace. The analyzed factors were Cobb angles, vertebral tilt angles, coronal decompensation, apical vertebral translation, apical vertebral rotation, lateral trunk shift, rib vertebral angle difference, pelvic tilt, and lumbar-pelvic relationship. Katz et al. concluded that patients with a double curve pattern in which the thoracic curve is over 35° Cobb and the lumbar-pelvic relationship is higher than 12° were significantly more likely to show curve progression. They also found that in-brace correction of at least 25% in double curves significantly increased the likelihood of success. Landauer et al. [38] predicted a final average curve correction of 7° in a child at growth when an in-brace correction of 40% could be reached with a Chêneau-type brace. Finally, Castro [39] concluded that brace treatment was not recommended in patients whose curves did not correct at least 20% in a TLSO. Most of the papers on braces that can be classified into the TLSO group have reported historically higher in-brace corrections in comparison with the Milwaukee brace, including the Chêneau-type brace.

The Boston brace has been considered the gold standard of the so-called TLSOs. It is definitely the most popular among scoliosis specialists around the world. Thus, it is obligatory for the authors of this paper to justify their gradual withdrawal from the Boston concept in favor of the Chêneau concept. Early studies on the Boston brace have reported about in-brace corrections of 50 to 60% [40]. Later, Uden et al. compared the in-brace correction of the Boston thoracic brace without superstructure (41%) with the Milwaukee brace (10%) [41]. In its already classical paper, Emans et al. also published a "mean better in-brace correction" of 51% [42]. The results of this last study showed that the Boston brace produced better in-brace corrections in single curves with the apex lower than T8, something also observed in other TLSOs. McCollough et al., reporting on the outcomes of the Miami brace, found that the initial correction was 36% in thoracic curves, 56% in thoracolumbar, and 63% in lumbar [43]. Double major curves showed an initial correction of around 37–38% for both curves, lumbar and proximal. At that time, popular opinion indicated that the Milwaukee brace was the choice for thoracic scoliosis with the apex at T8 or higher as well as for double curves with the thoracic apex cranial to T9. Conversely, a preliminary study from Laurnen et al. [44] showed the higher efficacy of the Boston brace compared with the Milwaukee, even for thoracic scoliosis with the apex at T8 and T7. The authors of this study strongly recommended locating the main thoracic pad pushing on the ribs from above but reaching the apex, in combination with a counter pad extended more cranially to the upper ribs on the concave thoracic side. Jonasson-Rajala et al. [45] and, later, Périé D et al. [46] also reported on the importance of the upper extension in order to create a three-point system to more efficiently correct the scoliosis at the main thoracic region. Also in the old study from Emans et al., the result for scoliosis with the apex lower than T7 was similar no matter if it was added to a superstructure or not [42]. The principle of "pushing at the apical level on the convexity of the main thoracic curve," in combination with other forces, was also supported by Wynarsky and Schultz [47] and Aubin et al. [48, 49]. Thus, at least these two theoretical biomechanical principles, both present in the original Chêneau concept, eventually found full support in external evidence. However, sometimes theory goes one way and its practical application goes a different one. We still see many Boston braces fitted incorrectly in accordance with this principle, a fact that is clearly detrimental to the efficiency of the Boston concept. Unfortunately, we also see many Chêneau-type braces clearly failing on this principle.

The earliest results with the Chêneau-type brace were published in Germany. Hopf and Heine [50] report the outcomes of 52 patients treated with a Chêneau-type brace between 1979 and 1980. The mean initial in-brace correction, including single thoracic, single lumbar, and combined curves, was 41%. Weiss and Deez-Kraus [51] reported an initial in-brace correction of 39% for the main thoracic curve and 58% for the lumbar curve. Rigo et al. [52] presented a preliminary mean in-brace correction of 34%. Finally, Liljenqvist et al. [53] achieved a mean in-brace correction of 36%. In a further study, Rigo et al. [54] showed a mean in-brace correction of 31% for the major angle and 26% for the secondary angle, and also reported an initial in-brace axial rotation correction of 22% for the major angle.

Comparing the in-brace correction of this series with those related to the Boston brace, a logical question would be: why continue using this theoretically more complex concept when the Boston concept offered an existing good-to-excellent in-brace correction with the added benefit of a theoretically better standard?

First, it would be a mistake to consider external evidence in only one sense—the in-brace correction of the Cobb angle—when the series are hardly comparable.

In-brace correction depends on many factors; some related to the brace but others related to the patient. Flexibility is one of, if not the most important, factors. Weiss has discussed his experience with an 11-year-old girl treated with one of his versions of the Chêneau-type brace, the Chêneau light® brace [55]. With a Cobb angle of 38° at the start of treatment, she was over-corrected and, after 2 years, had a Cobb angle of 19° with part-time bracing (16 h), which was sufficient to halt further progression. Thus, theoretically, any significant difference when comparing in-brace correction from two different studies could be due to both brace quality and patient quality. The ideal way to make studies comparable would be to match age, gender, and initial Cobb angle as well as curve pattern distribution and flexibility in each determined curve pattern. Thus, in-brace correction as an indicator in comparing brace quality between two different or similar brace concepts should only be partially considered, unless the methodology is strictly comparable.

On the other hand, when considering the discussion above, a significant increase of the in-brace correction reported by the same team over two different periods of time could be considered a good indicator of improved brace quality during the "learning curve" process after transitioning from one brace concept to a different one. Maruyama reported the outcomes of a first series of patients treated with a Rigo-Chêneau brace. His in-brace correction was similar to the first series reported by other authors in their preliminary series [56]. However, the pioneers of the Chêneau brace concepts have gradually increased the percentage of in-brace correction, suggesting that the correction and subsequent improved end results could be due to enhanced brace quality gained from clinical experience. We recently compared the in-brace correction of our own handmade braces (positive moulds corrected personally by the main author MR) with those from a CAD CAM system producing braces from models included in a library of pre-corrected moulds [57]. In this study, a group of 27 patients (26 female) with a mean age of 11.8 years (±2.1), Risser sign of 0.2 (±0.6), and an initial Cobb angle in the major curve of 33° (±7.2), all with no previous treatment and treated with a handmade brace, was compared with a matched group of 41 patients (39 female) treated with the CAD CAM system. In-brace correction—53% in the handmade group and 52.6% in the CAD CAM group—was not significantly different for the major curve. However, 53% is significantly higher than our first in-brace correction of 34% reported in 1995. The in-brace correction achieved with the CAD CAM version has been independently reported as 43, 42, 48, and 37% for thoracic, lumbar, major, and minor curves, respectively, in a group of 147 patients; a sub-group of patients fulfilling the more restrictive SOSORT criteria reportedly achieved corrections of 54, 59, 61, and 52% for thoracic, lumbar, major, and minor curves, respectively [58]. Notwithstanding, as discussed previously, the Chêneau-type brace is not just an orthopedic product but also a brace concept that is permanently evolving in pursuit of the highest possible standard. Brace design can suffer relevant changes and still be respectful to the original concept and theoretical principles. We presented a study comparing two different designs to treat the A1 curve type [59]. The A1 curve type is characterized by a long thoracic curve extending into the lumbar region, with a low apex in the main thoracic region (T9–T11). The study concluded that an over-corrected translation between the pelvis, including the coupled low lumbar region, and the main thoracic region significantly increased the correction when compared to the previously used classical design. The classic brace was built with a fully closed pelvic section, while the modern brace leaves one side totally open. A comparison of the in-brace correction in two similar groups of patients diagnosed with this A1 curve pattern showed a highly significant increase in-brace correction treated with the modern design in comparison with the group treated with the classic design (76.6 versus 45.3%, $p < .001$).

With this perspective, the fact that our own reported initial in-brace correction was not reaching 50% did not force us to give up. The main reason that we changed from the standard concepts used in Spain (Milwaukee, Boston, and Lyon) to the Chêneau concept around 1989 was the observed correlation between the use of the standard braces and the thoracic and lumbar morphological and functional flat back syndrome. Knowledge about the 3D nature of idiopathic scoliosis and its application in scoliosis treatment became very popular among scoliosis surgeons at that time. Jean Dubousset, in his already classic lecture entitled "Importance of the three-dimensional concept in the treatment of scoliotic deformities" (at the Montreal International Symposium on 3D Scoliotic Deformities joined with the VIIth International Symposium on Spinal Deformity and Surface Topography), pointed out the cause-effect relationship between the use of the Milwaukee, Boston, and Lyon braces and flat back syndrome [12]. This relationship has been confirmed and reported primarily by populations treated with the Boston brace [48, 49, 60–62], but this undesirable effect is also produced by other brace concepts, including the Chêneau-type brace. However, according to Dubousset, the only braces in use at the beginning of the 1990s that had the potential to correct scoliosis in 3D

were the 3D brace from Graf and Dauny and the Chêneau brace. All these combined arguments, external evidence, and preferences of some relevant clinicians reinforced our attraction to the Chêneau-type brace and forced us to gradually abandon other brace concepts. However, as discussed previously, the standard of the Chêneau-type brace is poor and, in spite of the claim made by the first promoters, the potential to correct in 3D has been studied rarely. Three-dimensional correction makes reference to (1) frontal plane component, the lateral curvature as measured by the Cobb angle; (2) transversal plane component, the axial rotation of the apical vertebrae, as measured by different methods; and (3) sagittal plane component, related to a highly variable amount of altered spinal geometries impossible to measure with a single angle, which "should be decreased or increased." In other words, in a progressive scoliosis, the torsional phenomenon gradually increases the lateral translation in the frontal plane, with the consequent increase of the Cobb angle; it also gradually increases the axial rotation, no matter which angle might be measured. Thus, reducing those angles is a direct action of the brace correction that can be easily assessed. However, in the sagittal plane, there is no single angle in the lateral radiograph to be decreased or increased always in the same direction for all the cases, which could be used to show the capability of the brace to correct in this plane. Sagittal parameters can be individually assessed according to pelvic incidence; sagittal values will need to be decreased in some cases and increased in others but this should be taken in consideration when designing studies. When we talk about a correction of the flat back component, what are we talking about? Morphological as well as geometrical lordotization of the main thoracic spine most likely happens in most cases of thoracic scoliosis; however, in a variable way and, depending on the orientation of the "plane of maximum deformity," it is only sometimes visible in the lateral radiograph. The "paradoxical kypho-scoliosis," a hyper-rotated lordo-scoliosis with a paradoxical kyphotic geometry in the lateral radiograph, although most typically related to severe "early onset scoliosis," is also observed in adolescent idiopathic scoliosis (AIS) with a relatively mild Cobb angle and a very low morphological lordotic component. Also this should be taken in consideration when designing studies.

Very few studies report on the in-brace correction of the axial rotation. We showed an initial in-brace correction of the axial rotation in the major curve of 22% [54]. Later, in the comparison study of two brace designs—classical and open pelvis—to treat A1 type, the percentage of correction or the axial rotation (Perdriolle) was 29% for the classical design and 59% for the new open pelvis design [59].

The general claim about the Chêneau-type brace correcting flat back syndrome is not adequately supported by external evidence of quality. Cahuzac JP et al. presented outcomes in 161 patients treated with a Chêneau-Toulouse-Münster (CTM) brace. In this study, 55% of patients were pre-pubertal at the initiation of treatment and the initial main Cobb angle of 27.5° was reduced to 22.5° at the end of treatment, with 70% of the patients stabilized or improved, and 30% showing some progression [63]. The sagittal angle between T4 and T12 decreased during the treatment and returned to the initial value at the end of treatment, concluding that the "thoracic lordosis" was temporary modified by the brace. However, these results are hardly interpretable according to the previous discussion related to the sagittal regional or sub-regional values. Other studies have shown also the tendency to reduce the kyphotic angle at the main thoracic region [64–66]. However, the Chêneau-type brace design used in these studies could be significantly different to the design described in this current paper. As mentioned previously, the pelvic section of the brace is not built in retroversion, as defined in old brace concepts and seen in some Chêneau versions, but maintains a physiological anterior inclination. The Milwaukee concept, as well as the first-generation Boston brace, was based on the popular principle of "obliteration of the sagittal postural curvatures to achieve a better correction of the pathological lateral deviation." A better understanding of the 3D nature of idiopathic scoliosis proved this principle incorrect, as it has been associated, in many cases, with an undesirable secondary flat back effect, in both the lumbar and thoracic regions [67]. Pelvis retroversion was considered the first step in the application of this principle due to its delordosant effect on the lumbar spine. Abdominal ventral pressure to ensure the delordosant effect was also very popular among orthotists. Soon after the introduction of the first-generation Boston brace, Willner [60, 61] emphasized the importance of reduction of the lumbar lordosis in the correction of the lumbar scoliosis. J. Chêneau was very critical of this very popular principle, recommending from the very beginning against unselective abdominal pressure and pelvis retroversion, but many orthotists used it in the past and continue to use it when constructing their braces under the name of Chêneau. Later, in a study of the 3D immediate effect of the Boston brace on the scoliotic lumbar spine, Labelle et al. [62] showed that the brace produced a distraction of the lumbar spine similar to that produced by the Harrington instrumentation by correcting the frontal plane deformity at expenses of a significant reduction of the physiological

lumbar lordosis. They were not able to demonstrate any significant effect on rotation of the apical vertebra or "detorsion." Modern Boston brace has abandoned the principle of pelvis retroversion and delordosis but still uses the unselective abdominal pressure. We must admit that at the current state of the art of the Chêneau-type brace, the principle of constructing the pelvis section with a physiological anterior inclination of the pelvis and physiological lumbar sagittal profile with selective abdominal expansion-pressure is subjective but not based on objective assessment. Notwithstanding, the concept of physiological pelvis anterior inclination is not a general one but has a high individual variability. Pelvis indexes (pelvic incidence; sacral slope, and pelvic tilt), in relationship with the sagittal geometry of the spine, more or less recoverable in the brace depending on the lordotic morphological component, could be used as a guide to define the amount of inclination the pelvic section of the brace should have case by case. We are now developing on this issue but cannot offer any information yet aside of the already explained three versions according to a normal, high, or low individual pelvic incidence.

Thus, the question about whether using Chêneau principles in brace construction can prevent the flat back or not is still open. In a relatively old study, we analyzed the 3D geometry of the spine in a group of patients treated with the first version of the Chêneau-type brace [68] and, although a significant number of patients showed improved sagittal alignment during brace treatment, some patients had what could be considered deterioration of the sagittal profile. From this experience, some significant changes were introduced in the brace design to prevent deterioration and further clinical observation supported the idea that a well-designed brace can prevent the deterioration of the morphological lordotization of the thoracic spine; further studies are necessary to support this statement. A recent study from Lebel et al. [69], comparing 3D effect from classical TLSO and Chêneau-type brace, has shown that only the Chêneau-type brace is able to reduce rotation of the apical vertebra. Coronal and sagittal correction did not differ significantly when comparing both brace concepts. The authors used EOS technology for spinal 3D reconstruction, but again here, we have no idea about which type of sagittal design they applied to their Chêneau-type version.

Although the end results were reported in some of the old series [50], more recent series support the effectiveness of the Chêneau-type brace when similar standards are observed. In 2003, two papers from independent centers with similar protocols in conservative management combining the Chêneau-type brace and Schroth scoliosis-specific exercises showed comparable effectiveness in

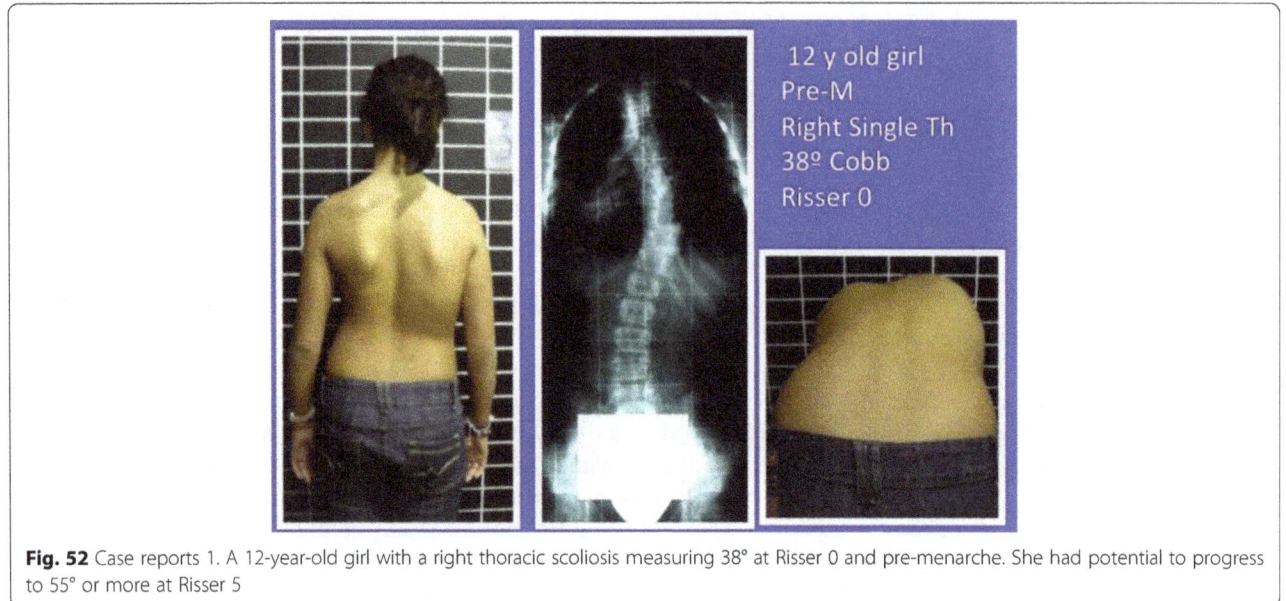

Fig. 52 Case reports 1. A 12-year-old girl with a right thoracic scoliosis measuring 38° at Risser 0 and pre-menarche. She had potential to progress to 55° or more at Risser 5

preventing surgery. In a retrospective study, which included 343 patients (females only) with a mean Cobb angle of 33.4° treated with a Chêneau-type brace between 1993 and 1996, Weiss et al. found that only 12% of all patients underwent surgery [70]. All the patients were at least 15 years of age at the time they were last investigated. In the second study, Rigo et al. retrospectively analyzed the outcome in patients treated with a Rigo-Chêneau-type brace [71]. The objective was to determine whether a center with an active policy of conservative management had a lower prevalence of surgery compared with a center that had a non-intervention policy. The study included 106 braced patients who were at least 15 years of age at last review. Ultimately, only 14% (in a worst case analysis of all the intents to treat, including non-compliance and considering lost patients as failures) of braced patients underwent

spinal fusion, which was statistically significantly lower than the 28% reported by the center with the policy of non-intervention.

Later, Weiss HR et al. [72] compared two brace concepts: the Chêneau-type brace (at that time, according to Rigo-Chêneau principles) and the soft brace concept, SpineCor. They compared the survival rates of the two different brace concepts with respect to curve progression and duration of treatment during pubertal growth spurt in two cohorts of patients. All girls in the study were pre-menarchial with the first clinical signs of maturation (Tanner 1–3). Twelve girls with an initial mean Cobb angle of 21.3° were treated with the SpineCor, compared to 15 girls matched in age with an initial mean Cobb angle of 33.7°. During the pubertal growth spurt, most of the patients (11 out of 12) with the

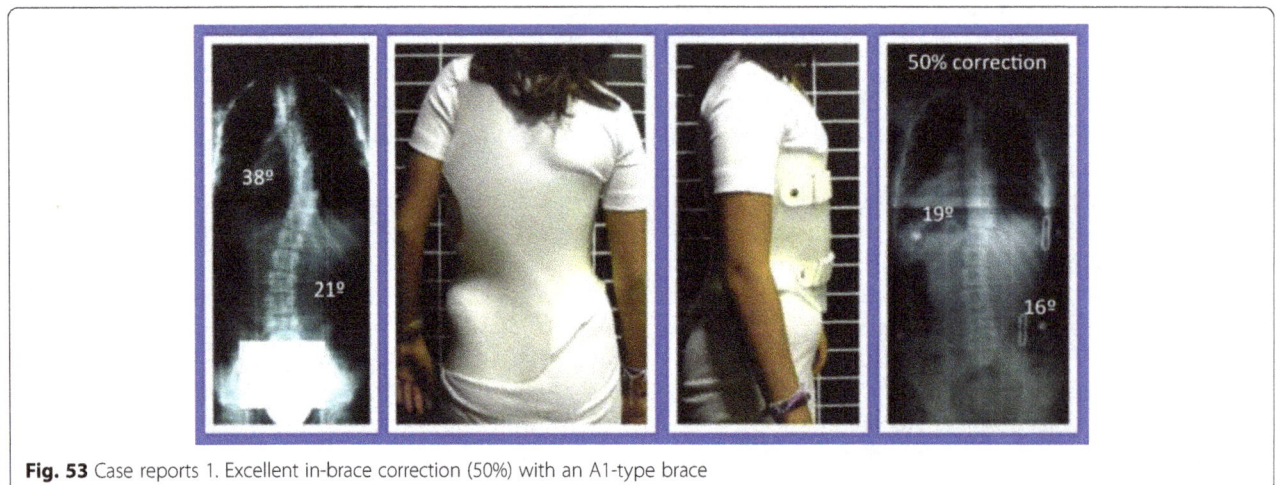

Fig. 53 Case reports 1. Excellent in-brace correction (50%) with an A1-type brace

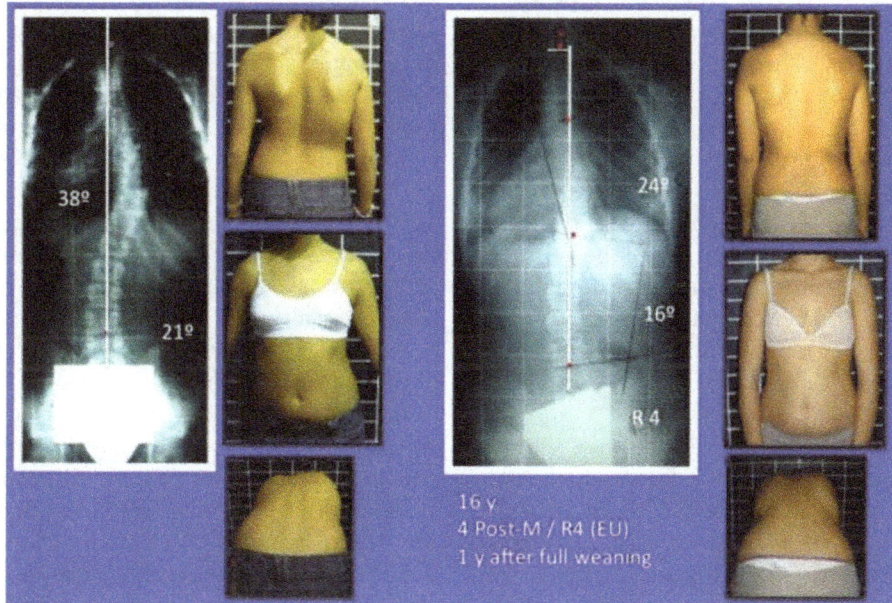

Fig. 54 Case reports 1. End result 1 year after full weaning. The girl had a stable curve of 24° (initial curve 38°) at Risser 4 (16 years of age). Clinical improvement is also noticeable

SpineCor progressed clinically and radiologically. Progression was halted after the patients transitioned from the SpineCor to the Chêneau-type brace in seven of the progressive cases. The sample treated initially with the Chêneau-type brace showed no progression. After 24 months of treatment time, 73% of the patients with a Chêneau-type brace and 33% of the patients with the SpineCor were still under treatment with their original brace concepts. After 42 months of treatment, 80% of the patients with the Chêneau-type brace and 8% of the patients with the SpineCor survived with respect to curvature progression.

Cinnella et al. [73] presented at the SOSORT meeting in Lyon a retrospective series of 152 patients treated with a Chêneau-type brace, with a minimum of 20 months of follow-up (mean 56 months). At the end of treatment, the authors observed an average initial curve improvement of 23.3%. At follow-up, they observed an average improvement of 15% from the beginning of treatment. In this study, however, the protocol was different to further published series because 79% of the population was previously treated with a cast. Thus, we are not adding this to the rest of the series discussed in the paper.

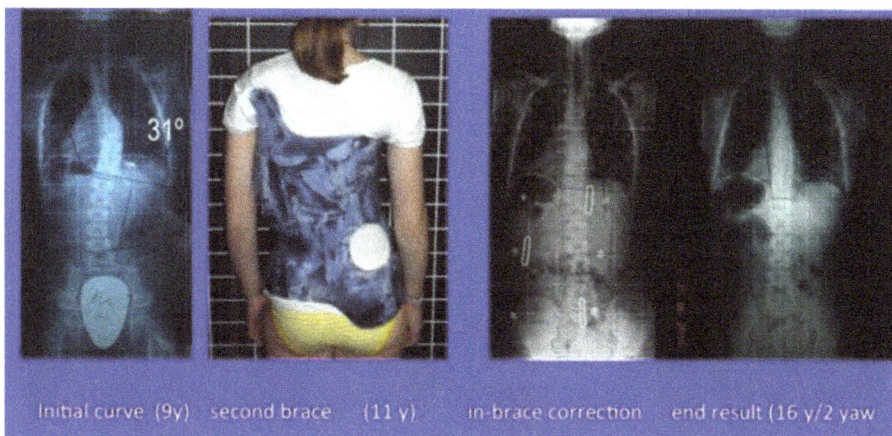

Fig. 55 Case reports 2. A 9-year-old girl showing an excellent end result 2 years after full weaning. She was treated with a C1-type brace and PSSE

Zaborovska-Sapeta et al. [74] conducted a prospective observational study according to SOSORT and SRS recommendations. The study included 79 patients with initial Cobb angles between 20° and 45°, no previous treatment, Risser 4 or higher at final evaluation, and a minimum 1-year follow-up after weaning from the brace. Results showed that 25% of all patients improved, 23% were stable, 39% progressed below 50°, and 13% progressed beyond 50°. This study suggested that conservative treatment with the Chêneau-type brace and physiotherapy (again, with similar brace standards and similar treatment approaches) can change the natural history of scoliosis, as 48% of patients did not progress.

Another retrospective cohort study from Ovadia et al. [75] was preformed to identify factors that could predict the therapeutic success or failure of the Rigo-Chêneau brace. Ninety-three patients with an average age of 13 years, Cobb angle of 32°, and Risser 1 were followed. All patients were treated with a Rigo-Chêneau-type brace during a mean treatment period of 36 months, and all had a 2-year follow-up after the termination of brace treatment. The authors concluded that the treatment was successful in 84% of patients, which indicates that the brace provides excellent clinical results in the treatment of mild to moderate AIS. Patients also showed a significant reduction of the angle of trunk rotation, suggesting the ability of the brace to correct the 3D trunk deformity, confirming initial observations about clinical improvement [68, 76]. Correction of the 3D trunk deformity can be assessed by using surface topography [68] as well as radiological indexes like the rib index from Grivas [77], although this last has not been used yet in patients treated with a Chêneau-type brace.

More recently, Rivett et al. [78] analyzed the effect of compliance to a Rigo System Chêneau brace and a specific exercise program on idiopathic scoliosis curvature, and compared the quality of life (QoL) and psychological traits of compliant and non-compliant subjects. Fifty-one subjects, all girls aged 12–16, with Cobb angles 20–50° participated in the study. Subjects were divided into two groups, according to their compliance, at the end of the study. The compliant group wore the brace 20 or more hours a day and exercised three or more times per week. The non-compliant group wore the brace less than 20 h a day and exercised less than three times per week. Cobb angle, vertebral rotation, Scoliometer reading, peak flow, QoL, and personality traits were compared between groups. The compliant group wore the brace 21.5 h per day and exercised four times a week, and significantly improved in all the measures compared to the non-compliant subjects, who wore the brace 12 h per day, exercised 1.7 times per week and

significantly deteriorated ($p < .0001$). The major Cobb angle in the compliant group improved 10.19° (±5.5) and deteriorated 5.52° (±4.3) in the non-compliant group. Compliant group had a significantly better QoL than the non-compliant subjects. The compliant subjects were significantly more emotionally mature, stable, and realistic than the non-compliant group ($p < .05$). The conclusion of this study was that good compliance of the RSC brace and a specific exercise regime resulted in a significant improvement in curvature, while poor compliance resulted in progression. A poorer QoL in the non-compliant group possibly was caused by personality traits of the group, being more emotionally immature and unstable. Other aspects of QoL like function have not been studied. Based on the theoretical principles of this brace, users claim about no deterioration of breathing function, but we do not know any study supporting this.

As discussed previously, different brace concepts cannot fairly be compared to current state-of-the-art concepts. Thus, the old statement about the best brace being managed with the highest experience by a particular multidisciplinary team could still be defended, at least in terms of patient safety. However, once the efficacy of bracing has been strongly supported, further studies are necessary to demonstrate the ability of a particular brace concept to correct scoliosis in 3D and whether or not 3D in-brace correction is a factor when predicting the success of bracing.

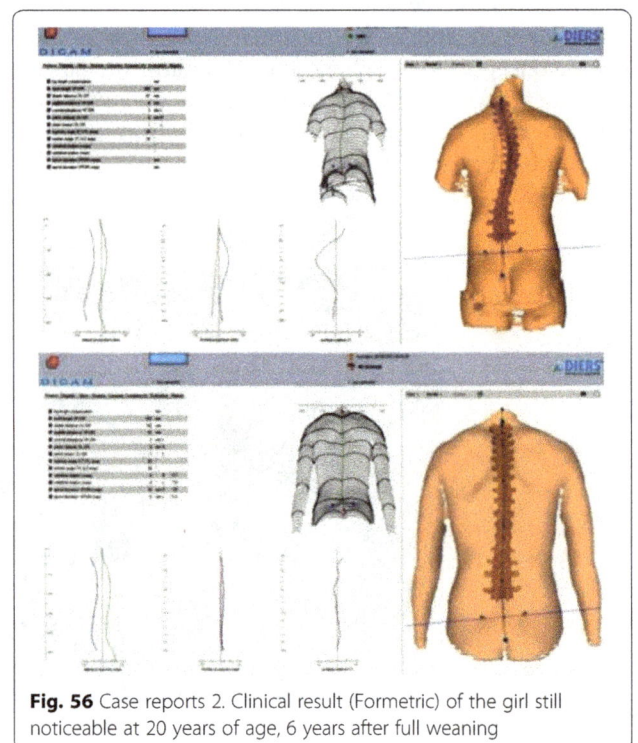

Fig. 56 Case reports 2. Clinical result (Formetric) of the girl still noticeable at 20 years of age, 6 years after full weaning

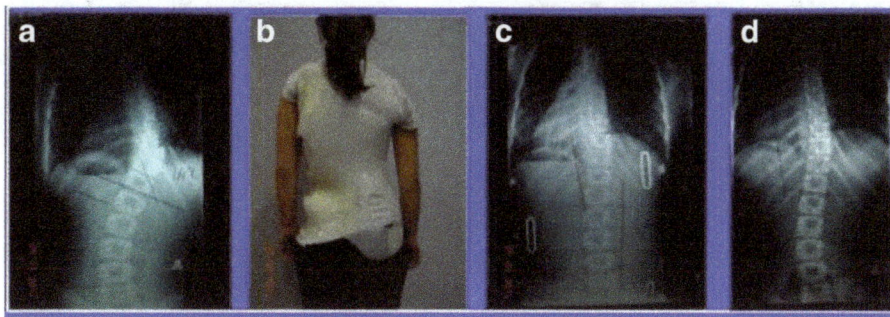

Fig. 57 Case reports 3. A 9-years-old girl (menarche at 10 years of age) treated with an A2-type brace (**b**) after being diagnosed with a right convex thoracic scoliosis measuring 44º Cobb (**a**). After excellent in-brace correction (**c**), she showed a short-term correction, out of brace (**d**), which allow us to recommend her for early weaning

The theoretical disadvantage of the Chêneau-type concept of bracing is the complexity of its principles and fabrication, which has been associated with poor standards. By summarizing previously reported studies and providing supporting published data, this paper attempts to raise awareness and education to improve the future standard of the Chêneau concept. Nevertheless, the fact that consistent and comparable results are reported by at least five independent centers using similar standards cannot be ignored.

Case reports
Case reports 1
This reports the final radiological and clinical result in a 12-year-old girl diagnosed with adolescent idiopathic scoliosis, 1 year after finishing treatment. She was still pre-menarche at diagnosis and initiation of treatment. Clinical presentation was like 3C and a radiograph confirmed a right long-low thoracic scoliosis measuring 38° Cobb and rotation degree $II^{1/2}$ according to Nash and Moe, and Risser 0. Curve pattern and "transitional point offset" were compatible with A1 type. Initial clinical and radiological presentation is shown in Fig. 52. Being closed to 40° Cobb before reaching Risser 1, the potential for progression of a thoracic scoliosis is reaching Risser 5 with a scoliosis over 55° [79]. Based on prognosis she was recommended to go under full-time bracing and PSSE according to BSPTS-Schroth principles. Figure 53 shows the girl just after first fitting, once the brace was finished, and before adaptation. The same figure shows also the first radiograph in brace with an excellent correction of 50% of the Cobb angle and a mild but relevant correction of the rotational component. She wore the brace full-time for 2 years and one additional year only at night. Figure 54 shows her radiograph 1 year after full weaning, at 16 years of age, Risser 4 (European scale), 4 years after menarche. A well-balanced scoliosis measuring 24° thoracic and 16° lumbar, with no structural

proximal curve and just a mild imbalance at T1 was confirmed. Rib cage appeared perfectly balanced on the pelvis. She had her first menstruation few months after starting treatment, still at 12 years of age. Clinical result is also noticeable when looking at both back asymmetry and postural balance in the frontal plane. Angle of trunk inclination (ATI) measured in forward bending from sitting position came down from 14° to 7° (50% correction). Sagittal photos were not documented but a photo from dorsal does not show any deterioration of the morphological flat back. She continued practicing her exercises during the year after full weaning.

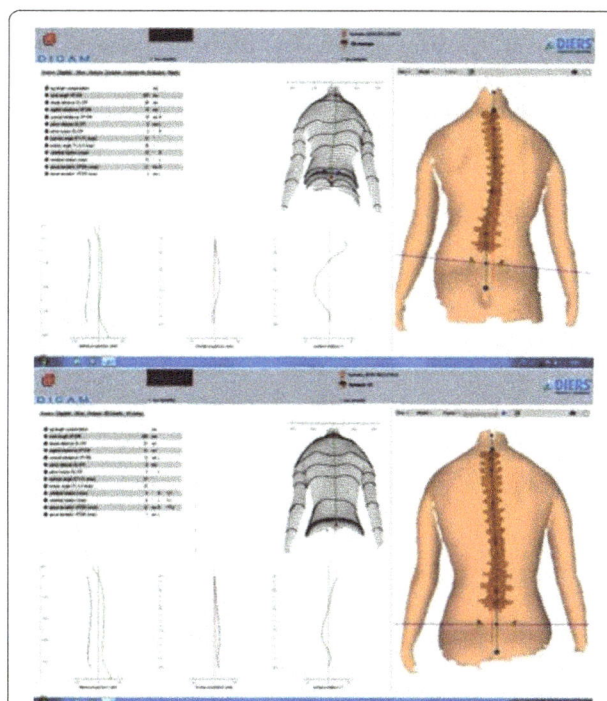

Fig. 58 Case reports 3. Clinical improvement (Formetric®) after 3 years of treatment (1 year full-time + 2 years nighttime)

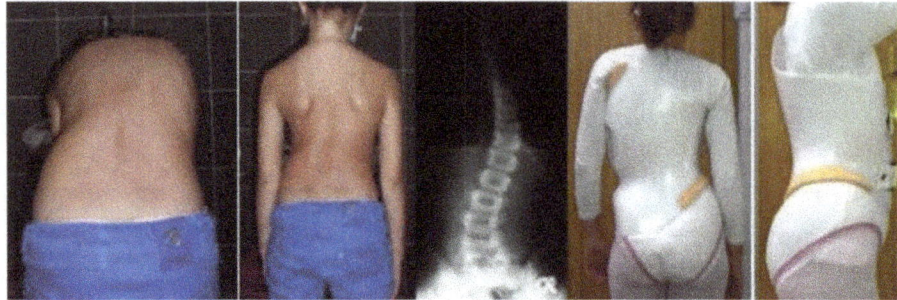

Fig. 59 Case reports 4. An 8-year-old girl treated initially with an A2-type brace by the junior author MJ. One year after initiation of treatment she showed some clinical and radiological changes (Fig. 60). The girl is still under treatment

Case reports 2

This reports the final radiological result in a 9-year-old girl diagnosed with late-onset juvenile idiopathic scoliosis. She had a clinical presentation like 3C (A2 type) and radiograph showed a single right thoracic scoliosis measuring 31° Cobb. We made a first C1-type brace (at that time still with pelvis closed) with an in-brace correction of around 50% (in-brace Cobb angle was 15°). Prescription was "full-time." She was also recommended to start physiotherapy scoliosis-specific exercises (PSSE) according to Barcelona School (BSPTS), based on Schroth principles. After 1 year of treatment, she was fitted in a second brace due to growth and development showing an in-brace Cobb angle of 7°. The girl was then 11 years old at Risser 0 and had pre-menarche status. She continued wearing the brace full-time. Her menarche was at 12 years of age. She continued wearing the brace full-time (>20 h) until 13 years of age, and due to an excellent clinical result, with a total reduction of the ATI from 9° to 0°, she was recommended to go under

"nighttime" regimen. Total weaning was at 14 years of age. A final radiograph was ordered when she was 16 years of age, 2 years after weaning, showing a very mild right thoracic curve measuring 10° Cobb, at Risser 5. Figure 55 shows the radiological result. Figure 56 shows the esthetic improvement 4 years after her last radiograph, at 20 years of age. Due to the consistent clinical improvement, no radiograph was then prescribed. Her spine looked rectilinear with insignificant right/left asymmetries and a relatively preserved sagittal profile, with a mild lumbar hypo-lordosis and thoracic hypo-kyphosis, but still into the normal range for the Formetric values, with no clinically relevant change in comparison with the initial profile, if perhaps a very mild ventral imbalance.

Case reports 3

This reports the initial in-brace correction and short-term results in a 9-year-old girl initially diagnosed with juvenile idiopathic scoliosis. Although the initial Cobb

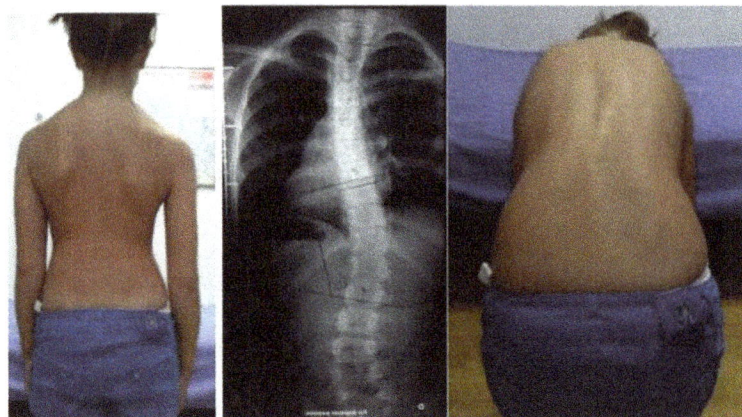

Fig. 60 Case reports 4. One year after initiating treatment with an A1-type brace, this girl showed a change in the curve pattern, which was considered to be relevant for this brace concept. The long-low thoracic curve (apex T10) combined with a hidden proximal curve (A1 with D mod), changed to a high thoracolumbar curve (apex disc T11–T12 with aplasia of the 12 rib) combined with a high thoracic curve. She was treated then with a B2-type brace as shown in Fig. 61. The girl is still under treatment

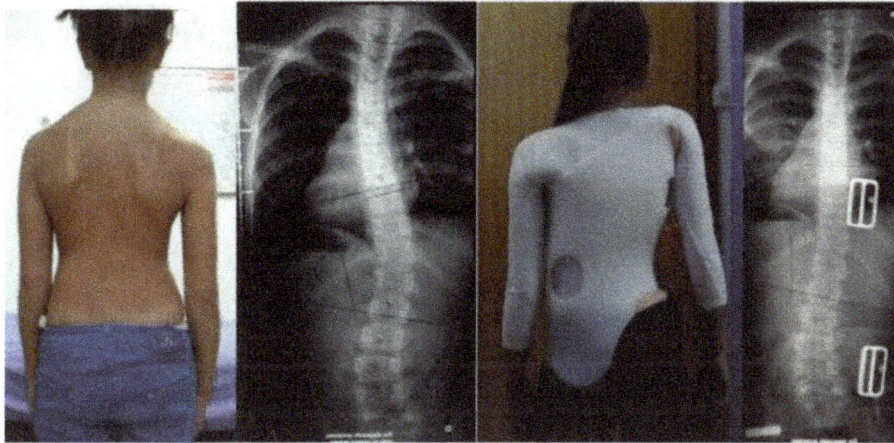

Fig. 61 Case reports 4. Excellent in-brace correction with a B2-type brace in a girl who was previously treated with an A2-type brace, which was associated with a change in the curve pattern. The girl is still under treatment

angle was 44° and she was 9 years of age, she had menarche at 10 years of age, few months after coming for her first consultation, so her evolution and potential for progression was expected to be like AIS. She was recommended for bracing immediately and was fitted with an A2-type brace. The Cobb angle in-brace (1 month of adaptation after reaching full-time) was 13° (70% in-brace correction) and consequently was strongly recommend wearing the brace in a full-time regimen (>20 h). She practiced also PSSE according to BSPTS regularly and was controlled every 6 months. Due to an excellent clinical response with a total correction of the back asymmetry (Formetric ®) and a very significant reduction of the ATI, she was recommended for partial early weaning, going under a "nighttime regimen" after she showed a significant correction of the Cobb angle in an out-brace radiograph, taken after 1 week using the brace only at night, and 8 h after she took of the brace in the morning. The radiograph showed a Cobb angle of 16°. Two years later she still showed a highly consistent improvement of the back asymmetry with a practical inversion of the expected asymmetry for a right thoracic scoliosis/left lumbar. She was then recommended to stop bracing. Her last radiograph, 3 months after total weaning, shows a quasi-stable situation with a scoliosis still under 20°. Final result will be assessed in a new radiograph 2 years after weaning in 2017. Figure 57 shows the radiological results. Figure 58 shows the clinical changes by surface topography. The asymmetry remained inverted after 2 years of nighttime brace (and just 1 year of full-time bracing). Sagittal profile shows a relatively disharmonic configuration with lower lumbar lordosis/upper thoracic kyphosis and a hypo-kyphotic/hypo-lordotic configuration in the main thoracic and upper lumbar region, but not different to the initial profile. The girl presents a mild sagittal imbalance, but she is doing well in terms of QOL.

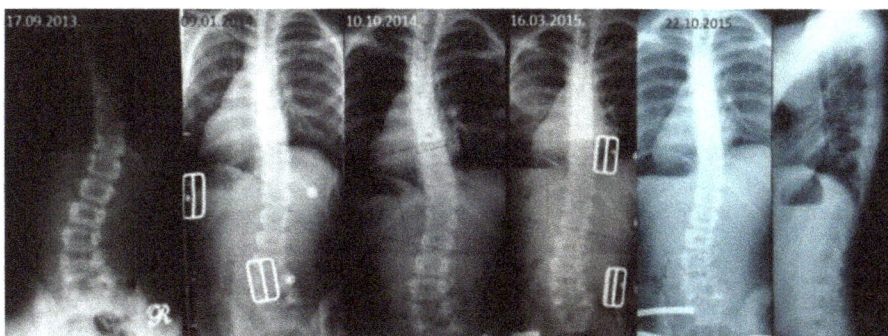

Fig. 62 Case reports 4. Radiological evolution from the initial presentation on September 2013, in-brace correction (A1-type brace); 1 year later, out the brace; in-brace correction in her second brace (B2 type) and out the brace on October 2015, 2 years after initiation of treatment. The lateral projection shows a normal sagittal configuration. The girl is still under treatment

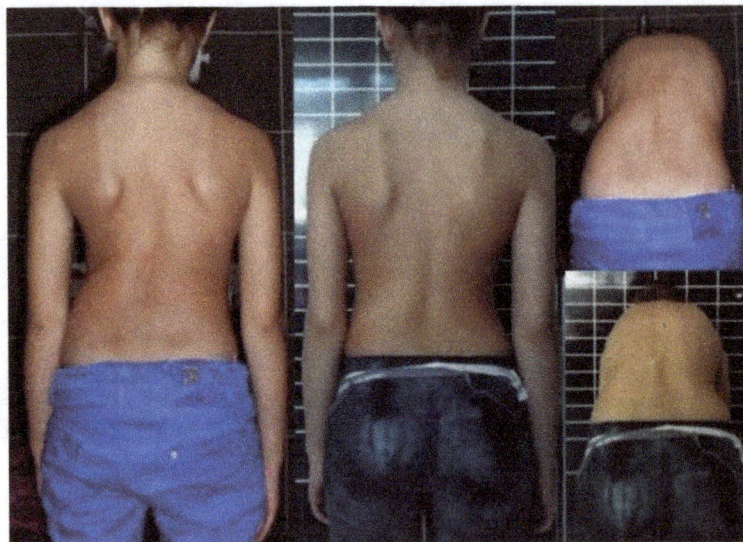

Fig. 63 Case reports 4. Short-term clinical result, 2 years after initiation of the treatment, first with an A1-type brace and later with a B2-type brace. Brace had to be remade after a change in the curve pattern. The girl is still under treatment

Case reports 4

This reports about a change in the curve pattern observed after 1 year of treatment with an A1-type brace, and the short-term radiological and clinical result in an 8-year-old girl treated by the junior author MJ. The girl was diagnosed with juvenile idiopathic scoliosis at 8 years of age. Clinical and radiological criteria were for A1 type: long-low thoracic curve combined with a hidden proximal thoracic curve (not visible on the radiograph due to bad quality, but clinically) (Fig. 59). She was then treated with an A1-type brace showing an excellent in-brace correction. One year later she had changed her curve pattern. The right long-low thoracic curve became a border case after a caudal migration of the apex to the disc T11–T12, combined with a high main thoracic rather than proximal thoracic curve (Fig. 60). We decided to change her brace design using a B2-type brace, which was made and adapted again by the second author MJ. The in-brace correction was also excellent in the B2-type brace ad clinical improvement after 1 year and half of treatment was also noticeable (Figs. 61, 62 and 63). The girl is still under treatment. The change in curve pattern is not a rare event in early onset scoliosis but in late onset, when using a hyper-corrective brace.

Conclusions

The Chêneau-type brace according to Rigo principles and classification is a 3D corrective device able to provide excellent in-brace correction as well as radiological and cosmetic end results. This paper offers a vast description of the applied corrective principles as well as a short revision of the specific classification, with the ambitious objective of improving the observed poor standard of the classically called Chêneau brace.

Abbreviations

3D: Tridimensional; BSPTS: Barcelona Scoliosis Physical Therapy School; BUFA: Bundesfaschule für Orthopadie Technik; CSL: Central sacral line; CTM: Chêneau-Toulouse-Münster; HRQL: Health-related quality of life; PSSE: Physiotherapy scoliosis-specific exercises; RASO: Relative anterior spinal overgrowth; SOSORT: International Society on Orthopaedic and Rehabilitation Treatment; TLS: Toracolumbosacral; TP: Transitional point

Acknowledgements

The authors are thankful to Luke Stikeleather for copyediting the final paper.

Funding

None.

Authors' contributions

MR is the main author of this paper and has contributed in the conception and design of it. To him belongs the intellectual property of the bracing concept as described in this paper. He has been fully involved in drafting the manuscript, preparing figures and case reports 1, 2, and 3. MJ is the second author of this paper and has contributed in the conception and design of it. She has been fully involved in drafting the manuscript and case reports 4. Both authors read and approved the final manuscript.

Competing interests

Manuel Rigo declares the next "Competing Interests":

1) Medical director of Rigo Quera Salvá S.L.P., a private institution for non-operative treatment of spinal deformities, which can be indirectly benefited by the publication of this paper.
2) Medical advisor of Ortholutions oHG (Rosenheim Germany) and Align Clinic (San Mateo, CA, USA), receiving consultation fees.
3) Lecturer in a course about Chêneau principles during the last 12 years, at the BUFA-Dortmund (Germany).
Mina Jelačić declares no competing interests.

Author details
[1]Elena Salvá Institute (Rigo Quera Salvá S.L.P.), Vía Augusta 185, 08021 Barcelona, Spain. [2]Specijalističa Ordinacija za fizikalnu medicine I rehabiliraciju "Ledja I vrat", Stojana Protića 48, Belgrade, Republic of Serbia.

References
1. Maruyama T, Grivas TB, Kaspiris A. Effectiveness and outcomes of brace treatment: a systematic review. Physiother Theory Pract. 2011;27(1):26–42.
2. Negrini S, Minossi S, Bettany-Saltikov J, Zaina F, Chockalingam N, Grivas TB, Kotwicki T, Maruyama T, Romano M, Vasiliadis ES. Braces for idiopathic scoliosis in adolescents. Spine. 2010;35(13):1285–93.
3. Weinstein SL, Dolan LA, Wright JG, Dobbs MB. Effects of bracing in adolescent with idiopathic scoliosis. N Engl J Med. 2013;369:1512–21.
4. Rigo M, Negrini S, Weiss HR, Grivas TB, Maruyama T, Kotwicki T, the members of SOSORT. SOSORT consensus paper on brace action: TLSO biomechanics of correction (investigating the rationale for force vector selection). Scoliosis. 2006;1:10.
5. Negrini S, Aulisa AG, Aulisa L, Circo AB, de Mauroy JC, Durmala J, Grivas TB, Knott P, Kotwicki T, Maruyama T, Minozzi S, O'Brien JP, Papadopoulos D, Rigo M, Rivard CH, Romano M, Wynne JH, Villagrasa M, Weiss HR, Zaina F. 2111 SOSORT guidelines: Orthopaedic and Rehabilitation treatment of idiopathic scoliosis during growth. Scoliosis. 2012;7:3.
6. Chêneau J. Corset-Chêneau. Manuel d'orthopédie des scolioses suivant la technique originale. Paris: Éditions Frison-Roche; 1994.
7. Weiss HR, Rigo M, Chêneau J. Praxis der Chêneau Korsettversorgung in der Skoliose-Therapie. Stuttgart: Thieme; 2000.
8. Weiss HR, Rigo M. The Chêneau concept of bracing – actual standards. Stud Health Technol Inform. 2008;135:291–302.
9. Rigo M, Weiss HR. The Chêneau concept of bracing – biomechanical aspects. Stud Health Technol Inform. 2008;135:303–19.
10. Rigo M, Villagrasa M, Gallo D. A specific scoliosis classification correlating with brace treatment: description and reliability. Scoliosis. 2010;5:1.
11. Negrini S, Grivas TB. Introduction to the "Scoliosis" Journal Brace Technology Thematic Series: increasing existing knowledge and promoting future developments. Scoliosis. 2010;5:2.
12. Dubousset J. Importance of the three-dimensional concept in the treatment of scoliosis deformities. Dansereau J ed. International Symposium on 3D Scoliotic Deformities joined with the VII International Symposium on Spinal Deformities and Surface Topography. Germany: Gustav Fisher Verlag; 1992. p. 302–11.
13. Raso VJ, Russell GG, Hill DL, Moreau M, MCivor J. Thoracic lordosis in idiopathic scoliosis. J Pediatric Orthop. 1991;11(5):599–602.
14. Raso VJ, Lou E, Hill DL, Mahood JK, Moreau MJ, Durdle NG. Trunk distorsion and idiopathic scoliosis. J Pediatric Orthop. 1998;18(2):222–6.
15. Guo X, Chau WW, Chang YL, Cheng JC, Burwell RG, Dangerfield PH. Relative anterior spinal overgrowth in adolescent idiopathic scoliosis – result of disproportionate endochondral-membranous bone growth? Summary of an electronic focus group debate of the IBSE. Eur Spine J. 2005;14(9):862–73.
16. Burwell RG, Dangerfield PH. Pathogenesis of progressive adolescent idiopathic scoliosis. Platelet activation and vascular biology in immature vertebrae: an alternative molecular hypothesis. Acta Orthop Belg. 2006;72(3):247–60.
17. Zhu F, Qiu Y, Yeung HY, Lee KM, Cheng JC. Histomorphometric study of the spinal growth plates in idiopathic scoliosis and congenital scoliosis. Pediatric Int. 2006;48(6):591–8.
18. Burwell RG, Dangerfield PH, Freeman BJ. Concepts on the pathogenesis of adolescent idiopathic scoliosis. Bone growth and mass, vertebral column, spinal cord, brain, skull, extra-spinal left-right skeletal length asymmetries, disproportions and molecular pathogenesis. Stud Health Technol Inform. 2008;135:3–52.
19. Chu WC, Lam WM, Ng BK, Tze-Ping L, Lee KM, Guo X, Cheng JC, Burwell RG, Dangerfield PH, Jaspan T. Relative shortening and functional tethering of the spinal cord in adolescent idiopathic scoliosis – Result of asynchronous neuro-osseous growth, summary of an electronic focus group debate of the IBSE. Scoliosis. 2008;3:8.
20. Burwell RG, Aujla RK, Freeman BJ, Dangerfield PH, Cole AA, Kirby AS, Polak FJ, Pratt RK, Moulton A. The posterior skeletal thorax: rib-vertebral angle and axial vertebral rotation asymmetries in adolescent idiopathic scoliosis. Stud Health Technol Inform. 2008;140:263–8.
21. Gu SX, Wang CF, Zhao YC, Zhu XD, Li M. Abnormal ossification as a cause the progression of adolescent idiopathic scoliosis. Med Hypotheses. 2009;72(4):416–7.
22. Liu Z, Tam EM, Sun GQ, Lam TP, Zhu ZZ, Sun X, Lee KM, Ng TB, Qiu Y, Cheng JC, Yeung HY. Abnormal leptin bioavailability in adolescent idiopathic scoliosis: an important new finding. Spine. 2012;37(7):599–604.
23. Schlösser TP, van Stralen M, Brink RC, Chu WC, Lam TP, Vincken KL, Castelein RM, Cheng JC. Three-dimensional characterization of torsion and asymmetry of the intervertebral disc versus vertebral bodies in adolescent idiopathic scoliosis. Spine. 2014;39(19):E1 159–166.
24. Stokes IA, Spence H, Aronsson DD, Kilmer N. Mechanical modulation of vertebral body growth. Implications for scoliosis progression. Spine. 1996;21(10):1162–7.
25. Burwell RG. Aetiology of idiopathic scoliosis: current concepts. Pediatr Rehabil. 2003;6(3-4):137–70.
26. Murray DW, Bulstrode CJ. The development of adolescent idiopathic scoliosis. Eur Spine J. 1996;5(4):251–7.
27. Duval-Beaupere G, Taussig G, Mouilleseaux B, Pries P, Mounier C. Prognostic factors for idiopathic scoliosis. Dansereau J ed. International Symposium on 3D Scoliotic Deformities joined with the VII International Symposium on Spinal Deformities and Surface Topography. Germany: Gustav Fisher Verlag; 1992. p. 211–6.
28. Legaye J, Orban C. Evolution of scoliosis by optical scanner I.S.I.S. Stud Health Technol Inform. 1995;15:415–21.
29. Bernhardt M, Bridwell KH. Segmental analysis of the sagittal plane alignment of the normal thoracic and lumbar spines and thoracolumbar junction. Spine. 1989;14(7):717–21.
30. Lehnert-Schroth C. Dreidimensionale Skoliosebehandlung. 6th ed. Stuttgart: Urban and Swarzer; 2000.
31. Moe JH, Kettleson D. Idiopathic scoliosis: Analysis of curve patterns and preliminary results of Milwaukee brace treatment in one hundred sixty-nine patients. J Bone Joint Surg Am. 1970;52(8):1509–33.
32. Working Group on 3-D Classification (Chair Larry Lenke, MD), and the Terminology Committee, March 2000. SRS Terminology Committee and Working Group on Spinal Classification Revised Glossary of Terms. http://www.srs.org/professionals/online-education-and-resources/glossary/revised-glossary-of-terms.
33. Rigo M, Quera-Salvá G, Villagrasa M, Ferrer M, Casas A, Corbella C, Urrutia A, Martínez S, Puigdevall N. Scoliosis intensive out-patient rehabilitation based on Schroth method. T.B. Grivas (Ed.) The Conservative Scoliosis Treatment. Stud Health Technol Inform. 2008;135:208–27.
34. Carr WA, Moe JH, Winter RB, Lonstein JE. Treatment of idiopathic scoliosis in the Milwaukee brace. J Bone Joint Surg Am. 1980;62(4):599–612.
35. Heine J, Gotze HG. Final results of the conservative treatment of scoliosis using the Milwaukee brace. Z Orthop Ihre Grenzgeb. 1985;123(3):56–62.
36. Noonan KJ, Weinstein SL, Jacobson WC, Dolan LA. Use of the Milwaukee brace for progressive idiopathic scoliosis. J Bone Joint Surg Am. 1996;78(4):557–67.
37. Katz DE, Durrani AA. Factors that influence outcome in bracing large curves in patients with adolescent idiopathic scoliosis. Spine. 2001;26(21):2354–61.
38. Landauer F, Wimmer C, Behensky H. Estimating the final outcome of brace treatment for idiopathic thoracic scoliosis at 6-month follow-up. Pediatr Rehabil. 2003;6(3-4):201–7.
39. Castro Jr FP. Adolescent idiopathic scoliosis, bracing and the Hueter-Volkmann principle. Spine J. 2003;3(3):180–5.
40. Watts HG, Hall JE, Stanish W. The Boston brace system for the treatment of low thoracic and lumbar scoliosis by use of a girdle without superstructure. Clin Orthop Relat Res. 1977;126:87–92.
41. Uden A, Willner S, Peterson H. Initial correction with the Boston thoracic brace. Acta Orthop Scand. 1982;53(6):907–11.

42. Emans JB, Kaelin A, Bancel P, Hall JE, Miller ME. The Boston bracing system for idiopathic scoliosis. Follow-up results in 295 patients. Spine. 1986;11(8):792–801.

43. MaCollough NC 3d, Schultz M, Javech N, Latta L. Miami TLSO in the management of scoliosis: preliminary results in 100 cases. J Pediatr Orthop. 1981;1(2):141–52.

44. Laurnen EL, Tupper JW, Mullen MP. The Boston brace in thoracic scoliosis. A preliminary report. Spine. 1983;8(4):388–95.

45. Jonasson-Rajala E, Josefsson E, Lundberg B, Nilsson H. Boston thoracic brace in the treatment of idiopathic scoliosis. Initial correction. Clin Orthop. 1984;183:37–41.

46. Périé D, Aubin CE, Petit Y, Beauséjour M, Dansereau J, Labelle H. Boston brace correction in idiopathic scoliosis: a biomechanical study. Spine. 2003;28(15):1672–7.

47. Wynarsky GT, Schultz AB. Optimization of skeletal configuration. Studies of scoliosis correction biomechanics. J Biomech. 1991;24(8):721–32.

48. Aubin CA, Dansereau J, Labelle H. Biomechanical simulation of the effect of the Boston brace on a model of the scoliotic spine and thorax. Ann Chir. 1993;47(9):881–7.

49. Aubin CE, Dansereau J, De Guise JA, Labelle H. Rib cage-spine coupling patterns involved in brace treatment of adolescent idiopathic scoliosis. Spine. 1997;22(6):629–35.

50. Hopf C, Heine J. Long-term results of conservative treatment of scoliosis using Chêneau brace. Z Orthop Ihre Grenzeb. 1985;123(3):312–22.

51. Weiss HR, Deez-Kraus K. Quality criteria of scoliosis bracing assessment of primary correction. Proceedings book of the 20th Annual Meeting of the British Scoliosis Society, Low Wood Hotel Windermere 23th-24th of March 1995;29.

52. Rigo M. The Chêneau brace. Preliminary results. Résonances Eur Rachis. 1995;8:3–10.

53. Liljenqvist U, et al. Conservative treatment of idiopathic scoliosis with the Chêneau brace. Zurich: Proceeding of the first combined meeting ESS-ESDS; 1998.

54. Rigo M, Quera-Salvá G, Puigdevall N, Martínez M. Retrospective results in immature idiopathic scoliosis patients treated with a Chêneau brace. Stud Health Technol Inform. 2002;88:241–5.

55. Weiss HR, Rigo M. Expert-driven Chêneau applications: description and in-brace corrections. Physiother Theory Pract. 2011;27(1):61–7.

56. Maruyama T. Early results of Rigo-Chêneau type brace treatment. Scoliosis. 2012;7 Suppl 1:O33.

57. Rigo M, Gallo D, Dallmayer R. In-brace correction of the Cobb angle with RSC-CAD CAM compared with 'hand made' from the original author. Scoliosis. 2010;5 Suppl 1:O68.

58. Gallo D, Wood G, Dallmayer R. Quality control of idiopathic scoliosis treatment in 147 patients while using the RSC brace. J Prosthet Orthot. 2011;23(2):69–77.

59. Rigo M, Gallo D. A new brace design to treat single long thoracic scoliosis. Comparison of the in-brace correction in two groups treated with the new and the classical models. Scoliosis. 2009;4 Suppl 2:O46.

60. Udén A, Willner S. The effect of lumbar flexion and Boston Thoracic brace on the curves in idiopathic scoliosis. Spine. 1983;8(8):846–50.

61. Willner S. Effect of the Boston thoracic brace on the frontal and sagittal curves of the spine. Acta Orthop Scand. 1984;55(4):457–60.

62. Labelle H, Dansereau J, Bellefleur C, Poitras B. 3-D study of the immediate effect of the Boston brace on the scoliotic lumbar spine. Ann Chir. 1992;46(9):814–20.

63. Cahuzac JP, Sales de Gauzy J, Kany J. Traitement de 161 scolioses idiopatique par le corset de C.T.M. In: Proceedings book od the 2nd Congreso Transpirenaico de Rehabilitación. Ed: ICS. Ciutat Sanitària I Universitaria de Bellvitge. L'Hospitalet, Barcelona 1993:55-56.

64. Périé D, De Gauzy S, Sévely A, Hobatho MC. In vivo geometrical evaluation of Cheneau-Toulouse_Munster brace effect on scoliotic spine using MRI method. Clin Biomech. 2001;16(2):129–37.

65. Schmitz A, Kandyba J, Jaeger U, Koenig R, Schmitt O. Brace effect in scoliosis in the sagittal plane – an MRI study. Z Orthop Ihre Grenzgeb. 2002;140(3):347–50.

66. Schmitz A, König R, Kandyba J, Pennekamp P, Schmitt O, Jaeger UE. Visualization of the brace effect on the spinal profile in idiopathic scoliosis. Eur Spine J. 2005;14(2):138–43.

67. Willers U, Normelli H, Aaro S, Svenson O, Hedlund R. Long-term results of Boston brace treatment on vertebral rotation in idiopathic scoliosis. Spine. 1993;18(4):432–5.

68. Rigo M. 3D correction of trunk deformity in patients with idiopathic scoliosis using Chêneau brace. Stud Health Technol Inform. 1999;59:362–5.

69. Lebel DE, Al-Aubaidi Z, Shin EJ, Howard A, Zeller R. Three dimensional analysis of brace biomechanical efficacy for patients with AIS. Eur Spine J. 2013;22(11):2445–8.

70. Weiss HR, Weiss G, Schaar HJ. Incidence of surgery in conservatively treated patients with idiopathic scoliosis. Pediatr Rehabil. 2003;6:111–8.

71. Rigo M, Reiter CH, Weiss HR. Effect of conservative management on the prevalence of surgery in patients with adolescent idiopathic scoliosis. Pediatr Rehabil. 2003;6:209–14.

72. Weiss HR, Weiss G. Brace treatment during pubertal growth spurt in girls with idiopathic scoliosis (IS) – A prospective trial comparing two different concepts. Pediatr Rehabil. 2005;8:199–206.

73. Cinnella P, Muratone M, Testa E, Bondente PG. The treatment of adolescent idiopathic scoliosis with Chêneau brace: long-term outcome. Scoliosis. 2009;4 Suppl 2:O44.

74. Zaborowska-Sapeta K, Kowalski IM, Kotwicki T, Protasiewicz-Faldowska H, Kiebzak W. Effectiveness of Chêneau brace treatment for idiopathic scoliosis: Prospective sturdy in 79 patients followed to skeletal maturity. Scoliosis. 2011;6:2.

75. Ovadia D, Eylon S, Mashiah A, Wientroub S, Lebel ED. Factors associated with the success of the Rigo System Chêneau brace in treating mild to moderate adolescent idiopathic scoliosis. J Child Orthop. 2012;6:327–31.

76. Rigo M. Radiological and cosmetic improvement 2 years after brace weaning – a case report. Pediatr Rehabil. 2003;6:195–9.

77. Grivas TB. Rib Index. Scoliosis. 2014;9(1):20.

78. Rivett L, Stewart A, Potterton J. The effect of compliance to a Rigo System Cheneau brace and specific exercise programme on idiopathic scoliosis curvature: a comparative study: SOSORT 2014 award winner. Scoliosis. 2014;9:5.

79. Perdriolle R, Vidal J. Thoracic idiopathic scoliosis curve evolution and prognosis. Spine. 1985;10(9):785–91.

2

Curve progression after long-term brace treatment in adolescent idiopathic scoliosis: comparative results between over and under 30 Cobb degrees

Angelo G. Aulisa[1]* (iD), Vincenzo Guzzanti[1,2], Francesco Falciglia[1], Marco Galli[3], Paolo Pizzetti[1] and Lorenzo Aulisa[3]

Abstract

Background: The factors influencing curve behavior following bracing are incompletely understood and there is no agreement if scoliotic curves stop progressing with skeletal maturity. The aim of this study was to evaluate the loss of the scoliotic curve correction in patients treated with bracing during adolescence and to compare patient outcomes of under and over 30 Cobb degrees, 10 years after brace removal.

Methods: We reviewed 93 (87 female) of 200 and nine patients with adolescent idiopathic scoliosis (AIS) who were treated with the Lyon or PASB brace at a mean of 15 years (range 10–35). All patients answered a simple questionnaire (including work status, pregnancy, and pain) and underwent clinical and radiological examination. The population was divided into two groups based on Cobb degrees (< 30° and > 30°). Statistical analysis was performed to test the efficacy of our hypothesis.

Results: The patients underwent a long-term follow-up at a mean age of 184.1 months (±72.60) after brace removal. The pre-brace scoliotic mean curve was 32.28° (± 9.4°); after treatment, the mean was 19.35° and increased to a minimum of 22.12° in the 10 years following brace removal. However, there was no significant difference in the mean Cobb angle between the end of weaning and long term follow-up period ($p = 0.105$). The curve angle of patients who were treated with a brace from the beginning was reduced by 13° during the treatment, but the curve size lost 3° at the follow-up period.

The groups over 30° showed a pre-brace scoliotic mean curve of 41.15°; at the end of weaning, the mean curve angle was 25.85° and increased to a mean of 29.73° at follow-up; instead, the groups measuring ≤ 30° showed a pre-brace scoliotic mean curve of 25.58°; at the end of weaning, it was reduced to a mean of 14.24° and it increased to 16.38° at follow-up.

There was no significant difference in the mean progression of curve magnitude between the ≤ 30° and > 30° groups at the long-term follow-up.

Conclusions: Scoliotic curves did not deteriorate beyond their original curve size after bracing in both groups at the 15-year follow-ups. These results are in contrast with the history of this pathology that normally shows a progressive and lowly increment of the curve at skeletal maturity. Bracing is an effective treatment method characterized by positive long-term outcomes, including for patients demonstrating moderate curves.

Keywords: Brace treatment, Adolescent idiopathic scoliosis, P.A.S.B, Long term, Follow-up

* Correspondence: angelogabriele.aulisa@fastwebnet.it
[1]U.O.C. of Orthopedics and Traumatology, Children's Hospital Bambino Gesù, Institute of Scientific Research, P.zza S. Onofrio 4, 00165 Rome, Italy
Full list of author information is available at the end of the article

Background

Adolescent idiopathic scoliosis (AIS) is a three-dimensional spinal deformity that it is characterized by lateral curvature of the spine and vertebral rotation. The severity of AIS varies greatly, and not all the curves have a progression that requires treatment [1, 2].

The most common and conservative approach to treatment of AIS is using a brace to prevent the progression of curvature and in select cases, to obtain a partial recovery of the curve [3–7]. The efficacy of bracing is correlated with longer daily application time and to patient adherence to treatment plans [8–10]. Literature shows the factors that influence curve behavior following bracing are not fully understood, but they are crucial to the prognosis of patients with AIS [10, 11]. Moreover, there is no agreement if scoliotic curves stop progressing after bracing at skeletal maturity.

The aims of this study were:

- To evaluate the loss of the scoliotic curve correction at long term follow-up in a cohort of patients treated with bracing during adolescence;
- To compare the outcomes of sub-group patients: (1) Over and under 30 Cobb degrees at start of treatment, to determine whether the initial curve's gravity could influence long-term results; and (2) over and under 30 Cobb degrees at end of weaning.

Methods

Patient population

This is a retrospective study based on an ongoing database including 1512 patients treated for idiopathic scoliosis between 1980 and 2016. Informed consent was obtained by all participants. This study was conducted in accordance with the World Medical Association Declaration of Helsinki of 1975, as revised in 1983, and all the participants signed an informed consent to allow the use of clinical data for research purposes.

A total of 209 scoliotic patients treated with the progressive action short brace (PASB) or Lyon brace were contacted a minimum of 10 years from the end of treatment (range 10–35). Ninety-three patients (87 female) responded to the long-term follow-up examination.

All patients presented at the beginning of treatment, AIS, with curves ranging in magnitude between 20° and 55° Cobb. Age at the beginning of treatment was 10–14 years, with Risser scores between 0 and 2.

Bracing protocol

All patients were prescribed a full-time (i.e., maximum 22 h daily, minimum 18 h daily) brace. For the study, patients showing curve angles < 25°, progression was assessed using two consecutive radiographs taken at 6-month intervals. Progression was defined as an increase greater than 5° in

both curve magnitude (Cobb's method) and apical torsion (Perdriolle's method) in an immature skeleton. Weaning was started when ring-apophysis fusion [12] was seen on a laterolateral view radiograph and consisted of 2 to 4 h of bracing reduction at 4-month intervals. Short term follow-up was discontinued 5 years after brace removal. Radiology reports with measurements of the deformity were available for all patients.

Follow up after 10 years since brace removing

Ninety-three patients were evaluated at long-term follow-up. Demographic characteristics were obtained. Patients were observed in the standing erect position and during the forward bending test.

Full-length anteroposterior (AP) and lateral view standing radiographs were taken. The AP view was used to obtain the curve magnitude (CM, Cobb's method) and torsion of the apical vertebra (TA, Perdriolle's method) [13, 14]. Measurements were obtained by two independent observers (two senior surgeons) and the end vertebrae were preselected to reduce interobserver bias [14].

All patients answered a simple questionnaire:

- Work Status (yes or no, full or part-time)
- Pregnancy (yes or no, born children)
- Back Pain (yes or no)

Sub group analysis

The patients were divided in sub-groups based on Cobb degrees. Those with curves ≤ 30 Cobb degrees and those with curves > 30 Cobb degrees at the beginning of treatment and at end of treatment.

Statistical analysis

Standard statistical methods have been used for descriptive statistics. Normally distributed continuous variables were analyzed by using an independent sample t test. Changes in CM and TA from beginning to follow-up were assessed via one-way analysis of variance for repeated measures. Mean differences between time points and 95% confidence intervals were calculated. Correlations between changes in CM at the start of bracing, at the end of weaning, and at follow-up were determined via the Pearson test. All analyses were performed according to the intention-to-treat principle. All tests were two-sided, with significance set at a P value less than 0.05. Results are presented as mean ± standard deviation (SD).

Results

Demographics

Ninety-three patients (females: 87) with a mean age 32.58 (±5.2) years were studied. The mean pre-brace scoliotic curve was 32.28 (± 9.4) degrees, and the mean Perdriolle

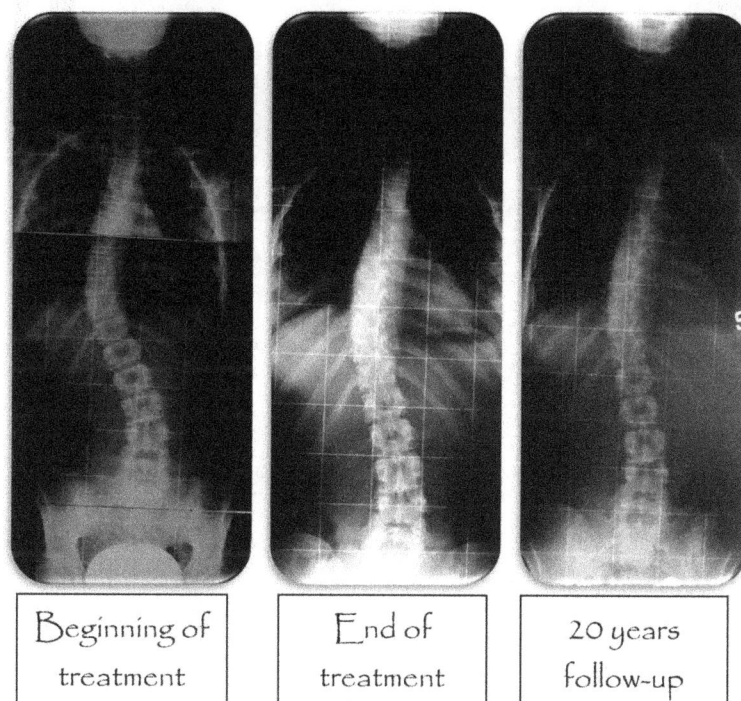

Fig. 1 Typical radiological trend in Cobb degrees of all samples

score of the apical vertebra of the scoliotic deformity was 13.86 (± 5.04).

Twenty-five patients had a thoracic curve, 40 a thoracolumbar or lumbar curve, and 28 had a double primary curve.

Fifty-three patients (57%) had pre-brace Cobb angle less than 30°, and 40 (43%) had a Cobb angle greater than 30°.

Mean time of brace application was 5.28 (±2.23) years. Patients underwent long-term follow-up at a mean of 15.33 (±5.22) years after brace removal.

Cohort results

In all 93 patients, the mean scoliotic curve was reduced of 13.41° (±8.1) at the end of weaning.

The mean pre brace Cobb angle of 32.17° (±9.12) was reduced to 19.39° (±10.8) following brace removal, it was 20.67° (±11.2) at the time of the short term follow-up (5 years) and increased to 22.12° (±12.11) at long-term follow-up. However, there was no significant difference in the mean Cobb angle between the end of weaning and long term follow up period ($p = 0.105$) (Fig. 1).

Seventy-three patients (78.5%) completed the long term follow up with less than 30°Cobb angle, 11 (11.8%) between 30 and 40° and nine (9.7%) with a Cobb angle greater than 40°. No patients at the long term follow-up demonstrated curve angles greater than 50°.

Comparison of ≤ 30° vs > 30° at begging of treatment

Fifty-three patients (57%) had curve with Cobb degrees ≤ 30° whereas 40 patients had a curve (43%) > 30°.

The group greater than 30° showed a pre-brace scoliotic mean curve of 41.15°; at the end of weaning, it was reduced to 25.85° and it increased to 29.73° at long-term follow-up; instead, the group < 30° showed a pre-brace scoliotic mean curve of 25.58°; at the end of weaning, it was reduced to 14.24° and it increased to 16.38° at long term follow-up (Table 1 and Fig. 2).

Significant differences were determined for CM across Cobb at beginning and at the end of weaning. Instead, insignificant differences were determined for CM between the end of weaning and the long-term follow-up period (Tables 2, 3).

Table 1 Demographic and radiological characteristics of the study sample

	Beginning of treatment (t_1)	End of treatment (t_2)	5 years follow-up (t_3)	10 years minimum follow-up (t_4)
Age (years)	11.1 ± 2.4	17.1 ± 2.0	22.1 ± 2.5	32.4 ± 5.1
Cobb degrees	32.28 ± 9.4	19.4 ± 10.8	20.7 ± 11.2	22.1 ± 12.1
Perdriolle degrees	13.9 ± 5.0	9.9 ± 6.2	10,1 ± 6.9	10.4 ± 6.2

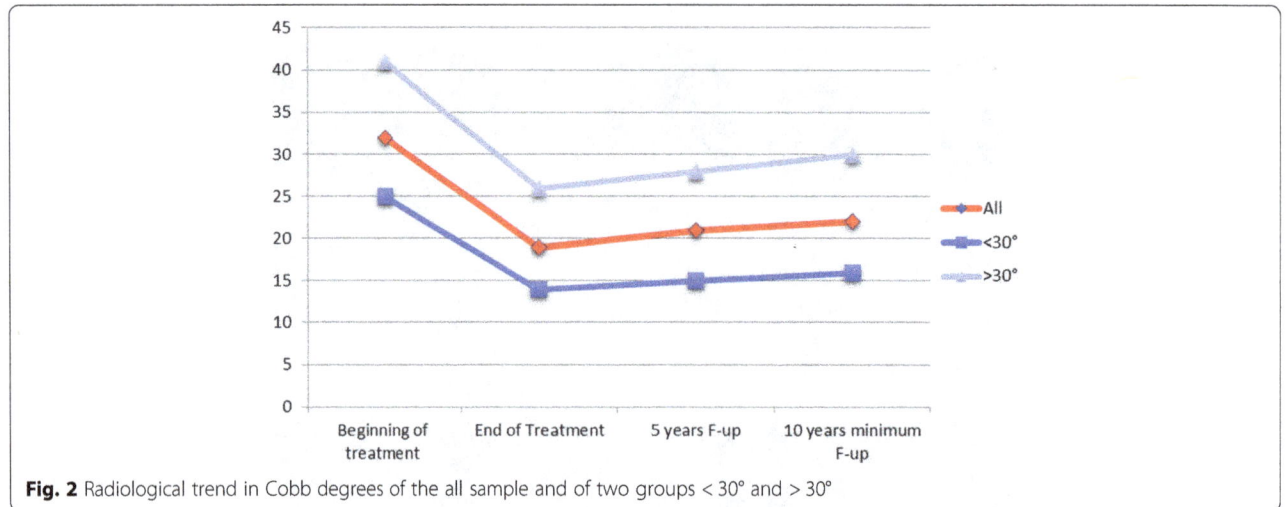

Fig. 2 Radiological trend in Cobb degrees of the all sample and of two groups < 30° and > 30°

The mean curve correction was 10.94° in the group with Cobb angles ≤ 30° and was 15.3° in the group with Cobb angles > 30°. There was no statistically significant difference in the mean curve correction between the two groups at short term follow-up (Fig. 1).

Long-term follow up revealed a moderate increase in the Cobb angle in both groups. The mean Cobb angle increase was 2.14° in the group with Cobb angles ≤ 30° and 3.88° in the group with Cobb angles > 30°. The difference between groups was not statistically significant ($p = 0.87$).

Comparison of ≤ 30° vs > 30° at end of treatment

Seventy five patients (81%) had curve angle ≤ 30°, whereas 18 patients (19%) had a curve angle > 30° at the end of conservative treatment.

The group greater than 30° showed a pre-brace scoliotic mean curve of 43.94°, at the end of weaning it was reduced to 34.89° and it increased to 38.39° at long term follow-up; instead the group < 30° showed a pre-brace scoliotic mean curve of 29.35°, at the end of weaning it was reduced to 15.05° and it increased to 18.21° at long-term follow-up. No significant differences were determined for CM between end of weaning and long-term follow up period.

Long term follow-up revealed a moderate increase in the Cobb angle in both groups. The mean Cobb angle increase was 3.16° in the group with Cobb angles ≤ 30° and 3.50° in the group with Cobb angles > 30°. Difference between groups was not statistically significant.

Demographics

Sixty-one patients were employed full-time, 19 were employed part-time, and 13 were unemployed. Twenty-one patients experienced pregnancy. Pain, related to instability of the spine, was present in 12 patients (3 cases were described as chronic).

Discussion

The main objective of this study was to evaluate the loss of correction at long term follow-up and to analyze our case series.

Past studies of AIS showed a progression of the curve also at the end of the growth, but the degree of progression was not clear. Weinstein reported that "even in progressive curves it cannot be predicted, for example, whether a progressive 30° curve's natural history would be to progress to 38° or to 78°" [15]. Instead, Bjerkreim [16] reported in his paper about the Progression in Untreated Idiopathic Scoliosis that curve progression was 3° per year before 20 of age and 1° per year after 20 years. Curves less than 40 degrees increased significantly less

Table 2 Differences in C_M across t_1–t_4 in < 30° as determined by one-way ANOVA with Bonferroni's post test

Cobb < 30°	Mean Diff,	t	P < 0.05	Summary	95% CI of diff
Beginning of treatment ($t1$) vs end of treatment ($t2$)	11.3	6.90	Yes	***	6.96 to 15.7
Beginning of treatment ($t1$) vs 5 years follow-up ($t3$)	10.5	6.49	Yes	***	6.16 to 14.7
Beginning of treatment ($t1$) vs 10 years minimum follow-up ($t4$)	9.21	5.72	Yes	***	4.92 to 13.5
End of treatment ($t2$) vs 5 years follow-up ($t3$)	−0,887	0.540	No	ns	−5.27 to 3.49
End of treatment ($t2$) vs 10 years minimum follow-up ($t4$)	−2.13	1.30	No	ns	−6.51 to 2.25
5 years follow-up ($t3$) vs 10 years minimum follow-up ($t4$)	−1.25	0.773	No	ns	−5.54 to 3.05

***significant
nsnot significant

Table 3 Differences in C_M across t_1–t_4 in > 30° as determined by one-way ANOVA with Bonferroni's post test

Cobb >30°	Mean Diff,	t	P < 0.05	Summary	95% CI of diff
Beginning of treatment (t1) vs End of treatment (t2)	15.3	7.36	Yes	***	9.75 to 20.9
Beginning of treatment (t1) vs 5 years follow-up (t3)	13.2	6.37	Yes	***	7.63 to 18.7
Beginning of treatment (t1) vs 10 years minimum follow-up (t4)	11.4	5.53	Yes	***	5.91 to 16.9
End of treatment (t2) vs 5 years follow-up (t3)	−2.15	1.04	No	ns	−7.71 to 3.40
End of treatment (t2) vs 10 years minimum follow-up (t4)	−3.88	1.87	No	ns	−9.43 to 1.67
5 years follow-up (t3) vs 10 years minimum follow-up (t4)	−1.73	0.835	No	ns	−7.24 to 3.79

***significant
ns not significant

than larger curves and curves measuring from 60° to 80° increased the most.

Unfortunately, there are a limited number of studies that support the corrective effect of bracing at the time of the long-term follow-up compared to the natural progression of untreated curves [17–21].

Pellios et al. [17] reported the long term results of 77 patients suffering from AIS at 25 years after Boston brace removal. The initial Cobb angle of 28.2° (±8.7) was reduced during brace application to 17.3° (±9.2) then increased at the 25 year follow-up to 25.4° (±13.8). The mean loss of correction at 25 years after brace discontinuation was 8.1°. Nachemson [20] confirmed similar long-term results of 109 patients, the mean loss of correction at 22 years after brace discontinuation was 7.9°. Lange et al. [21] showed better results in a similar study of 215 patients at 25 years after Boston brace removal. They reported the mean Cobb angle deterioration at the long term evaluation was 4.1° after brace removal.

In our study, the mean pre-brace Cobb angle of 32.17° (±9.12) was reduced during brace application to 19.39° (±10.8). It increased slightly at the short time follow-up to 20.67° (±11.2) and further increased at the 15-year follow-up to 22.12° (±12.11). However, the mean pre-brace Cobb angle was not significantly different at the 15-year follow-up, demonstrating stability with a loss of correction of 2.7°.

78.5% of our cohort completed the long-term follow up with less than 30° Cobb angle. Therefore, our results are slightly better than those published in the literature regarding the course of curve progression following brace removal. Bracing seems to be an effective treatment method, with good long-term results also shown in moderate curves.

Furthermore, the results from the subgroups at long-term follow-up revealed a slight increase in the Cobb angle in both groups. The increase was not significantly different at 15 years follow-up and the difference between groups, 2.14° (Cobb ≤ 30°) versus 3.88° (Cobb > 30°), was not statistically significant. These results are in contrast with past studies that showed a progressive increment of the curve at skeletal maturity in those that were classified as moderate [1, 22]. Reasons effecting the stability of the curve after the brace treatment were not clear from the results but may be related to stiffness of the treated curves.

Using collected demographic data, we found no significant difference in both pregnancy and pain between groups.

A limitation of our study was that the cohort is still young with a mean of 32 years. It would be useful to study patients older than 50 years, in which the degenerative processes of the spine are more evident and important. Even more interesting would be studying the behavior thoracolumbar curves; in fact, the three cases of chronic pain related to instability, due to rotational subluxation, were thoracolumbar curves.

Conclusions

The results demonstrate slight loss of correction 15 years post bracing. We found no difference in terms of long-term results and progression between patients with ≤ 30° vs > 30° Cobb angles. In conclusion, bracing could be effective for long-term in patients with adolescent idiopathic scoliosis.

Abbreviations
AIS: Adolescent idiopathic scoliosis; AP: Anterior-posterior; CM: Cobb's method; LL: Latero-lateral; PASB: Progressive action short brace; SOSORT: Society on Scoliosis Orthopedic and Rehabilitation Treatment; SRS: Scoliosis Research Society; TA: Perdriolle's method

Acknowledgements
None.

Funding
No funding was received.

Authors' contributions
AGA participated in the conception, design, coordination, acquisition, , analysis and interpretation of data, drafting of the manuscript, and performed the statistical analysis. PP, FF, MG, and VG helped to draft the manuscript. LA participated in the conception, design, coordination, and helped to draft the manuscript. All authors read and approved the final manuscript.

Competing interests
The authors declare that they have no competing interests.

Author details
[1]U.O.C. of Orthopedics and Traumatology, Children's Hospital Bambino Gesù, Institute of Scientific Research, P.zza S. Onofrio 4, 00165 Rome, Italy. [2]University of Cassino, 03043 Cassino, FR, Italy. [3]Department of Orthopedics, University Hospital "Agostino Gemelli", Catholic University of the Sacred Heart School of Medicine, 00168 Rome, Italy.

References
1. Weinstein SL, Ponseti IV. Curve progression in idiopathic scoliosis. J Bone Joint Surg Am. 1983;65(4):447–55.
2. Negrini S, Aulisa AG, Aulisa L, Circo AB, de Mauroy JC, Durmala J, et al. 2011 SOSORT guidelines: orthopaedic and rehabilitation treatment of idiopathic scoliosis during growth. Scoliosis. 2012;7(1):3.
3. Aulisa AG, Guzzanti V, Falciglia F, Giordano M, Marzetti E, Aulisa L. Lyon bracing in adolescent females with thoracic idiopathic scoliosis: a prospective study based on SRS and SOSORT criteria. BMC Musculoskelet Disord. 2015;16:316.
4. Negrini S, Marchini G, Tessadri F. Brace technology thematic series—the Sforzesco and Sibilla braces, and the SPoRT (symmetric, patient oriented, rigid, three-dimensional, active) concept. Scoliosis. 2011;6:8.
5. de Mauroy JC, Lecante C, Barral F, Pourret S. Prospective study and new concepts based on scoliosis detorsion of the first 225 early in-brace radiological results with the new Lyon brace: ARTbrace. Scoliosis. 2014;9:19.
6. Aulisa AG, Guzzanti V, Marzetti E, Giordano M, Falciglia F, Aulisa L. Brace treatment in juvenile idiopathic scoliosis: a prospective study in accordance with the SRS criteria for bracing studies—SOSORT award 2013 winner. Scoliosis. 2014;9:3.
7. Weinstein SL, Dolan LA, Wright JG, Dobbs MB. Effects of bracing in adolescents with idiopathic scoliosis. N Engl J Med. 2013;369(16):1512–21.
8. Aulisa AG, Giordano M, Falciglia F, Marzetti E, Poscia A, Guzzanti V. Correlation between compliance and brace treatment in juvenile and adolescent idiopathic scoliosis: SOSORT 2014 award winner. Scoliosis. 2014;9:6.
9. Weiss H-R, Goodall D. The treatment of adolescent idiopathic scoliosis (AIS) according to present evidence. A systematic review. Eur J Phys Rehabil Med. 2008;44(2):177–93.
10. Donzelli S, Zaina F, Negrini S. In defense of adolescents: they really do use braces for the hours prescribed, if good help is provided. Results from a prospective everyday clinic cohort using thermobrace. Scoliosis. 2012;7(1):12.
11. Zaina F, De Mauroy JC, Grivas T, Hresko MT, Kotwizki T, Maruyama T, et al. Bracing for scoliosis in 2014: state of the art. Eur J Phys Rehabil Med. 2014;50(1):93–110.
12. Bick EM, Copel JW. The ring apophysis of the human vertebra. J Bone Jt Surg Am. 1951;33(3):783–7.
13. Omeroğlu H, Ozekin O, Biçimoğlu A. Measurement of vertebral rotation in idiopathic scoliosis using the Perdriolle torsionmeter: a clinical study on intraobserver and interobserver error. Eur Spine J. 1996;5(3):167–71.
14. Morrissy RT, Goldsmith GS, Hall EC, Kehl D, Cowie GH. Measurement of the Cobb angle on radiographs of patients who have scoliosis. Evaluation of intrinsic error. J Bone Joint Surg Am. 1990;72(3):320–7.
15. Weinstein SL. Natural history. Spine. 1999;24(24):2592–600.
16. Bjerkreim I, Hassan I. Progression in untreated idiopathic scoliosis after end of growth. Acta Orthop Scand. 1982;53(6):897–900.
17. Pellios S, Kenanidis E, Potoupnis M, Tsiridis E, Sayegh FE, Kirkos J, et al. Curve progression 25 years after bracing for adolescent idiopathic scoliosis: long term comparative results between two matched groups of 18 versus 23 hours daily bracing. Scoliosis Spinal Disord. 2016;11:3.
18. Wiley JW, Thomson JD, Mitchell TM, Smith BG, Banta JV. Effectiveness of the boston brace in treatment of large curves in adolescent idiopathic scoliosis. Spine. 2000;25(18):2326–32.
19. Maruyama T. Bracing adolescent idiopathic scoliosis: a systematic review of the literature of effective conservative treatment looking for end results 5 years after weaning. Disabil Rehabil. 2008;30(10):786–91.
20. Danielsson AJ, Nachemson AL. Radiologic findings and curve progression 22 years after treatment for adolescent idiopathic scoliosis: comparison of brace and surgical treatment with matching control group of straight individuals. Spine. 2001;26(5):516–25.
21. Lange JE, Steen H, Gunderson R, Brox JI. Long-term results after Boston brace treatment in late-onset juvenile and adolescent idiopathic scoliosis. Scoliosis. 2011;6:18.
22. Tan K-J, Moe MM, Vaithinathan R, Wong H-K. Curve progression in idiopathic scoliosis: follow-up study to skeletal maturity. Spine. 2009; 34(7):697–700.

3

Is a persistent central canal a risk factor for neurological injury in patients undergoing surgical correction of scoliosis?

Steven Kyriacou[1]*[iD], Yuen Man[2], Karen Plumb[2], Matthew Shaw[1] and Kia Rezajooi[1]

Abstract

Background: Scoliosis patients with associated syringomyelia are at an increased risk of neurological injury during surgical deformity correction. The syrinx is therefore often addressed surgically prior to scoliosis correction to minimize this risk. It remains unclear if the presence of a persistent central canal (PCC) within the spinal cord also poses a similar risk. The aim of this study is to determine whether there is any evidence to suggest that patients with a PCC are also at a higher risk of neurological injury during surgical scoliosis correction.

Methods: Eleven patients with a PCC identified on pre-operative magnetic resonance imaging who had undergone correction of adolescent idiopathic scoliosis (AIS) over a 7-year study period at our institution were retrospectively identified. The incidence of abnormal intra-operative spinal cord monitoring (SCM) traces in this group was in turn compared against 44 randomly selected age- and sex-matched controls with no PCC who had also undergone surgical correction of AIS during the study period. Fisher's exact test was applied to determine whether there was a significant difference in the incidence of abnormal intra-operative SCM traces between the two groups.

Results: Statistical analysis demonstrated no significant difference in the incidence of abnormal intra-operative SCM signal traces between the PCC group and the control group.

Conclusions: This study demonstrates no evidence to suggest a PCC increases the risk of neurological complications during scoliosis correction. We therefore suggest that surgical correction of scoliosis in patients with a PCC can be carried out safely with routine precautions.

Keywords: Scoliosis, Persistent central canal, Syrinx

Background

One of the most devastating potential complications of scoliosis correction surgery is iatrogenic neurological injury [1, 2]. Numerous factors have been implicated as increasing the risk of such a complication including the presence of abnormalities within the spinal cord [3]. The incidence of spinal cord pathology in paediatric patients with scoliosis has previously been reported to be between 3 and 20%, with pre-operative magnetic resonance imaging (MRI) demonstrating various intra-spinal abnormalities including syringomyelia, Chiari malformation, diastematomyelia, tethered cord and spinal cord tumours [1, 4, 5]. The mechanism of neurological injury

arising from surgical correction of scoliosis can be from an instrument or implant striking the spinal cord, from a vascular injury related to the implant causing stretching or compression of vessels or from vascular compromise not directly related to the implant such as ischaemia secondary to hypotension [6].

Previous studies have demonstrated patients with spinal cord pathology undergoing surgical correction of scoliosis are at an increased risk of sustaining intra-operative iatrogenic neurological injury [1, 7–9]. However, to the authors' knowledge, there has not been a published study addressing the question as to whether the presence of a persistent central canal (PCC) also poses an increased risk of intra-operative neurological injury during surgical correction of scoliosis. The aim of this study is to therefore address this question.

* Correspondence: drstevenkyriacou@hotmail.co.uk
[1]Spinal Deformity Unit, Royal National Orthopaedic Hospital, Stanmore, UK
Full list of author information is available at the end of the article

Methods

The null hypothesis to be tested was defined as patients with a PCC are at an equal risk of developing intra-operative neurological complications during surgical correction of scoliosis as patients without a PCC.

In order to test this hypothesis, all patients who had undergone surgical correction of adolescent idiopathic scoliosis (AIS) over a 7-year period between June 2004 and October 2011 at our institution who had a co-existing PCC confirmed with routine pre-operative whole spine MRI were retrospectively identified using an electronic database and were included in the study. MRI was performed at 1.5 Tesla with a phased array coil, and image sequences included T1-weighted spin echo (SE) and T2-weighted fast SE (FSE) sagittal and axial images. All MRIs were reported by a consultant musculoskeletal radiologist.

A PCC was defined as a filiform or slit-like, centrally located, intra-medullary cavity of a maximum diameter of 4 mm [10] not communicating with the fourth ventricle and extending over at least two vertebral levels [11] in the absence of any co-existing neuro-axis abnormality (NAA) on neuro-radiological imaging potentially responsible for cerebrospinal fluid (CSF) flow disturbances, with no prior history of spinal trauma, spinal infections or previous spinal/neurosurgical intervention. Additional inclusion criteria was the use of intra-operative spinal cord monitoring (SCM) during the surgical correction of the spinal deformity.

Eleven patients in total met these criteria and were included in the study. Forty-four sex- and age-matched control group patients who had also undergone surgical correction of AIS during the same study period with no underlying NAA evident on pre-operative MRI screening were randomly selected from a list of 1150 patients using Stata/IC version 12 software (StataCorp, College Station, TX, USA). Therefore, in total, 55 patients were included in the study.

The pre- and post-operative neurological status as determined by clinical examination findings up to the time of 3-month outpatient follow-up, the type of deformity correction and the intra-operative SCM traces were identified in the medical records of each patient included in the study. The intra-operative SCM traces for each patient were analysed by the Department of Neurophysiology, with somato-sensory evoked potentials (SSEPs) being used throughout the surgery to monitor for potential neurological compromise. Deviation from baseline SCM traces was classified as either 'Green' (no trace change), 'Amber' (an event causing an indirect effect with partial trace change) or 'Red' (an event causing a direct effect with partial to complete trace loss).

The SCM equipment used to monitor intra-operative SSEPs during the study period were Nihon Kohden Neuromaster (Tokyo, Japan) and Nicolet Biomedical (Viking Madison, WI, USA).

In order to assess whether there was any significant difference in the incidence of abnormal intra-operative SCM traces between the PCC group and the control group, a Fisher's exact test was performed given the categorical nature of the data, again using Stata/IC version 12 software. In order to calculate a Fisher's exact test, a 2 × 2 contingency table was created using the results of the intra-operative SCM traces for each of the 55 patients included in the study. For the purposes of entering this data into the contingency table, the patients in the PCC group were subdivided into those with normal ('Green') and abnormal ('Amber' or 'Red') intra-operative SCM traces. The patients in the control group were similarly subdivided into those with normal and abnormal intra-operative SCM traces.

In addition to comparing the incidence of abnormal intra-operative SCM traces between the PCC and control group, a comparison was also made of the incidence of post-operative neurological deficit apparent on clinical examination between the two groups to assess for any difference.

Results

During the 7-year study period, 1161 AIS corrections were conducted out of which 11 patients met the criteria of having a PCC identified on pre-operative MRI. There was one male and ten females in the PCC group with an average age of 15.9 years (range 14–20). Only one patient in the PCC group had a pre-operative clinical neurological deficit in the form of mildly diminished sensation in the S1 distribution of the right foot with no associated motor weakness. No definite cause for this was demonstrated on pre-operative MRI and nerve conduction studies. Four patients in the PCC group underwent an anterior instrumented fusion (AIF), six patients underwent posterior instrumented fusion (PIF) and one patient underwent combined anterior release (AR) and PIF (Table 1 and Fig. 1).

There were 44 age- and sex-matched AIS controls. These included 4 males and 40 females with an average age of 15.9 years (range 14–20). Eleven patients in the control group underwent an AIF and 33 patients underwent a PIF (Table 2 and Fig. 2). No patient in the control group had a clinical neurological deficit pre-operatively.

In both the PCC and control group, baseline SSEPs were obtained for all patients. In the PCC group, no patient had an intra-operative deviation from the baseline traces, compared to four (9.1%) patients in the control group. These four patients all had a PIF procedure. Of these four patients, two patients had 'Amber' warning signal changes intra-operatively and two patients had 'Red' warning signal changes intra-operatively (Fig. 3). In all four control group patients who developed abnormal intra-operative SCM traces, the traces returned to normal when appropriate intra-operative measures were taken to reverse the precipitating factor such as reducing

Table 1 Demographic data and outcomes of patients in the PCC group

Patient number	Age	Sex	Surgery	Pre-operative neurological deficit	Post-operative neurological status	Intra-operative SCM traces
1	14	Female	AIF	None	Unchanged	
2	16	Female	PIF	None	Unchanged	
3	18	Female	PIF	Sensory	Unchanged	
4	16	Male	AIF	None	Unchanged	
5	20	Female	PIF	None	Unchanged	
6	15	Female	PIF	None	Unchanged	
7	20	Female	AR and PIF	None	Unchanged	
8	14	Female	AIF	None	Unchanged	
9	14	Female	AIF	None	Unchanged	
10	14	Female	PIF	None	Unchanged	
11	14	Female	PIF	None	Unchanged	

AIF anterior instrumented fusion, *PIF* posterior instrumented fusion, *AR* anterior release

the degree of distraction being applied to the spine. No patient in either the PCC or the control group had a new onset neurological deficit post-operatively evident on clinical examination.

The exact anatomical level of the PCC in each patient within the PCC group, the vertebral levels instrumented and the percentage deformity correction achieved were also recorded (Table 3). The PCC was found to be located either entirely or partially within the instrumented spinal levels in all patients within the PCC group. The average percentage deformity correction achieved was 70%.

Fisher's exact test did not demonstrate any statistically significant difference in the incidence of abnormal intra-operative SCM traces between patients in the PCC

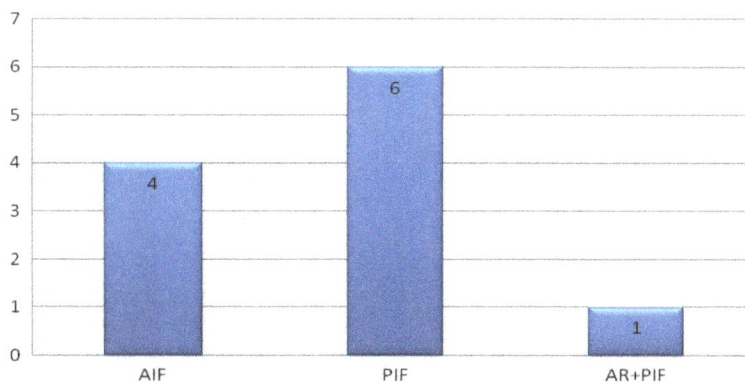

Fig. 1 Type of scoliosis correction surgery performed on the 11 patients in PCC group. *AIF*–Anterior Instrumented Fusion, *PIF*–Posterior Instrumented Fusion, *AR*-Anterior Release

Table 2 Demographic data and outcomes of patients in the control group

Patient number	Age	Sex	Surgery	Pre-operative neurological deficit	Post-operative neurological status	Intra-operative SCM traces
1	16	Male	PIF	None	Unchanged	Green
2	16	Male	AIF	None	Unchanged	Green
3	16	Male	PIF	None	Unchanged	Green
4	16	Male	PIF	None	Unchanged	Yellow
5	14	Female	PIF	None	Unchanged	Green
6	14	Female	AIF	None	Unchanged	Green
7	14	Female	PIF	None	Unchanged	Green
8	14	Female	PIF	None	Unchanged	Green
9	14	Female	PIF	None	Unchanged	Green
10	14	Female	PIF	None	Unchanged	Green
11	14	Female	PIF	None	Unchanged	Green
12	14	Female	AIF	None	Unchanged	Green
13	14	Female	PIF	None	Unchanged	Orange
14	14	Female	PIF	None	Unchanged	Green
15	14	Female	AR and PIF	None	Unchanged	Green
16	14	Female	AIF	None	Unchanged	Green
17	14	Female	AIF	None	Unchanged	Green
18	14	Female	PIF	None	Unchanged	Green
19	14	Female	PIF	None	Unchanged	Green
20	14	Female	PIF	None	Unchanged	Green
21	14	Female	PIF	None	Unchanged	Green
22	14	Female	PIF	None	Unchanged	Green
23	14	Female	AIF	None	Unchanged	Green
24	14	Female	AIF	None	Unchanged	Green
25	15	Female	AIF	None	Unchanged	Green
26	15	Female	PIF	None	Unchanged	Green
27	15	Female	PIF	None	Unchanged	Green
28	15	Female	PIF	None	Unchanged	Green
29	16	Female	PIF	None	Unchanged	Green
30	16	Female	AIF	None	Unchanged	Green
31	16	Female	PIF	None	Unchanged	Green
32	16	Female	PIF	None	Unchanged	Green
33	18	Female	PIF	None	Unchanged	Green
34	18	Female	PIF	None	Unchanged	Green
35	18	Female	PIF	None	Unchanged	Green
36	18	Female	AIF	None	Unchanged	Green
37	20	Female	PIF	None	Unchanged	Green
38	20	Female	PIF	None	Unchanged	Green
39	20	Female	PIF	None	Unchanged	Green
40	20	Female	PIF	None	Unchanged	Yellow
41	20	Female	PIF	None	Unchanged	Green
42	20	Female	PIF	None	Unchanged	Green
43	20	Female	PIF	None	Unchanged	Orange
44	20	Female	AIF	None	Unchanged	Green

AIF anterior instrumented fusion, *PIF* posterior instrumented fusion, *AR* anterior release

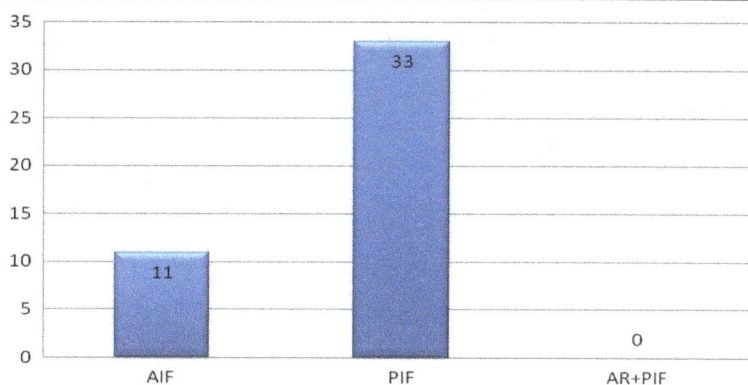

Fig. 2 Type of scoliosis correction surgery performed on the 44 patients in the control group. *AIF*–Anterior Instrumented Fusion, *PIF*–Posterior Instrumented Fusion, *AR*-Anterior Release

group and patients in the control group ($p = 0.5728$). The null hypothesis 'patients with a PCC are at an equal risk of developing intra-operative neurological complications during surgical correction of scoliosis as patients without a PCC' could therefore not be rejected.

Discussion

The central canal is an ependymal-lined structure in the spinal cord that extends inferiorly from the fourth ventricle to the conus medullaris [12]. Anatomical studies suggest the central canal is only seen in foetal and new-born spinal cords and undergoes age-related stenosis such that it is obliterated in the vast majority of adults [13–16]. In a PCC, a degree of age related stenosis has occurred such that the central canal no longer extends all the way from the fourth ventricle to the conus medullaris. A partial remnant may persist, however, as shown in autopsy studies, and although reported to be seen in only 1.5% of MRI studies of the spinal cord, it can

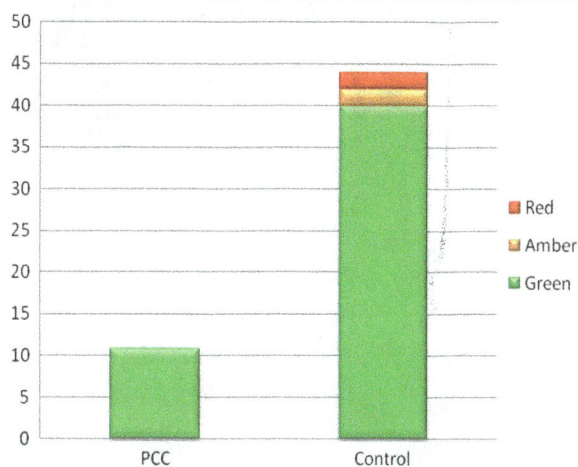

Fig. 3 Number of patients with normal (*green*), borderline (*amber*) or abnormal (*red*) spinal cord monitoring traces observed in the persistent central canal group (*left*) versus the control group (*right*)

normally be regarded as an incidental finding [10, 14, 15]. The 4 mm maximum diameter used to form our definition of a PCC is based on the paper by Petit-Lacour et al. [10] which was the first study published describing the visibility of the central canal on MRI. The central canal can communicate with the fourth ventricle beyond infancy, but this is uncommon and is usually associated with hydrocephalus which excludes it from being a PCC which is essentially idiopathic. The typical appearance of a PCC on T2-weighted coronal and axial spinal MRI is demonstrated in Figs. 4 and 5, respectively.

The term 'hydromyelia' is often used to refer to an ependymal-lined, CSF-filled spinal cord cavity which most likely represents persistence into adulthood of a foetal configuration of the anatomy of the central canal of the spinal cord [17]. Hydromyelia can therefore be used interchangeably with PCC as they represent the same entity, although it could be argued that calling it a 'persistent central canal' is a more literal description.

In contrast to syringomyelia, the literature defining a PCC and determining its clinical significance remains limited. There is currently no widely accepted definition of a PCC in the literature, and debate continues on the criteria for distinguishing between a PCC and syringomyelia. Syringomyelia tends to be used to refer to a CSF-filled cavity within the spinal cord which is surrounded by a wall comprised of glial cells (which therefore implies it is related to a pathological process) and may present with abnormal neurological signs and symptoms. The term PCC is generally used to refer to an ependymal-lined, CSF-filled cavity within the spinal cord. They are usually asymptomatic and have no identifiable underlying cause. Much of the confusion arises from the fact that in practice, it is often not possible to distinguish between the two radiologically and therefore the umbrella term 'syrinx' is applied despite the fact this encompasses more than one entity.

Table 3 Level of PCC, curve pattern, level of instrumentation and percentage deformity correction achieved in PCC patients

Patient number	Level of PCC	Curve pattern	Levels instrumented	Pre-operative Cobb angle	Post-operative Cobb angle	% correction
1	T3-L1	Thoraco-Lumbar	T11-L3	52	12	77
2	T3-T8	Thoracic	T2-T12	55	20	64
3	C5-L1	Thoracic	T2-L1	59	22	62
4	T8-T12	Thoraco-Lumbar	T11-L3	54	19	65
5	C4-T3	Thoracic	T2-L2	61	15	75
6	C6-T4	Thoracic	T2-L1	62	19	69
7	T3-T9	Thoracic	T2-L2	69	25	64
8	T7-L1	Thoraco-Lumbar	T11-L3	54	12	78
9	T5-T12	Thoraco-Lumbar	T12-L3	52	15	72
10	T6-L1	Thoracic	T2-L3	57	15	74
11	T4-T8	Thoracic	T2-L3	60	21	65

PCC persistent central canal, *C* cervical, *T* thoracic, *L* lumbar

Previous studies have recommended neurosurgical intervention should be performed prior to any orthopaedic procedure to reduce the higher risk of neurological injury associated with surgical correction of scoliosis in patients with neurological etiologies compared with patients with AIS [7–9, 18–24]. Whether or not a PCC should also be regarded as a risk factor for neurological injury during scoliosis correction is currently not clear and has to date not been addressed in the medical literature.

The general consensus is that a PCC may represent an anatomical variant with no identifiable underlying cause that is generally asymptomatic and most probably represents a different clinical entity from syringomyelia [11–13, 25]. Whether the presence of a PCC poses a risk of an individual ultimately developing syringomyelia in the future at present remains uncertain and open to discussion.

Of the 11 patients in the PCC group, all had 'adolescent idiopathic scoliosis', with the vast majority being female as would be expected in a group of patients with this condition. In order to minimise the risk of neurological injury during scoliosis correction, SCM is now routinely used during spinal deformity surgery and SSEPs represent the standard of care, their reliability in alerting the surgeon to a potential cord injury having been clearly established [26]. None of these patients had any intra-operative deviation from their baseline SCM traces or developed any postoperative neurological deficit as a complication of the surgical correction of their spinal deformity. There were no instances of any false negative SCM traces. When compared to their

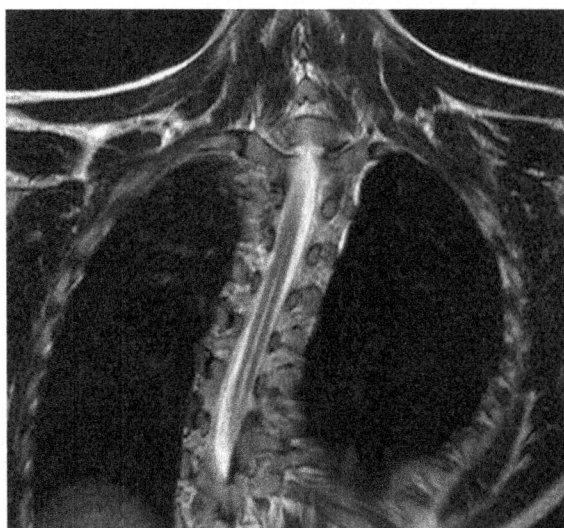

Fig. 4 Image demonstrating typical appearance of a persistent central canal on T2-weighted coronal MRI of the thoracic spine

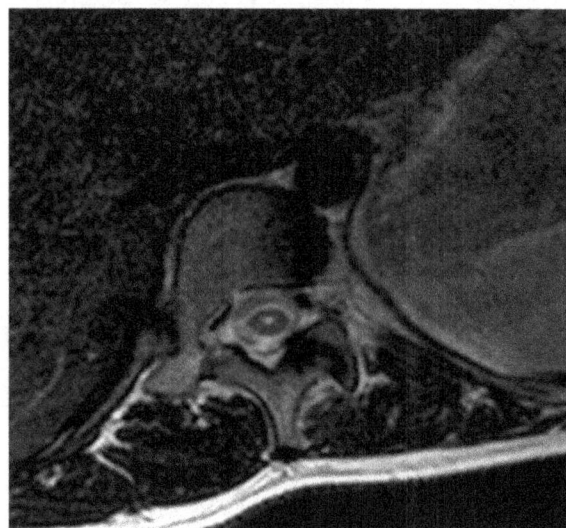

Fig. 5 Image demonstrating typical appearance of a persistent central canal on T2-weighted axial MRI of a thoracic spine segment

matched controls with regard to incidence of intra-operative deviation from baseline SSEPs, there was no statistically significant difference between the two groups ($p = 0.57$). Therefore, the null hypothesis could not be rejected, i.e. the presence of a PCC does not increase the risk of iatrogenic neurological injury during surgical correction of scoliosis.

The PCC was found to be located either entirely or partially within the instrumented spinal levels in all patients within the PCC group, and a satisfactory percentage curve correction was achieved in all 11 PCC patients. The absence of abnormal SCM traces in any of the 11 patients in the PCC group therefore cannot be attributed to either the PCC being anatomically remote to the level of instrumentation or be related to a minimal curve correction.

This study does have inherent weaknesses, the major one being the relatively small numbers involved. In order to increase the statistical power of the study, four times as many sex- and age-matched controls were included. However, the study spanned a 7-year period during which 1161 surgical scoliosis corrections were performed. This suggests that a PCC in a patient presenting with scoliosis is a rare finding, in the order of 0.95% in our study group. This is in a similar range to the 1.5% described by Petit-Lacour et al. [10], which at present remains the only published estimation of the prevalence of PCCs in the general population, based on a retrospective study of 794 whole spine MRI scans of patients who had initially been investigated for a variety of symptoms. Significantly increasing the numbers involved in our study would entail having to either lengthen the already considerable study period by a substantial amount of time or conduct a multicentre study, both of which have inherent difficulties.

Another weakness of this study is that it is retrospective and therefore has deficiencies inherent to all investigations of this nature. However, once again owing to the relative scarcity of PCCs, conducting a prospective study to address this research question is not practicable and is therefore very unlikely to ever be performed.

The significance of the results of this study relates to the fact that with the resolution of MRI scans progressively increasing and routine pre-operative MRI screening of all patients presenting with scoliosis becoming commonplace across a greater number of institutions, it is very likely that a growing number of patients with PCCs will be identified pre-operatively. At present, the pre-operative identification of a fluid collection within the spinal cord of a child with scoliosis but no other NAA often causes uncertainty for clinicians. The significance of such findings and the degree of additional risk of intra-operative neurological injury they may pose, if any, currently remains uncertain. Once identified, these patients are often pre-operatively referred for a neuro-surgical opinion on the appropriate management of these entities. At present, this remains largely unknown due to the absence of any literature to guide clinicians in these circumstances. This is therefore an issue this study may help to address.

Conclusion

Despite being based on relatively small numbers, our study does not provide any evidence to suggest that the presence of a PCC increases the risk of a neurological injury secondary to surgical correction of scoliosis. We therefore suggest that surgical correction of scoliosis in patients with a PCC can be carried out safely with routine precautions.

Abbreviations
AIF: Anterior instrumented fusion; AIS: Adolescent idiopathic scoliosis; AR: Anterior release; CSF: Cerebrospinal fluid; MRI: Magnetic resonance imaging; NAA: Neuro axis abnormality; PCC: Persistent central canal; PIF: Posterior instrumented fusion; SCM: Spinal cord monitoring; SSEPs: Somato-sensory evoked potentials

Acknowledgements
Not applicable.

Funding
There is no funding to be declared.

Authors' contributions
SK is the corresponding author who primarily wrote up the manuscript. YM made substantial contributions to the acquisition of data and its statistical analysis. KP made substantial contributions to the provision of data used in this study and its interpretation. MS and KR have all been involved in drafting the manuscript and revising it critically. All authors read and approved the final manuscript.

Competing interests
The authors declare that they have no competing interests.

Author details
[1]Spinal Deformity Unit, Royal National Orthopaedic Hospital, Stanmore, UK.
[2]The Royal National Orthopaedic Hospital, Stanmore, UK.

References

1.   El-Hawary R, et al. Spinal cord monitoring in patients with spinal deformity and neural axis abnormalities: a comparison with adolescent idiopathic scoliosis patients. Spine (Phila Pa 1976). 2006;31(19):E698–706.

2.   Sansur CA, et al. Scoliosis research society morbidity and mortality of adult scoliosis surgery. Spine (Phila Pa 1976). 2011;36(9):E593–7.

3.   Winter RB. Neurologic safety in spinal deformity surgery. Spine (Phila Pa 1976). 1997;22(13):1527–33.

4.   Gupta P, Lenke LG, Bridwell KH. Incidence of neural axis abnormalities in infantile and juvenile patients with spinal deformity. Is a magnetic resonance image screening necessary? Spine (Phila Pa 1976). 1998;23(2):206–10.

5.   Winter RB, et al. Magnetic resonance imaging evaluation of the adolescent patient with idiopathic scoliosis before spinal instrumentation and fusion. A prospective, double-blinded study of 140 patients. Spine (Phila Pa 1976). 1997;22(8):855–8.

6.   Mooney JF 3rd, et al. Neurologic risk management in scoliosis surgery. J Pediatr Orthop. 2002;22(5):683–9.

7.   Ozerdemoglu RA, Transfeldt EE, Denis F. Value of treating primary causes of syrinx in scoliosis associated with syringomyelia. Spine (Phila Pa 1976). 2003;28(8):806–14.

8.   Noordeen MH, Taylor BA, Edgar MA. Syringomyelia. A potential risk factor in scoliosis surgery. Spine (Phila Pa 1976). 1994;19(12):1406–9.

9.   Nordwall A, Wikkelso C. A late neurologic complication of scoliosis surgery in connection with syringomyelia. Acta Orthop Scand. 1979;50(4):407–10.

10. Petit-Lacour MC, et al. Visibility of the central canal on MRI. Neuroradiology. 2000;42(10):756–61.

11. Magge SN, et al. Idiopathic syrinx in the pediatric population: a combined center experience. J Neurosurg Pediatr. 2011;7(1):30–6.

12. Holly LT, Batzdorf U. Slitlike syrinx cavities: a persistent central canal. J Neurosurg. 2002;97(2 Suppl):161–5.

13. Roser F, et al. Defining the line between hydromyelia and syringomyelia. A differentiation is possible based on electrophysiological and magnetic resonance imaging studies. Acta Neurochir. 2010;152(2):213–9. discussion 219

14. Kasantikul V, Netsky MG, James AE Jr. Relation of age and cerebral ventricle size to central canal in man. Morphological analysis. J Neurosurg. 1979;51(1):85–93.

15. Milhorat TH, Kotzen RM, Anzil AP. Stenosis of central canal of spinal cord in man: incidence and pathological findings in 232 autopsy cases. J Neurosurg. 1994;80(4):716–22.

16. Yasui K, et al. Age-related morphologic changes of the central canal of the human spinal cord. Acta Neuropathol. 1999;97(3):253–9.

17. Vandertop WP. Syringomyelia. Neuropediatrics. 2014;45(1):3–9.

18. Sponseller PD. Syringomyelia and Chiari I malformation presenting with juvenile scoliosis as sole manifestation. J Spinal Disord. 1992;5(2):237–9. discussion 239-44

19. Emery E, Redondo A, Rey A. Syringomyelia and Arnold Chiari in scoliosis initially classified as idiopathic: experience with 25 patients. Eur Spine J. 1997;6(3):158–62.

20. Hanieh A, et al. Syringomyelia in children with primary scoliosis. Childs Nerv Syst. 2000;16(4):200–2.

21. Tomlinson RJ Jr, et al. Syringomyelia and developmental scoliosis. J Pediatr Orthop. 1994;14(5):580–5.

22. Farley FA, et al. Syringomyelia and scoliosis in children. J Pediatr Orthop. 1995;15(2):187–92.

23. Phillips WA, Hensinger RN, Kling TF Jr. Management of scoliosis due to syringomyelia in childhood and adolescence. J Pediatr Orthop. 1990;10(3):351–4.

24. Bradley LJ, et al. The outcomes of scoliosis surgery in patients with syringomyelia. Spine (Phila Pa 1976). 2007;32(21):2327–33.

25. Fischbein NJ, et al. The "presyrinx" state: a reversible myelopathic condition that may precede syringomyelia. AJNR Am J Neuroradiol. 1999;20(1):7–20.

26. Wilson-Holden TJ, et al. Efficacy of intraoperative monitoring for pediatric patients with spinal cord pathology undergoing spinal deformity surgery. Spine (Phila Pa 1976). 1999;24(16):1685–92.

4

Introversion, the prevalent trait of adolescents with idiopathic scoliosis: an observational study

Elisabetta D'Agata[1*], Judith Sánchez-Raya[2] and Juan Bagó[2]

Abstract

Background: A large number of studies about adolescents with idiopathic scoliosis focus on health-related quality of life (HRQOL). However, only a few articles aim at evaluating the personality of these patients. Therefore, the purpose of the present research is to assess the personality traits of adolescents with idiopathic scoliosis and their relationship with HRQOL.

Our hypothesis is that adolescents with idiopathic scoliosis present the principal personality trait of introversion, defined as self-reliance and inhibition in social relationships.

Methods: This was a cross-sectional study. The examined group consisted of 43 patients (only 4 boys), mean age = 14. 3 (SD = 2.23). On the day of the visit, HRQOL tools (Scoliosis Research Society-22 Questionnaire (SRS-22) and Trunk Appearance Perception Scale (TAPS)) and a personality test (16 Personality Factors-Adolescent Personality Questionnaire (16PF-APQ)) were completed; in addition, a posterior-anterior radiography was performed. Correlations among demographic and medical data and HRQOL and personality tests were assessed.

Results: Results for SRS-22 were as follows: Function 4.5 (SD = .4), Pain 4.3 (SD = .5), Self-image 3.6 (SD = .7), Mental Health 3.8. (SD = .7), and Subtotal 4.2 (SD = .7). Mean TAPS was 3.5 (SD = .6).

In personality, the lowest values were assessed for Extroversion ($M = 29.4$, SD = 24.7) and Self-reliance ($M = 71$, SD = 25.3). Independence was negatively related to Self-image ($r = -.51$), Mental Health ($r = -.54$), and Subtotal SRS-22 ($r = -.60$) ($p < .01$).

Conclusions: Adolescents with idiopathic scoliosis presented a common style of personality, characterized by social inhibition (introversion), preference for staying alone, and being self-sufficient (self-reliance).

Specific programs in promoting social abilities may help adolescent patients with idiopathic scoliosis in finding a way to express themselves and to become more sociable. Correlational studies between personality and HRQOL need to be performed to better understand these issues.

Keywords: Adolescent idiopathic scoliosis, Personality, Health related quality of life, Introversion, Psychology

Background

The medical profession is quickly going through a deep transformation as physicians move from managing acute diseases to chronic ones, such as idiopathic scoliosis. As a consequence, the need to adapt and redesign behavioral care models is increasing. The biopsychosocial model introduced by Engel [1] proposed a *human scientific approach*

---
* Correspondence: dagata.e@gmail.com
[1]Vall d'Hebron Research Institut, Passeig Vall d'Hebron, 119-129, 08035 Barcelona, Spain
Full list of author information is available at the end of the article

in medicine, involving the patient's perspective, and Balint opposed disease-oriented care to patient-centered medicine [2] in 1969.

As a result of this change, research in the field of idiopathic scoliosis in adolescence is mainly focused on assessing health-related quality of life (HRQOL) and especially body image during the delicate period of identity development [3].

As body image (measured by the Scoliosis Research Society-22 Questionnaire (SRS-22)) does not always correlate with the Cobb angle, researchers express a need to consider other variables that may influence body image perception in younger patients [4]. Furthermore, studies about the relationship between scoliosis and the mental conditions of patients are still unclear and inconclusive [5].

On the other hand, we have a proverbial sentence from the Canadian-born physician Osler: "It is much more important to know what sort of patient has the disease than what sort of disease a patient has," and that point of view is still considered progressive in today's hospital world [6]. So, it seems important to know the patients' personalities in order to improve healthcare and to enhance patient-doctor communication. In fact, patient-centered communication has been extensively considered as a crucial component of high-quality healthcare, as the interactions during the medical encounter improve the patients' ability to remember doctors' recommendations, to achieve satisfaction, and to improve adherence to treatment [7]. As a consequence, in order to know patients' personalities in depth, interesting studies about the relationships between diseases and behavior patterns are emerging for cardiac disease [8–11], cancer [12–15], fibromyalgia [16], etc.

Nevertheless, few studies about patients with scoliosis and personality traits have been performed. A high level of introversion was assessed in a preoperative sample and changed after surgery [17]; Misterska et al. [5] found a high level of self-criticism in a sample of non-operated patients compared with a healthy control group. Furthermore, a certain tendency to isolation or shyness and an almost total absence of aggressive expression were assessed [18].

According to Eysenck [19], introverts are governed by inhibition and restraint while extroverts are governed by expressiveness, impulsivity, and other-directedness. Moreover, introversion is related to an internalizing coping style: internalizers are generally shy, retiring, self-critical, withdrawn, constrained, over-controlled, self-reflective, worried, and inhibited. On the other hand, extroversion is related to an externalizing coping style: externalizers are commonly impulsive, action oriented, gregarious, aggressive, hedonistic, stimulation seeking, and lacking in insight [20].

From the previously mentioned research in the scoliosis field [17, 18] and from our clinical practice, we hypothesize that adolescents with idiopathic scoliosis would present a common personality trait of introversion unrelated to the magnitude of scoliosis, to their body image, or to the type of treatment they were following. Then, as a second objective, we assessed the relationship between personality and HRQOL.

Method
Procedure
This is a cross-sectional study approved by the Clinical Research Ethics Committee. Patients who visited the outpatient consulting clinic of our institution were recruited

consecutively for 1 year. Inclusion criteria for this study were diagnosis of idiopathic scoliosis; age between 10 and 19; absence of intellectual disability, brain injury, or acute/severe psychiatric disorder (e.g., psychosis); non-operative treatment (brace, physiotherapy, or observation); and consent to participate.

A psychologist administered all of the tests individually. For each patient, a posterior-anterior radiography of the full trunk in the standing position was taken, and later, a physician visited the patient and measured the magnitude of the largest curve.

The patients were divided into two groups: braced and not treated. Despite the instruction to wear a brace, those who declared not to be compliant belonged to the second group of "no treatment."

Questionnaires
All the patients completed a sociodemographic questionnaire, SRS-22, Trunk Appearance Perception Scale (TAPS), and 16 Personality Factors-Adolescent Personality Questionnaire (16PF-APQ).

The *sociodemographic questionnaire* was performed to collect generic data, such as name, age, sex, and kind of treatment.

SRS-22 [21] is used to assess HRQOL and has five domains (pain, function/activity, self-image, mental health, and satisfaction with treatment). The satisfaction with treatment domain was not measured as it was not related with the aim of the research. The total score is calculated from the average of each of the mean domain scores and can range from 1 (worst HRQOL) to 5 (best HRQOL). The original questionnaire has good psychometric properties: internal consistency (Cronbach's α = .86), reliability (r = .9), and concurrent validity (r = .7). The original English version has been translated and adapted into many languages, including Spanish. The Spanish version [22] presented satisfactory test-retest reliability (ICC = .9), internal consistency (Cronbach's $\alpha \geq$ .7), and convergent validity (r = .84).

TAPS [23] includes three sets of drawings corresponding to the three views of the trunk: from the back, in a forward bending position, and from the front. Each drawing is rated from 1 (most deformity) to 5 (no deformity), and an average score (the sum of the values of the three drawings divided by 3) between 1 and 5 is obtained. The scale has good reliability (Cronbach's α = .89, test-retest = .92) and validity (convergent validity, r = .52; discriminant validity, r = −.55).

16PF-APQ [24] is a self-reported personality inventory, validated for adolescents from 12 to 19 years of age. It collects valuable information regarding the young people's personal style, their problem-solving abilities, and favorite work activities. It consists of 161 items and takes 45–60 min to complete. The items are distributed as follows (Table 1): 135 items belong to 16 primary scales, 11 items to problem solving (a short measure of general reasoning ability), and 15 to work activity preferences (a measure of six career-interest variables). All the scales are bipolar. The 15 personality scales are further organized into five global scales: Extraversion (Warmth, Liveliness, Social Boldness, Vigilance, Privateness, and Self-reliance), Anxiety (Emotional Stability, Vigilance, Apprehension, and Tension), Tough-mindedness (Warmth, Sensitivity, Abstractedness, and Openness to Change), Independence (Dominance, Liveliness, Social Boldness, Vigilance, Openness to Change, and Tension), and Self-control (Warmth, Liveliness, Rule-Consciousness, Vigilance, Openness to Change, and Perfectionism). The test was adapted to a Spanish version [25] and presented adequate psychometric properties: reliability values fluctuated between .58 and .80 for personality scales and between .42 and .70 for work activity preferences.

To evaluate the test, Tea Edition software was used. It transforms the raw scores into centiles as a function of the age and the sex; so, the values of the assessed sample correspond to the percentiles of the *normative population*.

Results between the 30th and 70th centiles group 40% of the cases. Values out of this range represent a moderate high/low score of these dimensions.

Data analysis
Descriptive data included mean (*M*) and standard deviation (SD). The sample was split into two groups in relation to the magnitude of Introversion-Extraversion. Then, differences between these two groups were assessed through the Mann-Whitney *U* test for magnitude of curve, Body Image SRS-22, TAPS and treatment.

To check a correlation between HRQOL and personality, a correlational analysis was performed using Spearman correlation coefficients. Statistical software was SPSS 18.0.

Table 1 Description of 16PF-APQ scale with its bipolar dimensions: 16 primary scales, 6 career preferences, and 5 global scales

Dimensions	Low range	Scales	High range
Primary scales	Reserved	Warmth (A)[a]	Warm-hearted
	Concrete	Reasoning (B)	Abstract
	Reactive	Emotional Stability (C)	Emotionally Stable
	Deferential	Dominance (E)	Dominant
	Serious	Liveliness (F)[a]	Enthusiastic
	Expedient	Rule-Consciousness (G)	Rule-conscious
	Shy, Timid	Social Boldness (H)[a]	Socially Bold
	Tough	Sensitivity (I)	Sensitive
	Trusting	Vigilance (L)[a]	Vigilant
	Practical	Abstractedness (M)	Abstracted
	Forthright	Privateness (N)[a]	Private
	Self-assured	Apprehension (O)	Apprehensive
	Traditional	Openness to Change (Q1)	Open To Change
	Group-orientated	Self-reliance (Q2)[a]	Self-reliant
	Tolerates Disorder	Perfectionism (Q3)	Perfectionist
	Relaxed, Placid, Patient	Tension (Q4)	Tense, High Energy
Career preferences	More interested in people	Manual Style	More interested in things
	Preference to be persuaded	Scientific Style	Preference in ideas
	Preference in structured tasks	Artistic Style	Preference in creativity
	Interested in objects	Helping Style	Interested in people
	Interested in help	Sales/Managerial Style	Preference in persuading others
	Preference ambiguity	Procedural Style	Interested in planning
Global scales	Introverted	Extraversion	Extraverted
	Low Anxiety	Neuroticism	High Anxiety
	Receptive	Tough-minded	Resolute
	Accommodating	Independence	Independent
	Unrestrained	Self-controlled	Self-controlled

Adapted from Schuerger, J.M. (2001) [20]
[a]Table primary scales belonging to Extraversion

Results

The study group consisted of 43 patients with idiopathic scoliosis. Thirty-nine were women. Mean age was 14.3 (SD = 2.2). Mean of the magnitude of the curve with the largest Cobb angle was 32.9 (SD = 10.8). Forty-nine percent of the patients were treated with a brace (braced group); 51% did not require any treatment (not-treated group).

The averages for all the domains of SRS-22 were the following: Function 4.5 (SD = .4), Pain 4.3 (SD = .5), Self-image 3.6 (SD = .7), Mental Health 3.8 (SD = .7), and Subtotal 4.2 (SD = .7). TAPS mean was 3.5 (SD = .6).

Moderately high values were Self-reliance (M = 71.3, SD = 25) for Primary Factors and Sales/Managerial Style for Career Preferences (M = 71.3, SD = 20.5); low values were assessed for Extraversion (M = 29.4, SD = 24.7) belonging to Global Factors (Table 2).

Almost half (49th %) of the sample had an extremely low Extraversion score, rating under < 20th percentile of the normative population (Table 3 and Fig. 1).

Furthermore, splitting the group in relation to Extraversion (first group ≤ 30; second group > 30), the two groups did not differ significantly for Cobb angle, Body Image Scale SRS-22, TAPS, and treatment (Table 4).

Then, assessing correlations among 16PF-APQ and SRS-22, significant values of correlations were found only for Rule-Consciousness, Independency, and Vigilance (Table 5); SRS-22 Function, Pain, Body Image, Mental Health, and Subtotal had negative correlations with Vigilance and Independency, while positive correlations with Rule-Consciousness. No significant correlations were found between 16PF-APQ and TAPS.

Table 2 16PF-APQ sample mean and standard deviations

Dimensions	Scales	Mean	SD
Primary scales	Warmth (A)	52.7	27.7
	Reasoning (B)	51.6	25.7
	Emotional Stability (C)	55.6	28
	Dominance (E)	66.8	27.2
	Liveliness (F)	46.5	27
	Rule-Consciousness (G)	64.5	29
	Social Boldness (H)	43.2	30
	Sensitivity (I)	50.7	27.7
	Vigilance (L)	64	27.5
	Abstractedness (M)	48.6	26.7
	Privateness (N)	65	26
	Apprehension (O)	52.5	32
	Openness to Change (Q1)	52.9	32
	Self-reliance (Q2)	71.3[a]	25
	Perfectionism (Q3)	44	29
	Tension (Q4)	53.6	30
Career preferences	Manual Style	56.4	28.6
	Scientific Style	49.5	26.9
	Artistic Style	60.9	31.4
	Helping Style	55.3	27.4
	Sales/Managerial Style	71.3[a]	20.7
	Procedural Style	44.3	33.4
Global scales	Extraversion	29.4[a]	24.7
	Neuroticism	46.8	32.9
	Tough-minded	51.5	31.7
	Independence	56.6	31.3
	Self-controlled	50.8	30.0

[a]Values < 30th and values > 70th

Table 3 Frequencies and cumulative percentages for extraversion value

Extroversion	Frequency sample	Cumulative percent
1	2	5.4
2	4	16.2
3	1	18.9
4	1	21.6
7	1	24.3
8	1	27.0
10	1	29.7
11	2	35.1
16	1	37.8
17	2	43.2
18	1	45.9
19	1	48.6[a]
24	1	51,4
27	1	54.1
30	1	56.8
31	1	59.5
39	1	62,2
40	1	64.9
41	3	73.0
43	1	75.7
46	1	78.4
55	1	81.1
56	2	86.5
59	1	89.2
66	1	91.9
75	1	94.6
84	2	100
Total	37	100

[a]50th percentile of sample

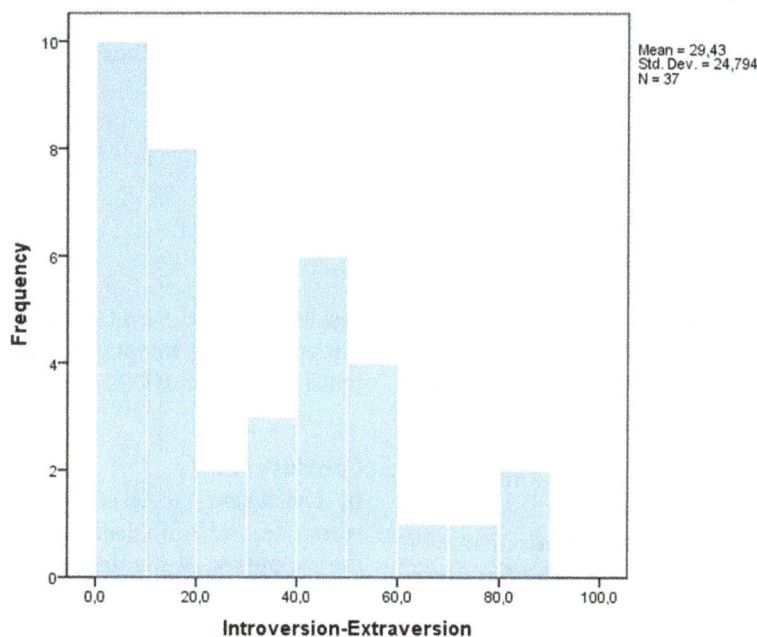

Fig. 1 Graph of frequency distribution of the bipolar dimension: Introversion-Extraversion

Discussion

As the new patient-centered medicine and the biopsychosocial model are gaining importance, HRQOL assessment, especially the measure of body image, has been used to assess adolescents with scoliosis. Furthermore, to study these patients in depth and to improve a doctor-patient communication, personality is measured in scoliosis patients. Besides, through the literature about personality studies and the observation of adolescents with idiopathic scoliosis in the outpatient clinic, a common psychological pattern of internalization has been assessed. So, as first aim, with the use of 16 Personality Factors-Adolescent Personality Questionnaire (16PF-APQ), the hypothesis of introversion was evaluated. Later, it was interesting to study HRQOL and to relate it with personality. For this second objective, a correlational study between HRQOL and Personality was performed. SRS-22 was applied to assess HRQOL, as it is one of the most used tests for adolescents with idiopathic scoliosis.

The results underlined a specific behavior pattern as patients scored moderately high in introversion, confirming results from previous research [17, 18]. In fact, patients presented a specific profile, appearing self-reliant, that is, self-sufficient, with a preference for staying alone and taking decisions by themselves; the opposite would have been a group-orientated person, affiliative, with a preference for working with other people. Furthermore, the most highly rated career preference was the sales/*managerial* one. This career preference is related to an entrepreneurial style [25] and could be explained in this sample of introverted adolescents as a managerial attitude, related to self-reliance, leadership, and dominance.

No differences were assessed for scoliosis magnitude, treatment, and body image scales. This result could be explained in view of the fact that personality is a complex system influenced by a lot of determinants from biology to environment. No linear cause-effect relations between body image and personality could be applied to explain how image influences personality in scoliosis.

We consider these data important for clinical consultations. As introverted people are generally shy, introspective, and withdrawn, we advise healthcare professionals to take this personality style into account in addition to their coping style. The following useful tips [26] could be applied for the communications with these patients: (1) creating a calm and "safe" space where patients speak, protecting them from interferences (noise, mothers, other family members, etc.); (2) at the beginning of the conversation, asking open-ended questions, showing real interest in their life, not only about scoliosis and its treatment. In fact, the patient's silence challenges the doctor's commitment to see and treat the whole person and not only measuring radiographs and clinical parameters during the visit.

Table 4 Mann-Whitney *U* and significant differences for Cobb angle, Treatment, SRS-22 Body Image, and TAPS between the two subgroups of patients with low and high Introversion

	Cobb angle	Body Image Scale SRS-22	TAPS	Treatment
Mann-Whitney *U*	124.0	91.5	80.0	148.0
p (2-tailed)	.16	.09	.29	.44

Table 5 Spearman correlations coefficients between SRS-22 domains and 4 factors of 16PF-APQ

SRS domains		Function	Pain	Body Image	Mental Health	SubtotSRS-22
16PF-APQ	Rule-Consciousness	.35*	.44**	.40*	.30	.61**
		p = .03	p = .001	p = .01	p = .06	p = .000
	Independency	−.22 p = .21	−.34*	−.51**	−.54**	−.60**
			p = .04	p = .002	p = .001	p = .000
	Vigilance	−.3	−.33*	−.42** p = .007	−.36*	−.45**
		p = .7	p = .04		p = .02	p = .003

*$p < .05$; **$p < .01$

Taking coping style into account, doctors may advise patients to join some group activities, avoiding the possible tendency to stay at home studying all day. Indoor activities, such as using internet social networks, make social interactions much less threatening, but that is only communicating and not a real connection with the real world. In a determined moment, shy teens "have to log off the computer and log on life" [27]. Physiotherapy in a group could be useful as well as all kinds of activities allowing personal expression such as theater, free dance, or any group activities (scouting, trekking, etc.).

In the correctional study about Personality and HRQOL, Body Image, Mental Health domains, and the overall HRQOL had the highest ($r > .5$, $p < .01$) negative correlations with Independency while correlated positively with Rule-Consciousness. These correlations surprised us as intuitively we would think the opposite: the more the person is independent, the better Body Image, Pain HRQOL, and Mental Health s/he has. Interpreting the results, we have to take into account that independence is a proper theme in adolescence when teenagers struggle to grow up, find their identity, and become adults [28]. As a consequence, Independency and Rule-Consciousness are core themes for adolescents. An adolescent, who is developing his independence in the building of his identity, has more difficulties than an obedient adolescent in accepting his/her body image and with his/her mental health.

Furthermore, significative correlations between Vigilance and HRQOL, specifically Pain, Body Image, and Mental Health, were found. A vigilant person appears suspicious, jealous, or envious while his/her opposite is a trusting person, who is collaborative, not competitive, and interested in the others. So, the correlation could be interpreted as follows: a vigilant person could suffer, comparing his/her body with the others and having more difficulties in accepting his/her body than a trusting person.

We suggest taking account of the results of adolescents' Body Image and Mental Health in SRS-22; also, other variables, such as *Independence, Rule-Consciousness*, and *Vigilance*, may influence them.

However, this study lacks a control group of patients without scoliosis. Further research will be needed to consider a control group of healthy adolescents not coming from the hospital and to enlarge the sample size;

besides, it would be interesting to repeat the study with a representative sample of adults, focusing on the relationship between HRQOL and personality.

Conclusions

In conclusion, adolescents with scoliosis were introverted and self-sufficient. Introversion did not differ for the magnitude of the deformity, for the brace treatment, or for the perception of the trunk. Adolescents with better Body Image and Mental Health were less vigilant but less Independent.

The assessment of the introversion trait should have a consequence in the planning of specific rehabilitation programs for the treatment of adolescents with scoliosis. Rehabilitation programs have to integrate physiotherapy exercises with psychosocial activities. These last activities help adolescents in expressing themselves and sharing their experiences with the others, in order to create interests beyond their inner world and improve their social relationship.

Abbreviations
16PF-APQ: 16 Personality Factors-Adolescent Personality Questionnaire; HRQOL: Health-related quality of life; SRS-22: Scoliosis Research Society-22 Questionnaire; TAPS: Trunk Appearance Perception Scale

Acknowledgements
There was no acknowledgment for this study

Funding
There was no funding for this study.

Authors' contributions
ED has made substantial contributions to the conception and design, data measurement, recruitment of patients, data analysis, and interpretation and has been involved in drafting the manuscript. JSR has made substantial contributions to the conception and design, acquisition of data, recruitment of patients, data analysis and interpretation, and drafting of the manuscript and given final approval of the version to be published. JB has revised it critically and gave important suggestions for intellectual contents. All authors read and approved the final manuscript.

Competing interests

The authors declare that they have no competing interests.

Author details

[1]Vall d'Hebron Research Institut, Passeig Vall d'Hebron, 119-129, 08035 Barcelona, Spain. [2]Vall d'Hebron Hospital, Passeig Vall d'Hebron, 119-129, 08035 Barcelona, Spain.

References

1. Engel GL. The need for a new medical model: a challenge for biomedicine. Science. 1977;196(4286):129–36.
2. Balint E. The possibilities of patient-centered medicine. JR Coll Gen Pract. 1969;17(82):269–76.
3. Klimstra TA, Hale WW, Raaijmakers QAW, Branje SJT, Meeus WHJ. Identity formation in adolescence: change or stability? J Youth Adolesc. 2010; doi:10.1007/s10964-009-9401-4.
4. Matamalas A, Bagó J, D'Agata E, Pellisé F. Body image in idiopathic scoliosis: a comparison study of psychometric properties between four patient-reported outcome instruments. Health Qual Life Outcomes. 2014; doi:10.1186/1477-7525-12-81.
5. Misterska E, Glowacki M, Harasymczuk J. Personality characteristics of females with adolescent idiopathic scoliosis after brace or surgical treatment compared to healthy controls. Med Sci Monit. 2010;16(12):CR606–15.
6. John M. From Osler to the cone technique. HSR Proc Intensive Care Cardiovasc Anesth. 2013;5(1):57–8.
7. Suarez-Almazor ME. Patient-physician communication. Curr Opin Rheumatol. 2004;16(2):91–5. Review. PubMed PMID: 14770091
8. Friedman M, Rosenman RH. Association of specific overt behavior pattern with blood and cardiovascular findings; blood cholesterol level, blood clotting time, incidence of arcus senilis, and clinical coronary artery disease. J Am Med Assoc. 1959; doi:10.1001/jama.1959.03000290012005.
9. Pedersen SS, Denollet J. Type D personality, cardiac events, and impaired quality of life: a review. Eur J Cardiovasc Prev Rehabil. 2003; doi:10.1097/01.hjr.0000085246.65733.06.
10. Condén E, Rosenblad A, Ekselius L, Aslund C. Prevalence of type D personality and factorial and temporal stability of the DS14 after myocardial infarction in a Swedish population. Scand J Psychol. 2014; doi:10.1111/sjop.12162.
11. Staniute M, Brozaitiene J, Burkauskas J, Kazukauskiene N, Mickuviene N, Bunevicius R. Type D personality, mental distress, social support and health-related quality of life in coronary artery disease patients with heart failure: a longitudinal observational study. Health Qual Life Outcomes. 2015; doi:10.1186/s12955-014-0204-2.
12. Batselé E, Denollet J, Lussier A, Loas G, Vanden Eynde S, Van de Borne P, Fantini-Hauwel C. Type D personality: application of DS14 French version in general and clinical populations. J Health Psychol. 2016; doi:10.1177/1359105315624499.
13. Zhang J, Fang L, Zhang D, Jin Q, Wu X, Liu J, et al. Type D personality is associated with delaying patients to medical assessment and poor quality of life among rectal cancer survivors. Int J Color Dis. 2016; doi:10.1007/s00384-015-2333-4.
14. Husson O, Vissers PAJ, Denollet J, Mols F. The role of personality in the course of health-related quality of life and disease-specific health status among colorectal cancer survivors: a prospective population-based study from the PROFILES registry. Acta Oncol (Stockholm, Sweden). 2015; doi:10.3109/0284186X.2014.996663.
15. Chen J, Liu Y, Cai QQ, Liu YM, Wang T, Zhang K, et al. Type D personality parents of children with leukemia tend to experience anxiety: the mediating effects of social support and coping style. Medicine. 2015; doi:10.1097/MD.0000000000000627.
16. Van Middendorp H, Kool MB, van Beugen S, Denollet J, Lumley MA, Geenen R. Prevalence and relevance of type D personality in fibromyalgia. Gen Hosp Psychiatry. 2016; doi:10.1016/j.genhosppsych.2015.11.006.
17. Kasai Y, Morishita K, Kawakita E, Kondo T, Uchida A. Pre-and postoperative psychological characteristics in mothers of patients with idiopathic scoliosis. Eur Spine J. 2006; doi:10.1007/s00586-005-0007-6.
18. D'Agata E, Rigo M, Pérez-Testor C, Puigví NC, Castellano-Tejedor C. Emotional indicators in young patients with idiopathic scoliosis: a study through the drawing of human figure. Scoliosis. 2014; doi:10.1186/s13013-014-0024-5.
19. Eysenck HJ. The biological basis of personality. Springfield: Thomas; 1967.
20. Beutler LE, Moos RH, Lane G. Coping, treatment planning, and treatment outcome: discussion. J Clin Psychol. 2003;59:1151–67.
21. Asher M, Min Lai S, Burton D, Manna B. The reliability and concurrent validity of the scoliosis research society-22 patient questionnaire for idiopathic scoliosis. Spine. 2003; doi:10.1097/01.BRS.0000047634.95839.67.
22. Climent JM, Bago J, Ey A, Perez-Grueso FJS, Izquierdo E. Validity of the Spanish version of the Scoliosis Research Society-22 (SRS-22) Patient Questionnaire. Spine. 2005; doi:10.1097/01.brs.0000155408.76606.8f.
23. Bago J, Sanchez-Raya J, Perez-Grueso FJS, Climent JM. The Trunk Appearance Perception Scale (TAPS): a new tool to evaluate subjective impression of trunk deformity in patients with idiopathic scoliosis. Scoliosis. 2010; doi:10.1186/1748-7161-5-6.
24. Schuerger JM. 16PF Adolescent Personality Questionnaire. Champaign: Institute for Personality and Ability Testing; 2001.
25. Schuerger JM, Seisdedos CN. 16PF-APQ: Cuestionario de personalidad para adolescentes 16PF: manual. Madrid: TEA Ediciones; 2003.
26. Cain S. In: Ni PC, editor. Relationship communication success for introverts; 2017.
27. Carducci BJ. Shyness. A bold new approach. 1st ed. New York: HarperPerennial; 2000.
28. Spear LP. The adolescent brain and age-related behavioral manifestations. Neurosci Biobehav Rev. 2000; doi:10.1016/S0149-7634(00)00014-2.

5

Effectiveness of Schroth exercises during bracing in adolescent idiopathic scoliosis: results from a preliminary study

Kenny Yat Hong Kwan[1*], Aldous C.S. Cheng[2], Hui Yu Koh[1], Alice Y.Y. Chiu[2] and Kenneth Man Chee Cheung[1]

Abstract

Background: Bracing has been shown to decrease significantly the progression of high-risk curves to the threshold for surgery in patients with adolescent idiopathic scoliosis (AIS), but the treatment failure rate remains high. There is evidence to suggest that Schroth scoliosis-specific exercises can slow progression in mild scoliosis. The aim of this study was to evaluate the efficacy of Schroth exercises in AIS patients with high-risk curves during bracing.

Methods: A prospective, historical cohort-matched study was carried out. Patients diagnosed with AIS who fulfilled the Scoliosis Research Society (SRS) criteria for bracing were recruited to receive Schroth exercises during bracing. An outpatient-based Schroth program was given. Data for these patients were compared with a 1:1 matched historical control group who were treated with bracing alone. The assessor and statistician were blinded. Radiographic progression, truncal shift, and SRS-22r scores were compared between cases and controls.

Results: Twenty-four patients (5 males and 19 females, mean age 12.3 ± 1.4 years) were included in the exercise group, and 24 patients (mean age 11.8 ± 1.1 years) were matched in the control group. The mean follow-up period for the exercise group was 18.1 ± 6.2 months. In the exercise group, spinal deformity improved in 17% of patients (Cobb angle improvement of ≥ 6°), worsened in 21% (Cobb angle increases of ≥ 6°), and remained stable in 62%. In the control group, 4% improved, 50% worsened, and 46% remained stable. In the subgroup analysis, 31% of patients who were compliant (13 cases) improved, 69% remained static, and none had worsened, while in the non-compliant group (11 cases), none had improved, 46% worsened, and 46% remained stable. Analysis of the secondary outcomes showed improvement of the truncal shift, angle of trunk rotation, the SRS function domain, and total scores in favor of the exercise group.

Conclusion: This is the first study to investigate the effects of Schroth exercises on AIS patients during bracing. Our findings from this preliminary study showed that Schroth exercise during bracing was superior to bracing alone in improving Cobb angles, trunk rotation, and QOL scores. Furthermore, those who were compliant with the exercise program had a higher rate of Cobb angle improvement. The results of this study form the basis for a randomized controlled trial to evaluate the effect of Schroth exercises during bracing in AIS.

Keywords: Schroth, Scoliosis-specific exercise, Adolescent idiopathic scoliosis, Bracing, Curve progression, Conservative management

* Correspondence: kyhkwan@hku.hk
[1]Department of Orthopaedics and Traumatology, Li Ka Shing Faculty of
Medicine, The University of Hong Kong, Pokfulam, Hong Kong
Full list of author information is available at the end of the article

Background

The aim of treatment of adolescent idiopathic scoliosis (AIS) is to prevent curve progression to 50°, beyond which there is a risk of continued progression in adulthood. Surgery is therefore usually recommended if the curve reaches 50° during adolescence. Treatment with rigid bracing has recently been shown in the Bracing in Adolescent Idiopathic Scoliosis Trial (BRAIST) to decrease significantly the progression of high-risk curves to the threshold for surgery [1] and is the most widely accepted form of treatment for the prevention of curve progression worldwide. Nonetheless, the rate of treatment success was reported to be 72%, suggesting a proportion of patients will still need to undergo surgery despite bracing.

The standard of care for non-operative management of scoliosis varies widely between North America and Europe [2, 3], and the use of physiotherapy scoliosis-specific exercises (PSSE) is not universally established or accepted. Exercise therapy is well-received by patients and parents [4], and several systematic reviews and randomized controlled trials have reported the positive effects of PSSE on slowing curve progression, improving cosmetic appearance, and quality of life (QOL) outcomes [5–7]. Nonetheless, these studies consisted of a heterogeneous population receiving mixed treatment regimens, various stages of skeletal maturity, and non-standardized outcome measures. Thus, the effect of PSSE on curve progression in the clinical scenario where the curves are at the highest risk of progression has remained unclear.

The Schroth method is the most widely studied and used PSSE approach. It consists of three-dimensional principles of correction, namely auto-elongation, deflection, derotation, rotational breathing, and stabilization [8]. It uses specific rotational angular breathing for vertebral and rib cage derotation, with muscle activation and mobilization. It emphasizes postural corrections throughout the day to change habitual postures and improve alignment, pain, and progression. The Schroth method exercises are curve pattern specific and can be applied in ordinary daily activity, thereby allowing the patients to spend more time in leisure activities and to live a normal life [9].

The Society on Scoliosis Orthopaedic and Rehabilitation Treatment (SOSORT) guidelines recommend the use of PSSE as a stand-alone therapy, add-on to bracing, and during the postoperative period [2]. Romano et al. [10] found that exercises produced a significant increase in the mechanical forces exerted at rest by the fiberglass brace in AIS patients. The positive effects of PSSE can exert its maximal clinical benefit if it improves the outcome of bracing in patients with the highest risk for progression. An improvement of the treatment success of bracing will decrease the rate of surgical interventions in AIS patients.

Therefore, the aim of this study was to assess prospectively the effect of Schroth exercise on curve progression, appearance, and QOL in AIS patients with high-risk curves during bracing.

Methods

Study design

A prospective, historical cohort-matched study was conducted. The study was done in compliance with the principles of Good Clinical Practice and the Declaration of Helsinki. The local Institutional Review Board approved the study protocol (Reference Number: UW 17-136). All patients' parents or legal guardians gave written informed consent.

Patient enrolment

Consecutive patients with AIS who met the Scoliosis Research Society (SRS) criteria for bracing [11] and received bracing were enrolled for the study. Inclusion criteria were as follows: age of 10 to 15 years, skeletal immaturity (defined on the Risser scale [12] as 0–2 inclusively or R6 U5 score or below on the Distal Radius Ulna Classification [13]), a Cobb angle for the largest curve of 25° to 40° [14], and ability to attend all the physiotherapy sessions. Exclusion criteria were diagnoses other than AIS, disabilities or systemic illnesses preventing exercise performance, and any other previous treatment for AIS.

Study interventions

All patients received a rigid underarm orthosis (Fig. 1), prescribed to be worn for a minimum of 18 h per day. The SOSORT Management for bracing guidelines for the physicians, orthotists, and physiotherapists were followed [15].

Schroth-certified therapist was involved and provided all the therapy sessions. No other treatments were advised during the study period.

Experimental group

The Schroth exercise intervention consisted of an individualized 8-week outpatient program that included four initial private training sessions, once every 2 weeks, where exercises were taught to the patient and their caregivers. A home exercise program was instituted thereafter, and patients were required to return for supervised sessions once every 2 months. Exercises were given in a pamphlet with a description of the corrective movements required, the curve type for which they were recommended, and digital photos of all the exercises taken during their private sessions which they were expected to perform at home. Figure 2 illustrates a case example of a specific curve type and the exercises that were prescribed.

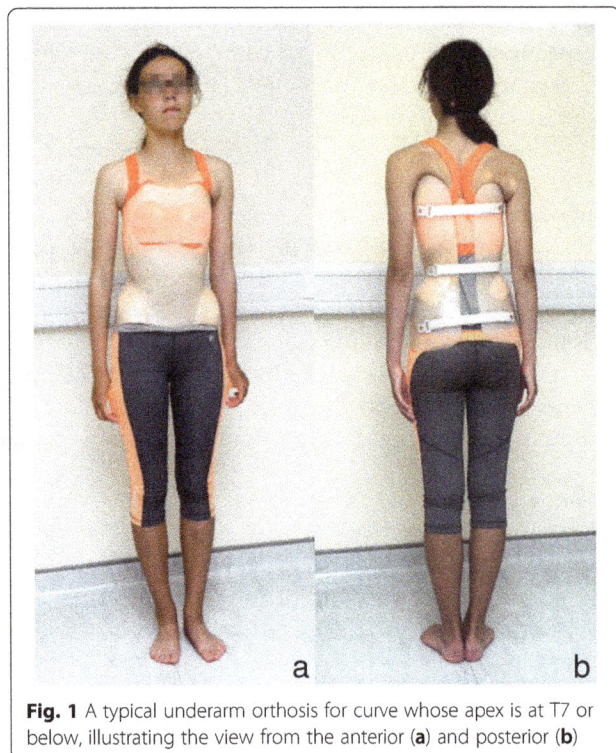

Fig. 1 A typical underarm orthosis for curve whose apex is at T7 or below, illustrating the view from the anterior (**a**) and posterior (**b**)

Compliance was monitored and verified daily by their caregivers and during the review sessions by the therapists. During these sessions, adequate exercise performance was assessed using a checklist. Attendance was calculated as a percentage of the prescribed visits attended and compliance as a percentage of the prescribed exercises completed to the therapists' satisfaction. Compliance was defined as > 80% of attendance of therapy sessions and completion of the prescribed home exercise program at least five out of 7 days per week.

Control group
A 1:1 historical cohort who was treated in the same institute with bracing only and matched for age, gender, skeletal maturity, and curve magnitude was used as a control group.

Outcome measures
The outcome measures were radiological deformities (primary outcome), clinical deformities, and QOL scores (secondary outcomes).

Cobb angles of all the major structural curves were measured on a standing posterior-anterior full-spine radiograph. Radiographic definitions of change were based on the SOSORT and SRS non-operative committee consensus

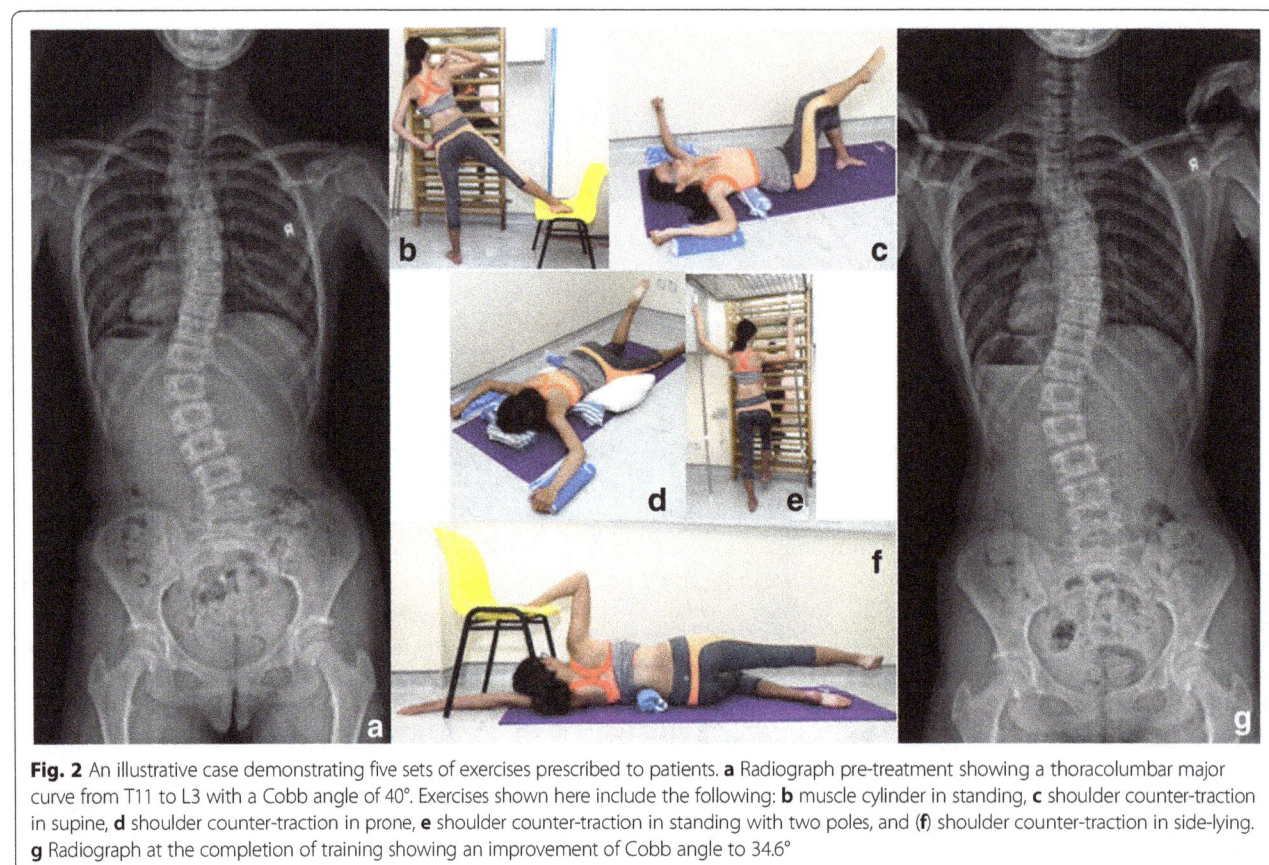

Fig. 2 An illustrative case demonstrating five sets of exercises prescribed to patients. **a** Radiograph pre-treatment showing a thoracolumbar major curve from T11 to L3 with a Cobb angle of 40°. Exercises shown here include the following: **b** muscle cylinder in standing, **c** shoulder counter-traction in supine, **d** shoulder counter-traction in prone, **e** shoulder counter-traction in standing with two poles, and (**f**) shoulder counter-traction in side-lying. **g** Radiograph at the completion of training showing an improvement of Cobb angle to 34.6°

[16]: improvement as 6° or more, unchanged as ± 5°, and progressed as 6° or more.

Clinical deformity was recorded in terms of truncal shift and angle of trunk rotation (ATR). The Bunnell scoliometer was used to measure the ATR, i.e., the angle between the horizontal plane and a plane across the posterior aspect of the trunk, of the hump in the main structural curve with the patient bending forward [17].

The SRS-22 questionnaire is a scoliosis-related QOL questionnaire that assesses five domains: function, pain, self-image, mental health (five questions each), and satisfaction with care (two questions). Each question is scored from 1 to 5, where 1 is the worst and 5 the best. The Chinese version was administered, which had been validated [18].

Adverse effects

Patients were asked to record any serious symptoms or events they experienced during the study.

Statistics

Student's paired t test ($p < 0.05$) was made for each of the outcome measures. Sub-analysis was performed within the experimental group to study the effects of compliance. The data were analyzed using SPSS 21.0 software.

Results

Subjects

Twenty-four (5 males and 19 females) were recruited into the experimental group, and 24 patients were matched in the control group. Both groups did not differ

Table 1 Baseline characteristics of the scoliosis-specific exercise and the historical-matched cohort groups

	SSE group	cohort group
Number of subjects	24	24
Age (mean/SD)	12.3 (10–14)/1.4	11.83 (10–14)/1.1
Gender (%)		
Female	79.2	79.2
Male	20.8	20.8
Risser sign at the start of treatment (%)		
0–1	54.2	79.2
2	29.2	16.7
≥3	16.6	4.2
Region of largest curve (%)		
Thoracic	20.8	33.3
Thoracolumbar/lumbar	79.2	66.7
Period of re-assessment/ months (mean/SD)	18.1/6.2	38.75/11

SSE scoliosis specific exercise, *SD* standard deviation

at baseline for age, gender, Risser sign, and magnitude of the main structural curves (Table 1). The mean age was 12.3 ± 1.4 years in the experimental group and 11.8 ± 1.1 years in the control group. The experimental and control groups had a mean follow-up period of 18.1 ± 6.2 and 38.8 ± 11 months, respectively.

Effects of the interventions

After training, the spinal deformity improved in 17% of the patients in the experimental group (Cobb angle decreases by 6° or more), worsened in 21% (Cobb angle increases by 6° or more), and remained stable in 62% (Cobb angle was ± 5°). In the control group, 4% improved, 50% worsened, and 46% remained stable.

After training, the mean ATR improved from 9.43° ± 3.27° to 8.45° ± 3.45°, although it did not reach statistical significance ($p = 0.08$), and it remained stable in the control group. There was no statistical significant difference in the mean truncal shift in the experimental and the control groups.

For the SRS-22 domains, high scores were noted at the baseline for both groups (mean of 4.25 ± 0.38 and 4.10 ± 0.52 out of 5). Statistical significant improvements were found in the experimental group in the function domain (4.60 ± 0.44 to 4.76 ± 0.33, $p = 0.05$) and the total score (4.25 ± 0.38 to 4.45 ± 0.34, $p = 0.04$) whereas changes in the other domains did not reach statistical significance. No significant changes were noted for the control group in any of the domains or the total score.

Effects of compliance

Brace compliance was rated as good in 70.8% in the experimental group and 79.2% in the historical cohort group. In the experimental group, 76.9% of patients who were compliant to the Schroth exercises had good bracing compliance, whereas only 63.6% of those who were non-compliant to the exercises had good bracing compliance.

In the experimental group, 13 patients were found to be compliant to Schroth exercises according to our definition above, and 11 patients did not meet this criterion. Compliance was strongly associated with curve improvement (31 vs 0%) and negatively associated with curve progression (0 vs 46%). Compliance was also positively associated with improvements in truncal shift from 11.87 ± 8.16 to 7.09 ± 6.41 mm ($p = 0.01$) and ATR from 10.15° ± 3.65° to 8.69° ± 3.01° ($p = 0.043$).

Adverse effects

No adverse effects were noted during the study period.

Discussion

This is the first prospective study investigating the effect of Schroth exercises on curve progression, topographical changes, and SRS-22 scores in AIS patients during bracing. The findings of this study show that Schroth exercises during bracing can increase the proportion of patients with Cobb angle improvement ≥ 6° by 6% compared with bracing alone. In addition, our results suggest that 20% more patients have improved Cobb angles of ≥ 6° if they are compliant with Schroth exercises during bracing compared with bracing alone. However, the outcomes of non-compliant patients were slight worse than the historical cohort, which might partly due to a worse compliance to brace treatment in this group.

Although previous studies have demonstrated the superiority of scoliosis-specific exercises in reducing curve progression, they were performed in a population undergoing conservative treatment for mild AIS only [19–23]. Furthermore, their data cannot be generalized to rehabilitation under other clinical scenarios, such as during bracing or after surgical correction. This preliminary study focused on a group of high-risk patients who were all treated with bracing. The usual intervention after treatment failure in these patients would be surgical correction and fusion and was recently reported in the BRAIST to be 25–28% [1]. Thus, any further treatment during bracing that can improve the outcome can lower the surgical rate. We show that the efficacy of bracing can be further improved by the addition of Schroth exercises with a strong compliance-response relationship.

Although there was a trend towards ATR reduction in the experimental group, it did not reach statistical significance in our study. All previous studies that reported ATR showed a decrease after scoliosis-specific exercises ranging from 0.33° to 4.23° [24, 25]. Schroth exercises have been shown to improve the cosmetic appearance in children, demonstrated in some studies to decrease the height of the hump [26], and improving waist asymmetry [27]. Although we cannot make a definite conclusion from our results, a more reliable and valid measure of objective cosmetic changes needs to be included in future studies.

The effect of the treatment on the SRS-22 scores shows that Schroth exercises improve the overall QOL in AIS patients during bracing. However, it is now increasingly noted that the SRS-22 questionnaire was designed to study the effects of surgery in AIS and suffers a ceiling effect in conservative treatments [7, 28, 29]. The high scores reported at the baseline therefore limit the ability of this questionnaire to measure large improvements. Different tools, such as SRS-7, Trunk Appearance Perception Scale (TAPS), Patient-Reported Outcomes Measurement Information System (PROMIS), and computer adaptive testing (CAT) instruments, may be administered together in future studies to detect clinically significant differences in their function and QOL. Currently, no alternative validated evaluating tools are available.

Our findings suggest that administering Schroth exercise program as an outpatient is feasible and has a reasonable compliance. These results are consistent with earlier findings that a physiotherapist-supervised Schroth exercise program is superior to a home-based program or no treatment [25]. In their study, the supervised program consisted of 18 sessions (1.5 h a day, 3 days a week) for 6 weeks. However, this would be too demanding for patients in this locality, and we predicted this would have deleterious effects on the study enrolment, the attendance, and compliance rate. We therefore modified the protocol to four sessions (1 h per session fortnightly) for 8 weeks. This was a compromise between maintaining adequate supervision and minimalizing disruption to the patients' and their families' lives.

The study has several limitations. First, it was a historical cohort comparison but every effort has been made to ensure the two groups are compatible by age, gender, and curve magnitude matching. However, there was a difference in the follow-up period between the two groups. At the time of analysis, all patients in the experimental group had a minimum of 12 months of follow-up, but some patients in the historical cohort had already completed treatment. Nonetheless, we felt this cohort provided a reasonable control since the only difference in intervention between the groups was the addition of Schroth training. Secondly, exercise compliance and adherence to treatment could not be fully assured, although the patients' diaries were checked, and full engagement of the caregivers ensured accurate data collection. Thirdly, although brace compliance between the two groups was comparable, sub-analysis based on exercise compliance found a difference in brace compliance between the groups and historical control. Hence, these results should be interpreted with caution. Fourthly, the therapists could not be blinded to the treatment group, although the analyses were done by an independent assessor. Finally, the sample size in the sub-analysis for compliance is small.

Conclusions

This is the first study to investigate the effects of Schroth exercises during bracing in patients with a high risk of curve progression. The findings from this preliminary study suggest that Schroth exercises during bracing can further improve the Cobb angle compared with bracing alone and compliance is associated with greater benefit. Based on the results of this study and using the current protocol, appropriate sample size calculation and attrition rate can be performed for a large-scale trial. Given the promising findings, a prospective, randomized-controlled trial to evaluate the effect of Schroth exercises during brace treatment in AIS patients is now warranted.

Abbreviations
AIS: Adolescent idiopathic scoliosis; ATR: Angle trunk rotation; BRAIST: Bracing in Adolescent Idiopathic Scoliosis Trial; CAT: Computer adaptive testing; PROMIS: Patient-Reported Outcomes Measurement Information System; PSSE: Physiotherapy scoliosis-specific exercises; QOL: Quality of life; SOSORT: Society on Scoliosis Orthopaedic and Rehabilitation Treatment; SRS: Scoliosis Research Society; TAPS: Trunk Appearance Perception Scale

Acknowledgements
Not applicable.

Funding
None declared.

Authors' contributions
KK conceived of the study, participated in the study design, and drafted the manuscript. ACSC performed the study and statistical analysis. HYK collected the data and participated in its design and coordination. AYYC participated in the study design and coordination. KC supervised the study and helped to draft the manuscript. All authors read and approved the final manuscript.

Competing interests
The authors declare that they have no competing interests.

Author details
[1]Department of Orthopaedics and Traumatology, Li Ka Shing Faculty of Medicine, The University of Hong Kong, Pokfulam, Hong Kong. [2]Department of Physiotherapy, Duchess of Kent Children's Hospital, Sandy Bay, Hong Kong.

References
1. Weinstein SL, Dolan LA, Wright JG, Dobbs MB. Effects of bracing in adolescents with idiopathic scoliosis. N Engl J Med. 2013;369(16):1512–21. https://doi.org/10.1056/NEJMoa1307337. PubMed PMID: 24047455; PubMed Central PMCID: PMC3913566
2. Kotwicki T, Durmala J, Czaprowski D, Glowacki M, Kolban M, Snela S, et al. Conservative management of idiopathic scoliosis—guidelines based on SOSORT 2006 consensus. Ortop Traumatol Rehabil. 2009;11(5):379–95. PubMed PMID: 19920281
3. Seifert J, Thielemann F, Bernstein P. Adolescent idiopathic scoliosis : guideline for practical application. Orthopade. 2016;45(6):509–17. doi:10.1007/s00132-016-3274-5. PubMed PMID: 27241514
4. Negrini S, Carabalona R. Social acceptability of treatments for adolescent idiopathic scoliosis: a cross-sectional study. Scoliosis. 2006;1:14. doi:10.1186/1748-7161-1-14. PubMed PMID: 16930488; PubMed Central PMCID: PMCPMC1560163
5. Negrini S, Antonini G, Carabalona R, Minozzi S. Physical exercises as a treatment for adolescent idiopathic scoliosis. A systematic review. Pediatric rehabilitation. 2003;6(3-4):227–35. doi:10.1080/13638490310001636781. PubMed PMID: 14713590

6. Romano M, Minozzi S, Zaina F, Saltikov JB, Chockalingam N, Kotwicki T, et al. Exercises for adolescent idiopathic scoliosis: a Cochrane systematic review. Spine. 2013;38(14):E883–93. doi:10.1097/BRS.0b013e31829459f8. PubMed PMID: 23558442. Epub 2013/04/06
7. Schreiber S, Parent EC, Moez EK, Hedden DM, Hill D, Moreau MJ, et al. The effect of Schroth exercises added to the standard of care on the quality of life and muscle endurance in adolescents with idiopathic scoliosis-an assessor and statistician blinded randomized controlled trial: "SOSORT 2015 Award Winner". Scoliosis. 2015;10:24. doi:10.1186/s13013-015-0048-5. PubMed PMID: 26413145; PubMed Central PMCID: PMCPMC4582716
8. Lehnert-Schroth C. Schroth's three dimensional treatment of scoliosis. ZFA (Stuttgart). 1979;55(34):1969–76. PubMed PMID: 547573
9. Berdishevsky H, Lebel VA, Bettany-Saltikov J, Rigo M, Lebel A, Hennes A, et al. Physiotherapy scoliosis-specific exercises—a comprehensive review of seven major schools. Scoliosis Spinal Disord. 2016;11:20. doi:10.1186/s13013-016-0076-9. PubMed PMID: 27525315; PubMed Central PMCID: PMCPMC4973373
10. Romano M, Carabalona R, Petrilli S, Sibilla P, Negrini S. Forces exerted during exercises by patients with adolescent idiopathic scoliosis wearing fiberglass braces. Scoliosis. 2006;1:12. doi:10.1186/1748-7161-1-12. PubMed PMID: 16859544; PubMed Central PMCID: PMC1578587. Epub 2006/07/25
11. Rowe DE. Idiopathic scoliosis, Scoliosis Research Society bracing manual. 2003.
12. Risser JC. The iliac apophysis; an invaluable sign in the management of scoliosis. Clin Orthop. 1958;11:111–9. PubMed PMID: 13561591
13. Luk KD, Saw LB, Grozman S, Cheung KM, Samartzis D. Assessment of skeletal maturity in scoliosis patients to determine clinical management: a new classification scheme using distal radius and ulna radiographs. Spine J. 2014;14(2):315–25. doi:10.1016/j.spinee.2013.10.045. PubMed PMID: 24239801
14. Richards BS, Bernstein RM, D'Amato CR, Thompson GH. Standardization of criteria for adolescent idiopathic scoliosis brace studies: SRS Committee on Bracing and Nonoperative Management. Spine. 2005;30(18):2068–75. discussion 76-7. PubMed PMID: 16166897
15. Negrini S, Grivas TB, Kotwicki T, Rigo M, Zaina F, international Society on Scoliosis O, et al. Guidelines on "Standards of management of idiopathic scoliosis with corrective braces in everyday clinics and in clinical research": SOSORT Consensus 2008. Scoliosis. 2009;4:2. doi:10.1186/1748-7161-4-2. PubMed PMID: 19149877; PubMed Central PMCID: PMCPMC2651850
16. Negrini S, Hresko TM, O'Brien JP, Price N, Boards S, Committee SRSN-O. Recommendations for research studies on treatment of idiopathic scoliosis: consensus 2014 between SOSORT and SRS non-operative management committee. Scoliosis. 2015;10:8. doi:10.1186/s13013-014-0025-4. PubMed PMID: 25780381; PubMed Central PMCID: PMCPMC4360938
17. Bunnell WP. An objective criterion for scoliosis screening. J Bone Joint Surg Am. 1984;66(9):1381–7. PubMed PMID: 6501335
18. Cheung KM, Senkoylu A, Alanay A, Genc Y, Lau S, Luk KD. Reliability and concurrent validity of the adapted Chinese version of Scoliosis Research Society-22 (SRS-22) questionnaire. Spine (Phila Pa 1976). 2007;32(10):1141–5. doi:10.1097/01.brs.0000261562.48888.e3. PubMed PMID: 17471100
19. Weiss HR, Weiss G. Curvature progression in patients treated with scoliosis in-patient rehabilitation—a sex and age matched controlled study. Stud Health Technol Inform. 2002;91:352–6. PubMed PMID: 15457754
20. Weiss HR, Weiss G, Petermann F. Incidence of curvature progression in idiopathic scoliosis patients treated with scoliosis in-patient rehabilitation (SIR): an age- and sex-matched controlled study. Pediatr Rehabil. 2003;6(1): 23–30. doi:10.1080/1363849031000095288. PubMed PMID: 12745892
21. Weiss HR, Klein R. Improving excellence in scoliosis rehabilitation: a controlled study of matched pairs. Pediatr Rehabil. 2006;9(3):190–200. doi:10.1080/13638490500079583. PubMed PMID: 17050397
22. Otman S, Kose N, Yakut Y. The efficacy of Schroth s 3-dimensional exercise therapy in the treatment of adolescent idiopathic scoliosis in Turkey. Saudi Med J. 2005;26(9):1429–35. PubMed PMID: 16155663
23. Monticone M, Ambrosini E, Cazzaniga D, Rocca B, Ferrante S. Active self-correction and task-oriented exercises reduce spinal deformity and improve quality of life in subjects with mild adolescent idiopathic scoliosis. Results of a randomised controlled trial. Eur Spine J. 2014;23(6):1204–14. doi:10.1007/s00586-014-3241-y. PubMed PMID: 24682356
24. Negrini S, Zaina F, Romano M, Negrini A, Parzini S. Specific exercises reduce brace prescription in adolescent idiopathic scoliosis: a prospective controlled cohort study with worst-case analysis. J Rehabil Med. 2008;40(6): 451–5. doi:10.2340/16501977-0195. PubMed PMID: 18509560

25. Kuru T, Yeldan I, Dereli EE, Ozdincler AR, Dikici F, Colak I. The efficacy of three-dimensional Schroth exercises in adolescent idiopathic scoliosis: a randomised controlled clinical trial. Clin Rehabil. 2016;30(2):181–90. doi:10.1177/0269215515575745. PubMed PMID: 25780260

26. Romano M, Negrini A, Parzini S, et al. Adolescent with 10 to 20 Cobb scoliosis during growth: efficacy of conservative treatments. A prospective controlled cohort observational study. Scoliosis. 2012;7:O50.

27. Watanabe K, Hosogane N, Chiba K, et al. Anterior chest hump in adolescent idiopathic scoliosis—questionnaire evaluation. Scoliosis. 2012;7:O11.

28. Negrini S, Donzelli S, Dulio M, Zaina F. Is the SRS-22 able to detect quality of life (QoL) changes during conservative treatments ? Stud Health Technol Inform. 2012;176:433–6. PubMed PMID: 22744547

29. Caronni A, Zaina F, Negrini S. Improving the measurement of health-related quality of life in adolescent with idiopathic scoliosis: the SRS-7, a Rasch-developed short form of the SRS-22 questionnaire. Res Dev Disabil. 2014; 35(4):784–99. doi:10.1016/j.ridd.2014.01.020. PubMed PMID: 24521663

6

Biomechanical effect of pedicle screw distribution in AIS instrumentation using a segmental translation technique: computer modeling and simulation

Xiaoyu Wang[1,2], A. Noelle Larson[3], Dennis G. Crandall[4], Stefan Parent[2], Hubert Labelle[2], Charles G. T. Ledonio[5] and Carl-Eric Aubin[1,2]*

Abstract

Background: Efforts to select the appropriate number of implants in adolescent idiopathic scoliosis (AIS) instrumentation are hampered by a lack of biomechanical studies. The objective was to biomechanically evaluate screw density at different regions in the curve for AIS correction to test the hypothesis that alternative screw patterns do not compromise anticipated correction in AIS when using a segmental translation technique.

Methods: Instrumentation simulations were computationally performed for 10 AIS cases. We simulated simultaneous concave and convex segmental translation for a reference screw pattern (bilateral polyaxial pedicle screws with dorsal height adjustability at every level fused) and four alternative patterns; screws were dropped respectively on convex or concave side at alternate levels or at the periapical levels (21 to 25% fewer screws). Predicted deformity correction and screw forces were compared.

Results: Final simulated Cobb angle differences with the alternative screw patterns varied between 1° to 5° (39 simulations) and 8° (1 simulation) compared to the reference maximal density screw pattern. Thoracic kyphosis and apical vertebral rotation were within 2° of the reference screw pattern. Screw forces were 76 ± 43 N, 96 ± 58 N, 90 ± 54 N, 82 ± 33 N, and 79 ± 42 N, respectively, for the reference screw pattern and screw dropouts at convex alternate levels, concave alternate levels, convex periapical levels, and concave periapical levels. Bone-screw forces for the alternative patterns were higher than the reference pattern ($p < 0.0003$). There was no statistical bone-screw force difference between convex and concave alternate dropouts and between convex and concave periapical dropouts ($p > 0.28$). Alternate dropout screw forces were higher than periapical dropouts ($p < 0.05$).

Conclusions: Using a simultaneous segmental translation technique, deformity correction can be achieved with 23% fewer screws than maximal density screw pattern, but resulted in 25% higher bone-screw forces. Screw dropouts could be either on the convex side or on the concave side at alternate levels or at periapical levels. Periapical screw dropouts may more likely result in lower bone-screw force increase than alternate level screw dropouts.

Keywords: Pedicle screw, Adolescent idiopathic scoliosis, Instrumentation, Biomechanical modeling, Simulation, Screw pattern, Screw density, Screw distribution

* Correspondence: carl-eric.aubin@polymtl.ca
[1]Department of Mechanical Engineering, Polytechnique Montréal, P.O. Box 6079, Downtown Station, Montreal, Quebec H3C 3A7, Canada
[2]Sainte-Justine University Hospital Center, 3175, Cote Sainte-Catherine Road, Montreal, Quebec H3T 1C5, Canada
Full list of author information is available at the end of the article

Background

Pedicle screw fixation has become the state-of-the-art instrumentation for the surgical treatment of adolescent idiopathic scoliosis (AIS), resulting in better deformity correction and lower revision surgery rates compared to hybrid or hook-rod constructs [1–3]. However, wide variation in clinical practice persists regarding the number and distribution of pedicle screws used, as well as the surgical techniques for the treatment of pediatric scoliosis.

Screw density is defined as the number of screws per level fused. There may be multiple clinical and biomechanical factors in determining screw density and distribution. Certain screw types and distributions are required in order to perform specific correction maneuvers, such as apical vertebral derotation and segmental vertebral derotation [4]. The effect of screw density depends also on the construct design. Some screw types and patterns tended to overconstrain the instrumented spine generating high (overconstraining) bone-screw forces in high-density screw constructs, such as monoaxial screws [5]; screws with multiple degrees of adjustability allowed the overconstraining effect to be reduced and segmental translation to be performed in a gradual and incremental way to lower the overall bone-screw force level [5, 6].

A structured literature review revealed that the mean reported screw density varies from 1.04 to 2.0, whereas the average curve corrections only varied from 64 to 70% [7]. Some surgeons routinely use two screws at every level fused where other surgeons may use up to 46% fewer screws [8, 9]. High screw density constructs have been associated with increased operative time, blood loss, radiation exposure, instrumentation costs, and risk of screw-related complications [10–14]. Constructs with fewer screws may have benefits for optimal use of health care resources [7, 8]. Some studies note improved percent correction of major coronal curve in the high screw density cohort [8, 9]; but, in other studies, no significant difference in outcome was found between the high and low screw density groups [10, 15, 16].

Until recently, studies of screw density have been underpowered, included hybrid constructs, or based on retrospective review of clinical data. Further, there is a lack of biomechanical data guiding screw number and placement. Thus, practice is mostly based on individual preferred technique, and scientific progress is limited by the inability to test alternative screw patterns on a given patient. In contrast to studies based on clinical data analysis, biomechanical studies using computerized patient-specific models allow the assessment and comparison of variable screw numbers and patterns with different correction techniques simulated for the same case. The objective of this study was to use computerized patient-specific spine models to biomechanically evaluate screw

dropouts at different regions in the curve for AIS correction to test the hypothesis that alternative screw patterns do not compromise anticipated correction in AIS when using segmental translation as the primary correction technique.

Methods

Numerical simulations of posterior spinal instrumentations were performed using computerized patient-specific biomechanical models of 10 AIS patients in order to assess the effect of screw density on curve correction and bone-screw forces. With the institutional review board approval, the cases were randomly selected from AIS patients having undergone instrumented spinal fusion at our university hospital center during the last 6 years. Clinical indices are provided in Table 1. Modeling and simulation details are presented in the following subsections.

Computerized patient-specific biomechanical spine model

Three-dimension (3D) spine geometry of the selected cases was built using calibrated preoperative coronal and lateral radiographs and 3D multi-view reconstruction techniques [17]. The process began with the identification of key anatomical landmarks of each vertebra, typically, the pedicles, vertebral endplate middle and corner points, and transverse and spinous process extremities. The 2D coordinates of these landmarks allowed the determination of their 3D coordinates in space, which was done using a self-calibration and optimization algorithm [17, 18]. The reconstruction process was completed by registering detailed vertebral models using the 3D coordinates of the key landmarks and a free form deformation technique [17, 18]. Average accuracies for pedicles and vertebral bodies were 1.6 mm (SD 1.1 mm) and 1.2 mm (SD 0.8 mm), respectively [18].

Vertebrae from T1 through L5 and the pelvis were modeled as rigid parts which were connected with multiple flexible elements respectively representing the biomechanical effect of the intervertebral disc, anterior longitudinal ligament (ALL), posterior longitudinal ligament (PLL), ligamentum flavum (LF), intertransverse ligament (ITL), facet joint capsule (FC), and interspinous ligament (ISL) combined with supraspinous ligament (SSL). Six translational springs were used to respectively represent (1) ALL, (2) PLL, (3) LF, (4) left ITL, (5) right ITL, and (6) the combined effect of ISL and SSL. The biomechanical behavior of the facet joints is more complex compared to the other intervertebral ligamentous elements; they were respectively represented with a six-dimensional general spring [19]. A primary general spring was used to represent the intervertebral disc to which the effect of all elements and factors which were not explicitly modeled in this study was incorporated by

Table 1 Clinical indices

Case no.		1	2	3	4	5	6	7	8	9	10
Sex		F	F	F	F	F	M	F	F	F	F
Age		14	16	19	17	14	15	16	15	15	14
Height (cm)		154	162	162	168	170	172	165	170	159	148
Weight (kg)		52	56	47	56	59	55	53	48	59	39
Lenke classification		1A	1A	3B	4A	3B	3C	1A	1A	3C	2A
MT superior end vertebra		T6	T6	T5	T5	T5	T7	T5	T4	T6	T5
Apical vertebra		T9	T11	T8	T8	T8	T10	T9	T8	T9	T9
Inferior end vertebra		T12	L2	T11	T11	T12	L1	L1	T12	T12	T11
PT Cobb	Preop.	32°	31°	39°	52°	31°	34°	28°	9°	40°	42°
	Left bending	22°	10°	12°	17°	24°	6°	20°	5°	15°	28°
	Right bending	35°	41°	42°	54°	35°	37°	32°	20°	41°	46°
MT Cobb	Preop.	55°	52°	58°	60°	64°	62°	44°	48°	67°	51°
	Left bending	59°	60°	63°	64°	65°	62°	73°	55°	63°	60°
	Right bending	29°	25°	29°	38°	50°	27°	10°	30°	35°	30°
MT AVR	Preop.	16°	17°	18°	19°	19°	20°	19°	18°	22°	19°
TL/L Cobb	Preop.	37°	37°	39°	30°	42°	48°	35°	39°	40°	32°
	Left bending	2°	5°	20°	9°	5°	30°	10°	10°	9°	2°
	Right bending	49°	50°	42°	40°	65°	50°	42°	45°	70°	49°
TL/L AVR	Preop.	5°	3°	7°	7°	3°	11°	6°	11°	9°	3°
Kyphosis	Preop.	7°	23°	37°	28°	22°	11°	20°	18°	7°	15°
Lordosis	Preop.	42°	37°	27°	45°	33°	15°	47°	40°	30°	32°
UIV		T4	T4	T4	T3	T3	T4	T4	T4	T3	T3
LIV		L2	L3	L1	L1	L1	L2	L2	L2	L2	L1

F female, *M* male, *PT* proximal thoracic, *MT* main thoracic, *TL/L* thoracolumbar/lumbar, *AVR* apical vertebral rotation, *UIV* upper instrumented vertebra, *LIV* lower instrumented vertebra

introducing weighting factors to the diagonal elements of its stiffness matrix, e.g., the rib cage increased the stiffness of the thoracic spine by 40, 35, and 31% respectively in flexion/extension, lateral bending, and axial rotation [20]. The multibody modeling elements are illustrated in Fig. 1.

The six translational springs were modeled as cable-like elements on the computer-aided engineering platform, Adams/View, Version MD Adams 2010 (MSC Software Corporation, Santa Ana, CA, USA). Their stiffness in compression were set to null and those in traction were adapted to the reported experiment results on cadaveric specimens, e.g., 23.6 N/mm (ALL), 24.9 N/mm (PLL), 32.6 N/mm (LF), 12.9 N/mm (ITL), and 32.1 N/mm (ISL combined with SSL) [21–23] for T6-T7 functional spinal unit. Instrumented posterior spinal fusion with pedicle screw fixation involves the removal of the facet joint capsules and the spinous process. The biomechanical effects of pedicle screw placement surgical procedure were modeled by removing the facet joint capsule and the interspinous model elements, whose mechanical properties were calibrated using experiment

data reported in the literature, i.e., osteotomies involved in pedicle screw placement procedure reduced the stiffness of a functional spine unit by 17% in axial rotation [24–27], 15% sagittal plane flexion [24, 28, 29], 3.8% in coronal plane bending [24], and 14% in axial compressive load [30–33]. The stiffness matrix of the primary general spring was calibrated such that the load-displacement simulations with the model of a functional spinal unit reproduced the reported load-displacement data [34–37]. All model element stiffness were further adjusted such that side bending simulations reproduced the Cobb angles measured on the patient's side bending radiographs using a similar optimization technique reported in [38, 39].

Biomechanical modeling and simulations of spinal instrumentation

Based on the actual instrumented fusion levels of the selected cases and the well-accepted alternative screw densities [4], five screw patterns were biomechanically evaluated on each case. The screw patterns were a reference screw pattern with bilateral screws at every level

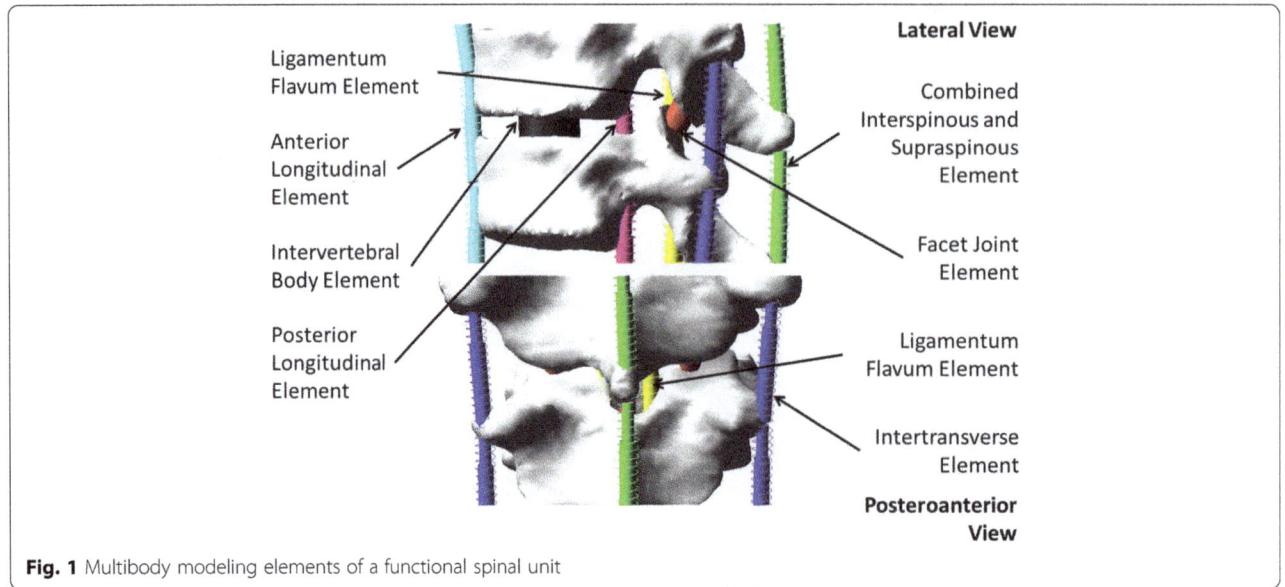

Ligamentum Flavum Element

Anterior Longitudinal Element

Intervertebral Body Element

Posterior Longitudinal Element

Lateral View

Combined Interspinous and Supraspinous Element

Facet Joint Element

Ligamentum Flavum Element

Intertransverse Element

Posteroanterior View

Fig. 1 Multibody modeling elements of a functional spinal unit

fused and four alternative patterns with mean 23% fewer screws (21 to 25%). Screw dropouts in the alternative patterns were respectively on the convex and concave sides and at alternate levels or periapical levels (Fig. 2). The modeled bone-screw connection and correction technique was based on polyaxial pedicle screws with dorsal height adjustability (4.5–5.5 mm diameters for the thoracic spine and 5.5–6.0 mm diameters for the lumbar spine) (Fig. 3) [6]. The screw kinematic design allows the translation of each pedicle screw toward the rod from any distance and at any angle, with the ability to rigidly lock the construct at any point between partial and complete corrections [6]. The simulated correction technique was simultaneous two-rod segmental translation. The biomechanical model of the rods was based on 5.5 mm Cobalt-chrome rods. The contouring angle of the convex rod was 25° as measured over the thoracic spinal segment, and the contouring angle of the concave rod was 35°. Modeling of instrumentation constructs, simultaneous two-rod segmental translation and the boundary conditions have been realized and validated in a previous study [6].

Results

The computed geometric indices from the reconstructed preoperative spine models and the simulated instrumented spine models are presented in Table 2. In the 40 simulations with the alternative screw patterns, the final simulated Cobb angle differences varied between 1° to 5° in 39 simulations and 8° in 1 simulation compared to the reference maximal density screw pattern. Thoracic kyphosis and apical vertebral rotation were within 2° of the reference screw pattern.

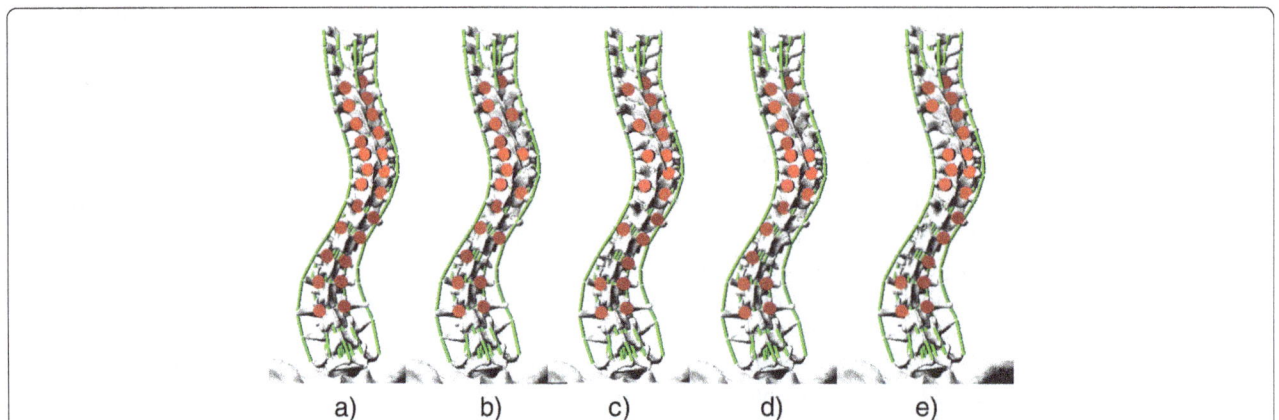

a)   b)   c)   d)   e)

Fig. 2 a Reference screw pattern (bilateral screws at every level fused). **b** Screw pattern with convex alternate screw dropouts. **c** Concave alternate screw dropouts. **d** Convex periapical screw dropouts. **e** Concave periapical screw dropouts

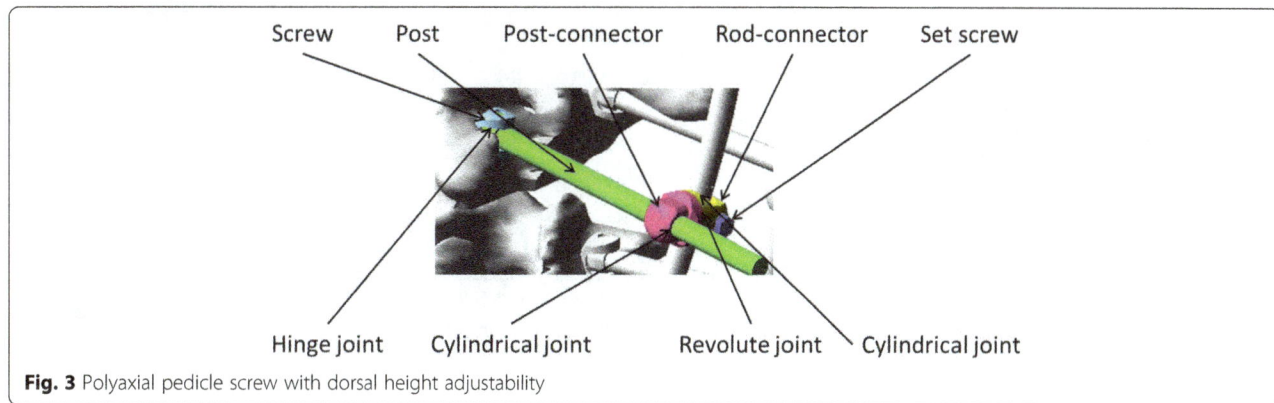

Fig. 3 Polyaxial pedicle screw with dorsal height adjustability

Average bone-screw force was computed for each simulation and the results are presented in Fig. 4. The overall bone-screw force was 76 ± 43 N (5–219 N) for the maximal density reference screw pattern. They were 96 ± 58 N (10–468 N), 90 ± 54 N (11–353 N), 82 ± 33 N (17–162 N), and 79 ± 42 N (7–222 N), respectively, for the four alternative screw patterns with screw dropouts at convex alternate levels, concave alternate levels, convex periapical levels, and concave periapical levels, which were respectively 26, 17, 7, and 4% higher than the reference screw pattern. Bone-screw forces for the alternative patterns were statistically higher than the reference pattern ($p < 0.0003$). Alternate dropout screw forces were higher than periapical dropouts ($p < 0.05$). There was no statistical bone-screw force difference between convex and concave alternate dropouts ($p > 0.28$). Although there was no statistical bone-screw force difference between convex and concave periapical dropouts ($p > 0.25$), the convex periapical screw dropouts had less impact on bone-screw force vector pattern in some

Table 2 Computed geometric indices from the reconstructed preoperative spine models and the simulated instrumented spine models

Case no.	1	2	3	4	5	6	7	8	9	10
Main thoracic Cobb angles										
Preop.	55°	52°	58°	60°	64°	62°	44°	48°	67°	51°
Pattern no. 1 (reference)	18°	10°	18°	14°	24°	21°	17°	15°	28°	17°
Pattern no. 2	18°	12°	22°	15°	25°	21°	17°	16°	29°	17°
Pattern no. 3	18°	10°	17°	22°	24°	21°	15°	16°	29°	17°
Pattern no. 4	16°	12°	20°	14°	24°	22°	16°	15°	30°	17°
Pattern no. 5	21°	9°	19°	19°	24°	21°	16°	15°	30°	17°
Thoracic kyphosis										
Preop.	7°	23°	37°	28°	22°	11°	20°	18°	7°	15°
Pattern no. 1 (reference)	27°	31°	33°	22°	24°	28°	29°	27°	24°	25°
Pattern no. 2	26°	30°	33°	20°	24°	28°	29°	27°	24°	25°
Pattern no. 3	27°	32°	33°	21°	23°	28°	29°	27°	24°	25°
Pattern no. 4	28°	31°	32°	22°	23°	28°	29°	27°	24°	25°
Pattern no. 5	26°	31°	33°	21°	24°	29°	29°	27°	24°	25°
Main thoracic apical vertebral rotation										
Preop.	16°	17°	18°	19°	19°	20°	19°	18°	22°	19°
Pattern no. 1 (reference)	15°	18°	18°	17°	17°	19°	18°	17°	20°	18°
Pattern no. 2	14°	18°	17°	16°	17°	19°	19°	17°	21°	19°
Pattern no. 3	15°	18°	18°	15°	17°	19°	17°	17°	20°	18°
Pattern no. 4	15°	18°	18°	17°	16°	19°	18°	17°	21°	19°
Pattern no. 5	14°	18°	19°	15°	17°	19°	17°	17°	20°	18°

Pattern no. 1 (reference): bilateral screws at every level fused; pattern no. 2: convex alternate screw dropouts; pattern no. 3: concave alternate screw dropouts; pattern no. 4: convex periapical screw dropouts; pattern no. 5: concave periapical screw dropouts

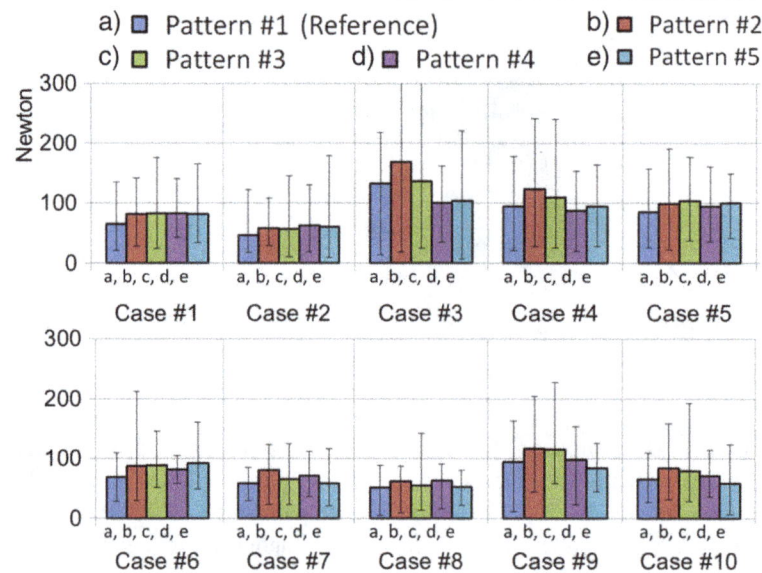

Fig. 4 Average (*bars* = min, max) bone-screw forces (pattern no. 1 (reference): bilateral screws at every level fused; pattern no. 2: convex alternate screw dropouts; pattern no. 3: concave alternate screw dropouts; pattern no. 4: convex periapical screw dropouts; pattern no. 5: concave periapical screw dropouts)

of the cases in both the coronal and the sagittal plane, i.e., bone-screw force vector pattern was the closest to the reference screw pattern. Bone-screw force vectors for a representative case are provided in Fig. 5.

Discussion

Comparing alternative screw patterns respectively with the maximal density reference screw pattern, differences in the final simulated MT Cobb angles, thoracic kyphosis, and apical vertebral rotation did not exceed 5° for all except one case. These differences are within the accepted systematic error found in clinical Cobb angle measurements [40]. The mean correction of each of the alternative screw pattern was within 2° of the mean correction of the reference screw pattern. Based on a previous study on 279 AIS patients [9] and a structured literature review on AIS instrumentations [7], the population mean of major curve Cobb angles was estimated to be 55° and the population mean of percent corrections of major curves was estimated to be 67% with a standard deviation of 14%. The correction difference to be detected was set to 5° (11% difference in percent correction). There was no statistical difference between the reference screw pattern and the alternative screw patterns in terms of percent corrections of major curves, with 5% of type I error and a statistical power of 70%.

Alternative screw patterns with fewer screws resulted in higher overall bone-screw forces. Previous studies showed that higher density screw patterns had usually higher bone-screw forces due to the overconstraining effect [41]. The difference can be attributed to differences between

the construct designs, type of screws, and simulated correction techniques. Higher bone-screw forces were generally associated with higher Cobb angles when percent corrections were similar; bone-screw forces in curves of higher Cobb angles may be more sensitive to screw density and distribution. The number of vertebrae in the major curve and the local shape of the curve seem to have an important effect on the average bone-screw force; higher forces were more seen in cases in which the major curves spanned fewer vertebrae and were more angular (Fig. 6). In other words, curves which span longer spinal segment and whose curvature does not varies significantly tend to have lower bone-screw forces. A sharp, short angular curve with a high local Cobb angle requires greater corrective forces to align the spine to the smoothly contoured spinal rods. Short, angular curves may therefore be more sensitive to screw density and distribution, which should be taken into consideration in addition to curve flexibility. Significantly higher bone-screw forces in some cases may be explained by the fact that the curve spanned a shorter spinal segment and was more angular (cases 3, 4, and 9). In the sagittal plane, the spinal profiles in some cases may have a better match with the rod shapes than in other cases, which should also have an impact on the final bone-screw forces. Screw density and distribution should therefore be determined by taking into account the local geometric characteristics of the curve in both the sagittal and coronal planes in addition to the curve type, deformity magnitude, and spinal stiffness.

In summary, with simultaneous two-rod segmental translation using polyaxial pedicle screws with dorsal

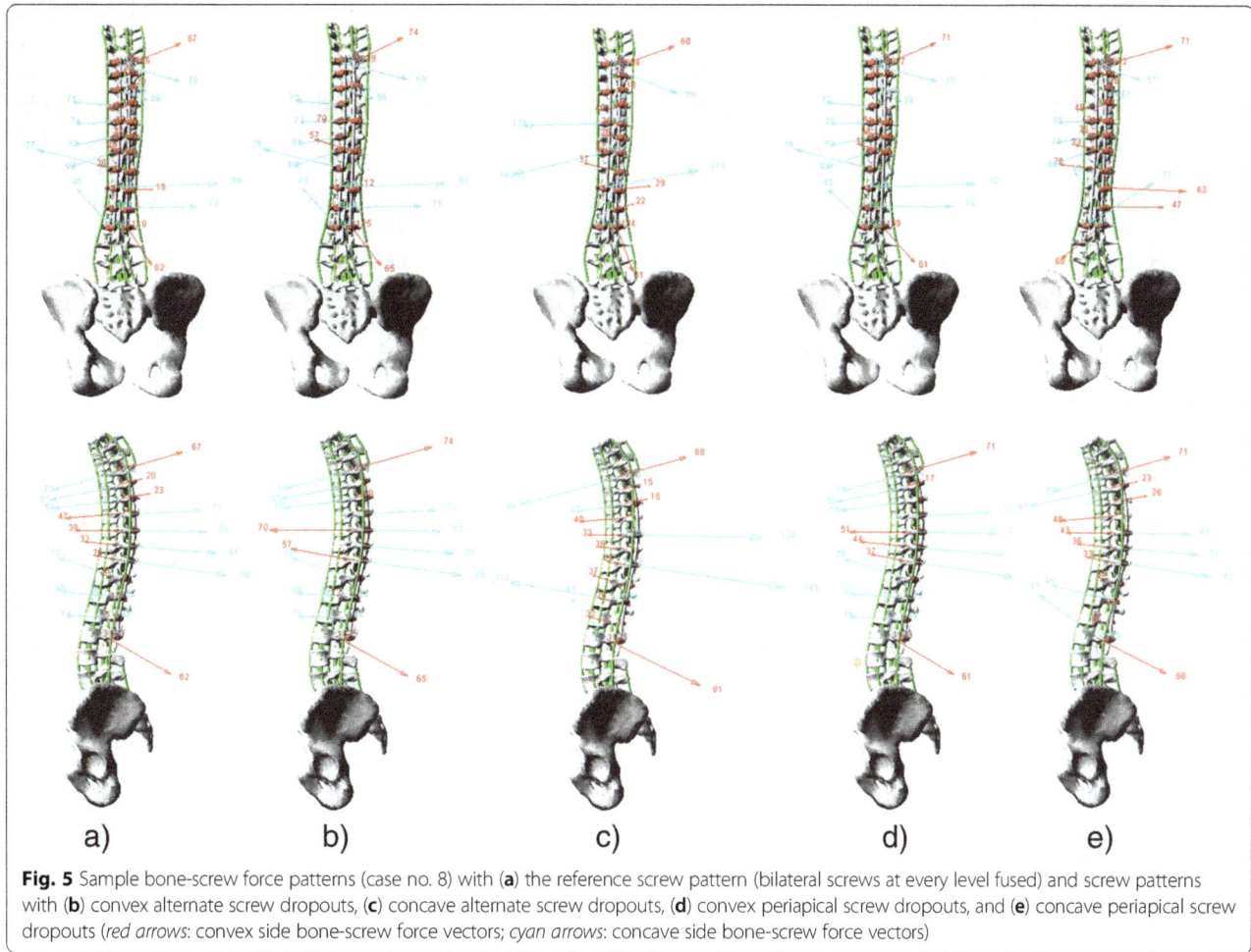

Fig. 5 Sample bone-screw force patterns (case no. 8) with (**a**) the reference screw pattern (bilateral screws at every level fused) and screw patterns with (**b**) convex alternate screw dropouts, (**c**) concave alternate screw dropouts, (**d**) convex periapical screw dropouts, and (**e**) concave periapical screw dropouts (*red arrows*: convex side bone-screw force vectors; *cyan arrows*: concave side bone-screw force vectors)

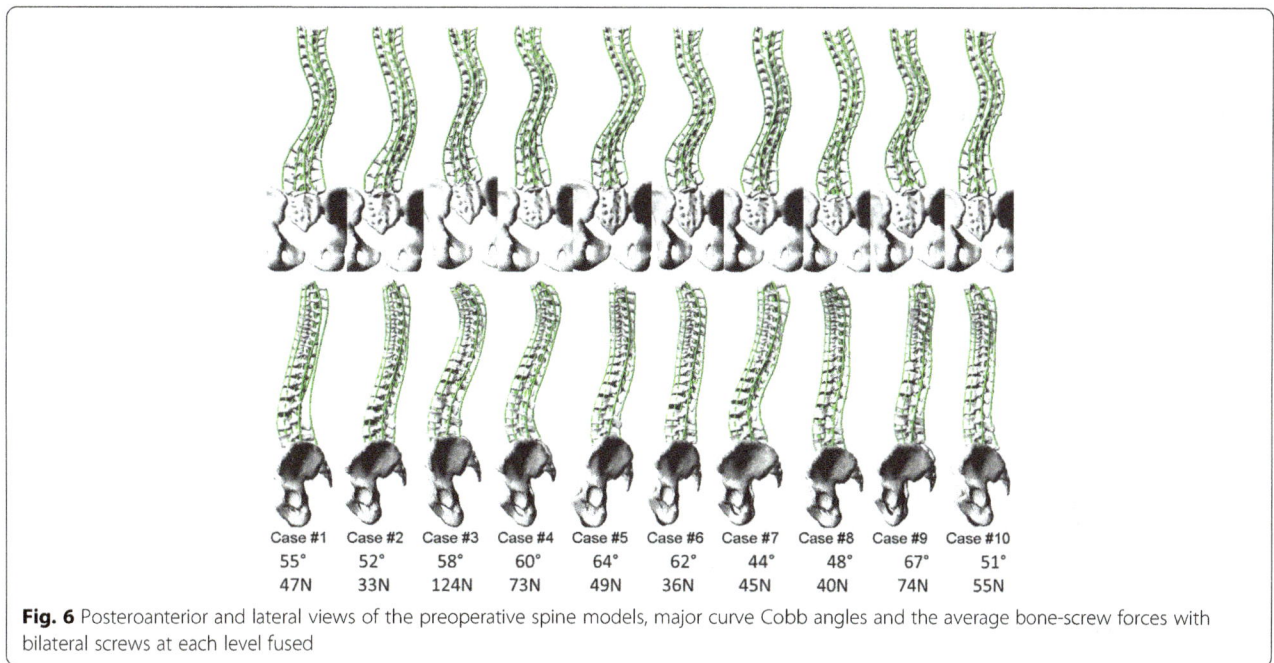

Case #1	Case #2	Case #3	Case #4	Case #5	Case #6	Case #7	Case #8	Case #9	Case #10
55°	52°	58°	60°	64°	62°	44°	48°	67°	51°
47N	33N	124N	73N	49N	36N	45N	40N	74N	55N

Fig. 6 Posteroanterior and lateral views of the preoperative spine models, major curve Cobb angles and the average bone-screw forces with bilateral screws at each level fused

height adjustability, there was no statistical difference between convex side screw dropouts and concave side screw dropouts. Periapical screw dropouts may more likely result in lower bone-screw force increase than alternate level screw dropouts. The number of vertebrae spanned by the major curve or the sharpness of the curve affects the bone-screw forces; screw dropouts should be reduced within short structural curves with high local curvature. Screw density and distribution should be determined by taking into account the local geometric characteristics of the curve in both the sagittal and coronal planes and the shape of the rods in addition to the curve type, deformity magnitude, and spinal stiffness.

Different correction techniques and instrumentation construct designs may have important roles in curve correction and bone-screw forces. Since the simulated correction technique was simultaneous two-rod segmental translation using polyaxial pedicle screws with dorsal height adjustability, findings in this study may not be directly applied to other techniques, types of screws, and construct designs. However, based on the fundamental laws of mechanics, for an equivalent curve correction, the overall effective corrective forces should be at an equivalent level independent of correction techniques and construct designs. Findings in this study provided therefore useful data on the overall effect of screw density and distribution. Knowledge of potential bone-screw forces in AIS instrumentation using alternative computer-simulated screw constructs can help surgeons select the best possible screw configuration specific for the patient. All bone-screw forces may not contribute to the actual curve correction due to the high mechanic complexity of the instrumented spine. Parts of the bone-screw forces are the "true corrective forces," which are necessary and sufficient to achieve the desired correction and the rest are overconstraining forces which are induced when forcing to ensure proper rod seating and locking at all pedicle screws as required by the construct design [42]. The effects of screw design, and density and distribution on true corrective forces and overconstraining forces need to be investigated with more AIS cases using various correction techniques and construct designs. Depending on the pedicle size of each individual patient, the pedicle screw diameter used varies among patients, which should be an important factor in determining the screw density and distribution and needs to be investigated.

This study is limited by the available experimental data to calibrate and describe the biomechanical properties of the scoliotic spine model. However, the modeling technique has been adapted to make the best of the available calibration data to meet the needs of this study. Some simplifications were made, such as modeling the vertebral bodies as rigid parts, limiting the model solving in the quasistatic domain, and approximating the intervertebral connection with limited number of elastic elements. Since the focus was on the overall comparative curve correction and bone-screw forces, these simplifications and approximations were considered as adequate for this study. To establish baseline data for screw density and distribution, studies through simulations using computerized biomechanical models should be combined with prospective clinical studies and biomechanical experiments. The computerized model will be refined and better calibrated using the more comprehensive clinical and experimental results and then used to perform more extensive studies which may not be possible in a clinical and experimental context.

Conclusions

Deformity correction can be achieved with 23% fewer screws than maximal density screw pattern, in which screw dropouts could be either on the convex side or on the concave side at alternate levels or at periapical levels. Using fewer screws resulted in higher average bone-screw forces. Findings in this study provided preliminary data on the effect of screw density and distribution. Further studies should be conducted on more screw densities and distributions using different correction techniques and different instrumentation in order to acquire comprehensive biomechanical knowledge to assist in individualized surgical treatment for AIS.

Abbreviations
3D: Three-dimension; AIS: Adolescent idiopathic scoliosis; ALL: Anterior longitudinal ligament; AVR: Apical vertebral rotation; FC: Facet joint capsule; ISL: Interspinous ligament; ITL: Intertransverse ligament; LF: Ligamentum flavum; LIV: Lower instrumented vertebra; MT: Main thoracic; PLL: Posterior longitudinal ligament; PT: Proximal thoracic; SD: Standard deviation; SSL: Supraspinous ligament; TL/L: Thoracolumbar/lumbar; UIV: Upper instrumented vertebra

Acknowledgements
The authors acknowledge the Natural Sciences and Engineering Research Council of Canada (Industrial Research Chair program with Medtronic of Canada) and the Scoliosis Research Society for providing financial supports. The authors acknowledge Julie Joncas for her efforts in the clinical data collection.

Funding
This study was financially supported by the Natural Sciences and Engineering Research Council of Canada (Industrial Research Chair program with Medtronic of Canada) and the Scoliosis Research Society.

Authors' contributions
XW and C-EA performed the study design, data collection and compilation, biomechanical modeling and simulations, result analysis, and manuscript drafting and revision. ANL and DGC all made substantial contributions to the study design, result analysis, and manuscript revision. SP, HL, and CGTL all made substantial contributions to the data collection, results analysis, and manuscript revision. All authors read and approved the final manuscript.

Competing interests
The authors declare that they have no competing interests.

Author details

[1]Department of Mechanical Engineering, Polytechnique Montréal, P.O. Box 6079, Downtown Station, Montreal, Quebec H3C 3A7, Canada. [2]Sainte-Justine University Hospital Center, 3175, Cote Sainte-Catherine Road, Montreal, Quebec H3T 1C5, Canada. [3]Department of Orthopedic Surgery, Mayo Clinic, 200 1st Street SW, Rochester, MN 55905, USA. [4]Sonoran Spine Center and Research Foundation, 1255 W Rio Salado Pkwy, Suite 107, Tempe, AZ 85281, USA. [5]Department of Orthopaedic Surgery, University of Minnesota, 2450 Riverside Avenue South, Suite R200, Minneapolis, MN 55454, USA.

References

1. Ledonio CG, Polly Jr DW, Vitale MG, et al. Pediatric pedicle screws: comparative effectiveness and safety: a systematic literature review from the Scoliosis Research Society and the Pediatric Orthopaedic Society of North America task force. J Bone Joint Surg Am. 2011;93:1227–34.

2. Lenke LG, Kuklo TR, Ondra S, et al. Rationale behind the current state-of-the-art treatment of scoliosis (in the pedicle screw era). Spine (Phila Pa 1976). 2008;33:1051–4.

3. Crawford AH, Lykissas MG, Gao X, et al. All-pedicle screw versus hybrid instrumentation in adolescent idiopathic scoliosis surgery: a comparative radiographical study with a minimum 2-year follow-up. Spine (Phila Pa 1976). 2013;38:1199–208.

4. Le Naveaux F, Aubin CE, Larson AN, et al. Key anchor points for specific correction maneuvers in Lenke 1 AIS: how important is the implant pattern design? In SRS ed. The 22nd International Meeting on Advanced Spine Techniques (IMAST). Kuala Lumpur, Malaysia, 2015.

5. Wang X, Aubin CE, Crandall D, et al. Biomechanical analysis of 4 types of pedicle screws for scoliotic spine instrumentation. Spine (Phila Pa 1976). 2012;37:E823–35.

6. Wang X, Aubin CE, Crandall D, et al. Biomechanical modeling and analysis of a direct incremental segmental translation system for the instrumentation of scoliotic deformities. Clin Biomech (Bristol, Avon). 2011;26:548–55.

7. Larson AN, Aubin CE, Polly Jr DW, et al. Are more screws better? A systematic review of anchor density and curve correction in adolescent idiopathic scoliosis. Spine Deformity. 2013;1:237–47.

8. Larson AN, Polly Jr DW, Diamond B, et al. Does higher anchor density result in increased curve correction and improved clinical outcomes in adolescent idiopathic scoliosis? Spine (Phila Pa 1976). 2014;39:571–8.

9. Le Naveaux F, Aubin CE, Larson AN, et al. Implant distribution in surgically instrumented Lenke 1 adolescent idiopathic scoliosis: does it affect curve correction? Spine (Phila Pa 1976). 2015;40:462–8.

10. Bharucha NJ, Lonner BS, Auerbach JD, et al. Low-density versus high-density thoracic pedicle screw constructs in adolescent idiopathic scoliosis: do more screws lead to a better outcome? Spine J. 2013;13:375–81.

11. Di Silvestre M, Parisini P, Lolli F, et al. Complications of thoracic pedicle screws in scoliosis treatment. Spine (Phila Pa 1976). 2007;32:1655–61.

12. Mac-Thiong JM, Parent S, Poitras B, et al. Neurological outcome and management of pedicle screws misplaced totally within the spinal canal. Spine (Phila Pa 1976). 2013;38:229–37.

13. Sugarman E, Sarwahi V, Amaral T, et al. Comparative analysis of perioperative differences between hybrid versus pedicle screw instrumentation in adolescent idiopathic scoliosis. J Spinal Disord Tech. 2013;26:161–6.

14. Ul Haque M, Shufflebarger HL, O'Brien M, et al. Radiation exposure during pedicle screw placement in adolescent idiopathic scoliosis: is fluoroscopy safe? Spine (Phila Pa 1976). 2006;31:2516–20.

15. Chen J, Yang C, Ran B, et al. Correction of Lenke 5 adolescent idiopathic scoliosis using pedicle screw instrumentation: does implant density influence the correction? Spine (Phila Pa 1976). 2013;38:E946–51.

16. Gotfryd AO, Avanzi O. Randomized clinical study on surgical techniques with different pedicle screw densities in the treatment of adolescent idiopathic scoliosis types Lenke 1A and 1B. Spine Deformity. 2013;1:272–9.

17. Cheriet F, Laporte C, Kadoury S, et al. A novel system for thE 3-D reconstruction of the human spine and rib cage from biplanar X-ray images. IEEE Trans Biomed Eng. 2007;54:1356–8.

18. Delorme S, Petit Y, de Guise JA, et al. Assessment of the 3-D reconstruction and high-resolution geometrical modeling of the human skeletal trunk from 2-D radiographic images. IEEE Trans Biomed Eng. 2003;50:989–98.

19. Jaumard NV, Welch WC, Winkelstein BA. Spinal facet joint biomechanics and mechanotransduction in normal, injury and degenerative conditions. J Biomech Eng. 2011;133:071010.

20. Watkins R, Watkins 3rd R, Williams L, et al. Stability provided by the sternum and rib cage in the thoracic spine. Spine (Phila Pa 1976). 2005;30:1283–6.

21. Myklebust JB, Pintar F, Yoganandan N, et al. Tensile strength of spinal ligaments. Spine (Phila Pa 1976). 1988;13:526–31.

22. Pintar FA. The biomechanics of spinal elements (ligaments, vertebral body, disc). Ann Arbor: Marquette University; 1986. p. 237.

23. Tong SY-P. A mechanical model of the normal human spine. Ann Arbor: University of Alberta (Canada); 1999. p. 164.

24. Holewijn RM, Schlösser TPC, Bisschop A, et al. How does spinal release and Ponte osteotomy improve spinal flexibility? The law of diminishing returns. Spine Deformity. 2015;3:489–95.

25. Wang C, Bell K, McClincy M, et al. Biomechanical comparison of Ponte osteotomy and discectomy. Spine (Phila Pa 1976). 2015;40:E141–5.

26. Wiemann J, Durrani S, Bosch P. The effect of posterior spinal releases on axial correction torque: a cadaver study. J Child Orthop. 2011;5:109–13.

27. Wollowick AL, Farrelly EE, Meyers K, et al. Anterior release generates more thoracic rotation than posterior osteotomy: a biomechanical study of human cadaver spines. Spine (Phila Pa 1976). 2013;38:1540–5.

28. Anderson AL, McIff TE, Asher MA, et al. The effect of posterior thoracic spine anatomical structures on motion segment flexion stiffness. Spine (Phila Pa 1976). 2009;34:441–6.

29. Panjabi MM, Hausfeld JN, White 3rd AA. A biomechanical study of the ligamentous stability of the thoracic spine in man. Acta Orthop Scand. 1981;52:315–26.

30. Adams MA, Hutton WC. The effect of posture on the role of the apophysial joints in resisting intervertebral compressive forces. J Bone Joint Surg (Br). 1980;62:358–62.

31. Pal GP, Routal RV. A study of weight transmission through the cervical and upper thoracic regions of the vertebral column in man. J Anat. 1986;148:245–61.

32. Pal GP, Routal RV. Transmission of weight through the lower thoracic and lumbar regions of the vertebral column in man. J Anat. 1987;152:93–105.

33. Yang KH, King AI. Mechanism of facet load transmission as a hypothesis for low-back pain. Spine (Phila Pa 1976). 1984;9:557–65.

34. Gardner-Morse MG, Stokes IA. Structural behavior of human lumbar spinal motion segments. J Biomech. 2004;37:205–12.

35. Panjabi MM, Brand Jr RA, White 3rd AA. Three-dimensional flexibility and stiffness properties of the human thoracic spine. J Biomech. 1976;9:185–92.

36. Panjabi MM, Brand Jr RA, White 3rd AA. Mechanical properties of the human thoracic spine as shown by three-dimensional load-displacement curves. J Bone Joint Surg Am. 1976;58:642–52.

37. Panjabi MM, Oxland TR, Yamamoto I, et al. Mechanical behavior of the human lumbar and lumbosacral spine as shown by three-dimensional load-displacement curves. J Bone Joint Surg Am. 1994;76:413–24.

38. Aubin CE, Labelle H, Chevrefils C, et al. Preoperative planning simulator for spinal deformity surgeries. Spine (Phila Pa 1976). 2008;33:2143–52.

39. Petit Y, Aubin CE, Labelle H. Patient-specific mechanical properties of a flexible multi-body model of the scoliotic spine. Med Biol Eng Comput. 2004;42:55–60.

40. Dang NR, Moreau MJ, Hill DL, et al. Intra-observer reproducibility and interobserver reliability of the radiographic parameters in the Spinal Deformity Study Group's AIS Radiographic Measurement Manual. Spine (Phila Pa 1976). 2005;30:1064–9.

41. Wang X, Aubin CE, Robitaille I, et al. Biomechanical comparison of alternative densities of pedicle screws for the treatment of adolescent idiopathic scoliosis. Eur Spine J. 2012;21:1082–90.

42. Wang X, Aubin CE, Labelle H, et al. Biomechanical analysis of corrective forces in spinal instrumentation for scoliosis treatment. Spine (Phila Pa 1976). 2012;37:E1479–87.

7

Functional outcome of non-surgical and surgical management for de novo degenerative lumbar scoliosis: a mean follow-up of 10 years

Sayf S.A. Faraj[1], Tsjitske M. Haanstra[1], Hugo Martijn[1], Marinus de Kleuver[2] and Barend J. van Royen[1*]

Abstract

Background: No studies have evaluated the long-term results of non-surgical and surgical management in de novo degenerative lumbar scoliosis (DNDLS). This study reports on the long-term functional outcome of patients being treated for DNDLS by non-surgical and surgical management.

Methods: This is a retrospective review of a single center database of DNDLS patients that underwent surgical or usual non-surgical management between 1996 and 2007. In a total of 88 patients, 50 (57%) underwent non-surgical and 38 (43%) surgical management. Baseline demographic, radiological-, clinical-, and surgical-related variables were collected. An Oswestry Disability Index (ODI) 2.0 questionnaire was sent to all patients after written informed consent.

Results: Twenty-nine of 88 patients participated in the study, 15 (52%) had undergone surgical and 14 (48%) non-surgical management with a mean follow-up of 10.9 years (range 8–15 years). There were no significant differences ($p > 0.05$) between non-surgical and surgical patients at baseline for age, body mass index, coronal Cobb angle, and clinical data. None of the non-surgical patients had undergone surgery during follow-up. In the surgical group, 40% had revision surgery. There was no significant difference in ODI total scores between groups at final follow-up ($p = 0.649$). A larger proportion of patients in the non-surgical group reported an ODI total score of ≤ 22, reflecting minimal disability (43 versus 20%; $p = 0.245$).

Conclusions: This is the first study that describes the long-term 10-year functional outcome of non-surgical and surgical management in a cohort of patients with DNDLS. No significant difference in functional outcome was found between groups after a mean follow-up of 10 years. Despite the significant potential for selection bias, these results indicate that non-surgical management of patients with DNDLS may lead to adequate functional outcome after long periods of time, with no crossover to surgery. Further study is warranted to define which patients may benefit most from which management regimen.

Keywords: De novo degenerative lumbar scoliosis, Adult scoliosis, Adult spinal deformity, Treatment, Surgical, Non-surgical, Functional outcome

* Correspondence: BJ.vanRoyen@vumc.nl
[1]Department of Orthopaedic Surgery, VU University Medical Center, De Boelelaan 1117, 1081HV Amsterdam, The Netherlands
Full list of author information is available at the end of the article

Background

De novo degenerative lumbar scoliosis (DNDLS) is a condition in which a lumbar scoliotic curve develops after the fifth decade as a result of degenerative changes of the spine [1]. DNDLS is generally moderately symptomatic, but it can result in severe back pain and neurological symptoms including leg weakness and numbness, thereby resulting into severe functional impairments [2–4]. The prevalence of DNDLS in the low back pain population has been reported to be 15% [5], and 68% in asymptomatic adults over the age of 60 years [6]. In light of the aging population, the prevalence of DNDLS will continue to increase [7, 8]. For this reason, the identification of proper ways of management has gained in urgency.

Non-surgical management of DNDLS with exercise therapy, the use of non-steroidal anti-inflammatory drugs, steroid injections, and narcotics has shown to be inadequate in providing relief of symptoms [9, 10]. As a result, a large subset of patients ultimately reach the point of undergoing lumbar spinal surgery, a decision that depends on progression of the deformity, neurological symptoms, functional limitations, and patient and surgeon preference [11, 12]. Despite the fact that these factors are patient-specific, surgical management is a generally accepted and a commonly performed intervention for this disorder. However, surgical treatment for DNDLS is known to be associated with high complication and revision rates [13].

Several studies have compared surgical with non-surgical management for DNDLS. Surgery has repeatedly been shown to be superior in relieving pain and improving function over a follow-up of 2 years [14–16]. However, emphasis on healthy and vital aging, in which elderly want to maintain their functional abilities, reflects the need to evaluate both management regimens after long periods of time. Even though surgery is widely used, to the best of our knowledge, no studies are available in the peer-reviewed literature that have evaluated both strategies over a long-term follow-up. The objective of this study is, therefore, to evaluate long-term functional outcome of surgical and non-surgical management in patients with DNDLS, exceeding a mean follow-up of 10 years. The focus will be patient centered, hence, using a validated patient-reported outcome measure to evaluate function.

Methods

Study design and patient population

This is a single-center observational cohort study of patients who presented between 1996 and 2007 with symptomatic DNDLS. Inclusion criteria were age ≥ 50 years and a Cobb angle of 10°–55° in the coronal plain with an apex of the main curvature located in the lumbar region (L1-L5). Patients with a history of juvenile, adolescent idiopathic scoliosis, neuromuscular spinal abnormalities, or metabolic spinal pathology were excluded. A total of 88 patients met the inclusion criteria. Baseline demographic and radiographic findings of this study population have been reported previously [17].

In this group of 88 patients, 50 (57%) underwent non-surgical and 38 (43%) underwent surgical management based upon a consent process between patient and surgeon and was ultimately guided by patient choice and surgeon preference. Patients being treated surgically underwent decompression, short fusion (≤ 3 levels), or long fusion (≥ 4 levels) with pedicle screw fixation. Standardized non-surgical management protocols were not used. Non-surgical management included exercise therapy if possible, steroid injections, and/or pharmacological treatments. The non-surgical management modality was left to the discretion of the treating physician and the patient. Baseline demographic variables included age, self-reported back pain (yes/no), radicular leg pain (yes/no), muscle weakness (yes/no), and numbness in the legs (yes/no). In addition, neurological examination was performed (i.e., straight leg raise test, patellar, Achilles, and plantar reflex). Finally, radiographic measures at initial presentation included Cobb angle, location of the apical vertebra, and side of convexity on coronal spine radiographs. Full-spine standing sagittal radiographs were not routinely performed (patient enrollment 1996–2007).

Data collection

Considering the relative old age of the study population at the current follow-up, a database search was performed in the national database registry for identification of patients that had passed away during follow-up. A Dutch translated and validated version of the Oswestry Disability Index (ODI) 2.0 was sent to eligible patients that had given their written informed consent [18]. In addition, patients were asked if they received (additional) spine surgery in our institution or elsewhere during follow-up. In case of no response, a reminder was sent after 4 weeks.

The ODI is a questionnaire that evaluates the limitations in functional status caused by low back pain. This outcome measure has been shown to be valid, reliable, and responsive in patients with low back pain and is often used in studies in the evaluation of degenerative spinal disorders [19]. The total sum score of the ODI ranges from 0 to 100; the higher the score, the higher the disability. An ODI total score between 0 and 20 reflects minimal disability, 21–40 moderate disability, 41–60 severe disability, 61–80 crippling back pain, and 81–

100 bed-bound patients [20]. ODI total score was compared between groups at final follow-up.

Recent study by Van Hooff et al. [21] reported that an absolute ODI score of ≤ 22 reflects an acceptable symptom state and should be considered as a criterion for treatment success in patients who had undergone surgery for degenerative disorders of the lumbar spine. Therefore, the number of patients reporting minimal disability, hence an "acceptable symptom state" (ODI score 0–22) versus severe disability (ODI score 40–100), were stratified according to management.

Statistical analysis

Data was checked for normal distribution of variables using the Shapiro-Wilk test. Baseline demographic, neurological, and radiographic values were compared between both groups using Student's t test in case of normal distribution of data, whereas a Mann-Whitney U test was performed when variables were non-normally distributed. Frequency analysis of categorical variables (ODI score 0–22 versus 40–100) was performed using a Fisher's Exact test. All statistical tests were performed with SPSS 22.0 IBM. Statistical significance was set at $p < 0.05$.

Results
Study population

Thirty (34%) of the 88 patients passed away during follow-up. Six patients' addresses were untraceable and one patient suffered from a stroke and was therefore not able to answer the questionnaire. Thus, 51 patients were eligible for this long-term follow-up study of which 29 (57%) agreed to participate. Of these 29 patients, 15 (52%) were treated surgically and 14 (48%) were managed non-surgically, with a mean age of 65.2 ± 8.2 (range, min–max 50–81 years) and a median Cobb angle of 19.0 (interquartile range 16.0–25.5°) at initial presentation. The total group consisted out of 22 (76%) females and 7 (24%) males. Mean follow-up was 10.9 ± 1.9 years (range 8–15 years). During follow-up, there was no crossover from non-surgical to surgical group. Baseline demographic, radiological, and clinical data is stratified according to group in Table 1. There was no significant difference between the two groups with regards to age ($p = 0.25$), body mass index (BMI) ($p = 0.79$), Cobb angle ($p = 0.37$), and years of follow-up ($p = 0.84$). Interestingly, the non-surgical group had a larger median coronal Cobb angle than the surgical group (21.0 versus 18.0; $p = 0.37$). With regard to clinical evaluation at initial presentation, all patients (100%) reported back pain and a high comparable number of patients in both groups reported radicular leg pain (79% versus 87%). Neurological symptoms during physical examination (straight leg raise test, patellar, Achilles, and plantar reflex), muscle weakness, and numbness in the legs were found in both groups (Table 1).

Management

Non-surgical management included exercise therapy if possible, steroid injections, and/or pharmacological treatments. All patients treated surgically underwent postero(lateral) lumbar fusion with pedicle screw fixation to restore coronal malalignment and stenosis. Details of surgical treatment are presented in Table 2 and Table 3. Nine (60%) patients underwent long fusion (≥ 4 levels) and six (40%) short fusion (≤ 3 levels). Six (40%) patients underwent additional decompression. Six patients (40%) in the surgical group had one or more revision surgeries during follow-up due to implant failure (3 patients), wound infection (1 patient), or recurrence of symptoms (2 patients). Revision surgery included, but was not limited to, screw replacement, (re-)decompression or extension of the fusion.

Functional outcome

In terms of total score of the ODI, there was no significant difference in the non-surgical versus the surgical group ($p = 0.649$). The non-surgical group had a mean ODI total score of 35.2 ± 26.9 (range 2.0–88.0) and the surgical group a mean ODI total score of 39.4 ± 21.6 (range 4.0–76.0), both groups reflecting an overall moderate disability (ODI range 21–40) [20].

The number of patients reporting minimal disability, hence a "satisfactory symptom state" (ODI total score 0–22) and severe disability (ODI total score 40–100), were stratified according to management in Table 4. More patients in the non-surgical group reported an ODI total score ≤ 22, reflecting minimal disability (43 versus 20%, $p = 0.245$); however, this difference was non-significant. In addition, no significant difference was found in the number of patients reporting severe disability ($p = 0.715$).

Discussion

In elderly patients, DNDLS significantly affects the overall health-related quality of life and is one of the most prevalent indications for reconstructive spinal surgery [22, 23]. It is important to compare the long-term results of surgical and non-surgical management in order to optimize clinical decision-making. Surgical decompression and spinal correction has shown to improve functional limitations in DNDLS, but long-term follow-up seldom exceeds 2 years. In the current literature, there are no studies that have evaluated both surgical and non-surgical strategies with long-term follow-up. This study provides the first long-term evaluation in functional outcome of non-surgical and surgically treated DNDLS patients. Notable, the purpose of the current analysis was not to suggest that one approach is uniformly superior to the other, but rather to report the functional outcome after long-term follow-up of two management strategies.

Table 1 Demographic, radiology, and clinical evaluation at baseline according to surgical and non-surgical management

	All	Non-surgical	Surgical	p value
Number of patients	29	14 (48%)	15 (52%)	
Female:Male	22:7	11:3	11:4	
Age at baseline, mean ± SD, (years)	65.2 ± 8.2	67.0 ± 8.8	63.5 ± 7.5	0.253
BMI, mean ± SD, (kg/m^2)	24.7 ± 3.8	24.3 ± 5.6	24.9 ± 3.2	0.790
Coronal Cobb angle, median [IQR], (°)	19.0 [16.0–25.5]	21.0 [16.0–30.0]	18.0 [16.0–22.0]	0.370
Follow-up time, mean ± SD, (years)	10.9 ± 1.9	10.3 ± 1.5	10.5 ± 1.4	0.836
Apical vertebra, (n)				
L1	2	2	0	
L2	12	5	7	
L3	12	6	6	
L4	3	1	2	
Convex side, (n)				
Right sided	14	10	4	
Left sided	15	4	11	
Back pain, n (%)	29 (100%)	14 (100%)	15 (100%)	
Radicular leg pain, n (%)	24 (83%)	11 (79%)	13 (87%)	
Right	11	7	4	
Left	5	1	4	
Left and right	8	3	5	
Not present	5	3	2	
Neurological symptoms[†], n (%)	4 (14%)	1 (7%)	3 (20%)	
Muscle weakness in the legs, n (%)	10 (34%)	6 (43%)	4 (27%)	
Right	4	2	2	
Left	3	2	1	
Left and right	3	2	1	
Not present	11	7	4	
Data not available	8	1	7	
Numbness in the legs, n (%)	3 (10%)	2 (14%)	1 (7%)	
Yes	3	2	1	
Not present	14	10	4	
Data not available	12	2	10	

Values of age, body mass index (BMI), Cobb angle, and follow-up time are expressed as the mean and standard deviation (normal distribution of data) or as the median and interquartile range [IQR] (non-normal distribution of data). Percentages are calculated from the total number of patients

P-value were calculated between non-surgical and surgical group using Student's t test (normal distribution of data) or Mann-Whitney U test (non-normal distributed data)

[†]Neurological symptoms evaluated during physical examination by straight leg raise test, patellar, Achilles, and plantar reflex

Despite weaknesses in the methodology (e.g., no baseline sagittal full-spine radiographs), the results of the present study seem to indicate that non-surgical managed patients seem to function reasonably after long periods of time, with surprisingly no crossover to surgery.

The findings of the present study seem somewhat contradictory compared to previous shorter term follow-up studies which have suggested that surgical management is superior to non-surgical management in terms of pain relief and improved function [11, 14–16]. In a retrospective study, Dickson et al. [24] compared 81 patients who underwent surgical treatment versus 30 patients that underwent non-surgical management. Patients in the surgical group demonstrated significantly more improvement of pain, fatigue, and disability over 5 years of follow-up, compared to the non-surgical managed group. However, the study by Dickson and colleagues had several limitations, including the use of the traditional Harrington distraction rod instrumentation and non-validated outcome measures. Smith et al. [16] offered perhaps the most complete assessment of the benefit of surgical treatment as compared to non-

Table 2 Characteristics of surgical cohort

Parameter	Value
Number of patients	15
Age at index surgery (years)	63.5 ± 7.5
Posterior-only approach	15 (100%)
Posterior instrumentation and fusion	15 (100%)
Number of levels fused, range (average)	2–8 (4.7)
UIV, range	T10-L4
LIV, range	L5-ilium
PLIF	2 (13.3%)
DLIF	2 (13.3%)
Decompression	6 (40%)

Value of age is expressed as the mean and standard deviation
UIV upper-most instrumented vertebra, *LIV* lower-most instrumented vertebra, *DLIF* direct lateral interbody fusion, *PLIF* posterior lumbar interbody fusion

surgical management in adult spinal deformity. In a multicentre prospective analysis, surgical and non-surgical treated patients were matched based upon similar radiographic and clinical features. The surgical treated group demonstrated significant improvements in Scoliosis Research Society-22 questionnaire (SRS-22), ODI, and Numeric Rating Scale (NRS) back and leg pain scores at 2 years follow-up, whereas the non-surgical cohort maintained the baseline level of pain and disability scores. However, whether 2-year outcome evaluation is adequate in adult spinal deformities is debatable [25]. Bridwell et al. [26] evaluated changes in radiographic and clinical outcome of primary adult scoliosis surgery after 2, 3, and 5 years' follow-up. In a multicentre prospective analysis, Bridwell

et al. [26] demonstrated that patients who experienced new complications (i.e., implant failure, infection, and proximal junctional failure) that were identified at final follow-up demonstrated significantly worse ODI and SRS total scores. For this reason, it is important to evaluate the durability of surgical and non-surgical management over longer term follow-up and to define which patients may benefit most from which treatment regimen.

In the present study, we sought to assess one important patient-reported outcome measure to provide insight in the long-term results of both management regimens. We chose to focus on the ODI as it is considered the gold standard to assess functional limitations caused by low back pain, a characterizing feature of DNDLS [20]. At initial presentation, all patients reported some degree of back pain; radicular leg pain was reported by 79% in the non-surgical group and 87% in the surgical group. In addition, a moderate number of patients demonstrated pre-treatment weakness in the legs in the non-surgical group and in the surgical group (43 and 27%, respectively) (Table 1). After a mean follow-up of 10 years, no significant difference was found in ODI scores between surgical and non-surgical management in DNDLS. Moreover, a higher proportion of patients report an acceptable symptom state (ODI total score 0–22) in the non-surgical group compared to the surgical group (43 versus 20%); however, this difference was non-significant ($p = 0.245$) (Table 4). Even though the studied patient cohort (e.g., relatively small Cobb angle, a high percentage of reported back

Table 3 Detailed surgical characteristics at baseline and whether patients underwent revision surgery during follow-up

Baseline						Follow-up
Patient no.	Gender	Age	Cobb (°)	Apical vertebra	Postero(lateral) fusion with pedicle screws	Revision surgery
1	M	71	26°	L2	Th11-S1+ decompression L3-L4	No
2	F	59	37°	L2	Th11-L5	No
3	M	63	18°	L2	L2-L5	Yes
4	F	50	42°	L2	Th10-S1	No
5	F	71	17°	L2	L3-L5 + decompression + DLIF	No
6	F	59	22°	L2	Th12-L5 + PLIF	No
7	F	67	16°	L2	L4-L5+ DLIF	Yes
8	M	66	17°	L3	Th11-S1	Yes
9	F	62	12°	L3	Th12-S1	No
10	M	68	10°	L3	Th12-L5 + decompression L2–3	Yes
11	F	55	22°	L3	Th12-S1	No
12	F	79	22°	L3	Th112-L5 + decompression L4-L5	Yes
13	F	62	19°	L4	L4-L5 + decompression L4-L5	Yes
14	F	66	14°	L4	L3-S1 + decompression L3- S1	No
15	F	54	18°	L3	L5-S1 + PLIF	No

DLIF diffuse lateral interbody fusion, *PLIF* posterior lumbar interbody fusion

Table 4 Number of patients reporting minimal disability (ODI score 0–22) versus severe disability (ODI score 40–100) after 10-year follow-up, stratified according to management

ODI total score	Non-surgical (14)	Surgical (15)	p value
score 0–22	6 (43%)	3 (20%)	0.245
score 40–100	7 (50%)	6 (40%)	0.715

ODI indicates Oswestry Disability Index; the range is 0–100, with higher numbers reflecting greater disability. ODI total score between 0 and 22 reflects minimal disability hence a "satisfactory symptom state" and an ODI total score 40–100 severe disability. Percentages are calculated from the total number of non-surgical ($n = 14$) and surgical ($n = 15$) patients. p values were calculated using Fisher's Exact Test

and leg pain, and pre-treatment neural comprise) in the present study is relatively comparable to previous studies demonstrating that surgical is superior to non-surgical management (Table 1), the results of the present study demonstrate that certain patients can benefit from non-surgical management for long periods of time (Table 4). Further study is warranted to determine which patients benefit most from which treatment regimen.

The results of the present study should be interpreted with some caution. The objective of the present study was to evaluate long-term functional outcome of both strategies, and thus, it was not designed to assess the gain in functional outcome over time, since it does not include ODI assessment at initial presentation. Despite great efforts to obtain the follow-up measures in both groups, many patients (34%) had passed away during follow-up or did not want to participate (25%). The difficulty of including non-surgical managed elderly patients in a follow-up study has previously been reported. Previous studies achieved a 2-year follow-up rate of 45–55% when including non-operative patients [15, 27]. The present study achieved a total follow-up rate of 57% (excluding deceased patients) after a mean follow-up exceeding 10 years. The major limitations of the present study are related to its potential for selection bias (despite the fact that we were not able to identify any significant differences between the groups), the relatively small follow-up rate, and the absence of data related to other forms of non-surgical management (protocols were not used) between baseline and follow-up that patients may have tried. Finally, the surgical correction of adult spinal deformity, including restoration of spinopelvic alignment and sagittal balance, is now better defined [28]. However, the present study could not take into account sagittal spinopelvic alignment due to the historic context of the cohort (patient enrolment 1996–2007) and the absence of lateral full-spine standing radiographs at initial presentation. For this reason, we cannot make direct conclusions regarding the long-term surgical outcome of restoring sagittal spinopelvic alignment. Whether restoring sagittal alignment will prove significant beneficial on the longer term will require further study and careful follow-up.

Conclusions

This is the first study that describes the long-term outcome of non-surgical and surgical management in patients with symptomatic DNDLS. For these relatively comparable cohorts of patients from a single institution and during the same time frame, we could not demonstrate a significant difference in ODI total score between surgical and non-surgical management after long-term follow-up exceeding 10 years. Despite methodological weaknesses, this study provides the first ever long-term evaluation in patient reported outcome of non-surgical and surgical treated symptomatic DNDLS patients. The results indicate that certain patients can benefit from non-surgical management after long periods of time. Further study is warranted to determine which patients benefit most from which treatment regimen.

Abbreviations
BMI: Body mass index; DNDLS: De novo degenerative lumbar scoliosis; NRS: Numeric Rating Scale; ODI: Oswestry Disability Index; SRS-22: Scoliosis Research Society-22 Questionnaire

Acknowledgments
The authors thank the assistance of Janneke Wilschut of the Department of Epidemiology and Biostatistics, VU University Amsterdam for her statistical support.

Funding
No funding was received for this work.

Authors' contributions
SF contributed to study design, data collection, data analysis, data interpretation, and writing of the manuscript. TH contributed to data analysis and data interpretation and critically reviewed the manuscript. HM contributed to the data collection, data interpretation, and writing of the manuscript. MdK contributed to data interpretation and wrote and critically reviewed the manuscript. BvR contributed to study design, data interpretation, and writing of the manuscript. All authors read and approved the final manuscript.

Competing interests
MdK reports on receiving compensation for being on the speakers' bureaus of DePuy and Medtronic and receiving non-study-related grant support from AO and the Scoliosis Research Society for clinical or research overseen by him. All remaining authors declare that they have no competing interests.

Author details
[1]Department of Orthopaedic Surgery, VU University Medical Center, De Boelelaan 1117, 1081HV Amsterdam, The Netherlands. [2]Department of Orthopedics, Radboud University Medical Center, Huispost 611, 6500HB Nijmegen, The Netherlands.

References

1. Aebi M. The adult scoliosis. Eur Spine J. 2005;14:925–48.
2. Smith JS, K-M F, Urban P, Shaffrey CI. Neurological symptoms and deficits in adults with scoliosis who present to a surgical clinic: incidence and association with the choice of operative versus nonoperative management—clinical article. J Neurosurg Spine. 2008;9:326–31.
3. Bess S, Boachie-Adjei O, Burton D, et al. Pain and disability determine treatment modality for older patients with adult scoliosis, while deformity guides treatment for younger patients. Spine (Phila Pa 1976). 2009;34:2186–90.
4. Longo DL, Ropper AH, Zafonte RD. Sciatica. N Engl J Med. 2015;372:1240–8.
5. Perennou D, Marcelli C, Herisson C, Simon L. Adult lumbar scoliosis. Epidemiologic aspects in a low-back pain population. Spine (Phila Pa 1976). 1994;19:123–8.
6. Schwab F, Dubey A, Gamez L, et al. Adult scoliosis: prevalence, SF-36, and nutritional parameters in an elderly volunteer population. Spine (Phila Pa 1976). 2005;30:1082–5.
7. United States Census Bureau 2014. http://www.census.gov/topics/ population/age-and-sex.html. Accessed 31 Dec 2016.
8. The Nationwide Inpatient Sample, US (2014) http://hcup-us.ahrq.gov/ nisoverview.jsp Accessed 11 Sept 2016.
9. Glassman SD, Berven S, Kostuik J, et al. Nonsurgical resource utilization in adult spinal deformity. Spine (Phila Pa 1976). 2006;31:941–7.
10. Ames CP, Scheer JK, Lafage V, et al. Adult spinal deformity: epidemiology, health impact, evaluation, and management. Spine Deform. 2016;4:310–22.
11. Smith JS, Shaffrey CI, Berven S, et al. Operative versus nonoperative treatment of leg pain in adults with scoliosis: a retrospective review of a prospective multicenter database with two-year follow-up. Spine (Phila Pa 1976). 2009;34:1693–8.
12. Glassman SD, Schwab FJ, Bridwell KH, et al. The selection of operative versus nonoperative treatment in patients with adult scoliosis. Spine (Phila Pa 1976). 2007;32:93–7.
13. Daubs MD, Lenke LG, Cheh G, et al. Adult spinal deformity surgery: complications and outcomes in patients over age 60. Spine (Phila Pa 1976). 2007;32:2238–44.
14. Smith JS, Shaffrey CI, Berven S, et al. Improvement of back pain with operative and nonoperative treatment in adults with scoliosis. Neurosurgery. 2009;65:84–6.
15. Bridwell KH, Glassman S, Horton W, et al. Does treatment (nonoperative and operative) improve the two-year quality of life in patients with adult symptomatic lumbar scoliosis: a prospective multicenter evidence-based medicine study. Spine (Phila Pa 1976). 2009;34:2171–8.
16. Smith JS, Lafage V, Shaffrey CI, et al. Outcomes of operative and nonoperative treatment for adult spinal deformity: a prospective, multicenter, propensity-matched cohort assessment with minimum 2-year follow-up. Neurosurgery. 2016;78:851–61.
17. de Vries B, Mullender MG, Pluymakers WJ, et al. Spinal decompensation in degenerative lumbar scoliosis. Eur Spine J. 2010;19:1540–4.
18. van Hooff ML, Spruit M, Fairbank JCT, et al. The Oswestry Disability Index (version 2.1a): validation of a Dutch language version. Spine (Phila Pa 1976). 2015;40:E83–90.
19. Fairbank JC, Couper J, Davies JB, O'Brien JP. The Oswestry low back pain disability questionnaire. Physiotherapy. 1980;66:271–3.
20. Fairbank JC, Pynsent PB. The Oswestry Disability Index. Spine (Phila Pa 1976). 2000;25:2940–52. discussion 2952
21. van Hooff ML, Mannion AF, Staub LP, et al. Determination of the Oswestry Disability Index score equivalent to a "satisfactory symptom state" in patients undergoing surgery for degenerative disorders of the lumbar spine-a Spine Tango registry-based study. Spine J. 2016;16:1221–30.
22. Healthcare Costs, Utilization Project. U.S. Department of Health and Human Services; 2013. Available at: https://www.hcup-us.ahrq.gov/; Accessed 28 July 2016.
23. Terran J, McHugh B, Fischer C, et al. Surgical treatment for adult spinal deformity: projected cost effectiveness at 5-year follow-up. Ochsner J. 2014; 14:14–22.
24. Dickson JH, Mirkovic S, Noble PC, et al. Results of operative treatment of idiopathic scoliosis in adults. J Bone Joint Surg Am. 1995;77:513–23.
25. Glassman SD, Schwab F, Bridwell KH, et al. Do 1-year outcomes predict 2-year outcomes for adult deformity surgery? Spine J. 2009;9:317–22.
26. Bridwell KH, Baldus C, Berven S, et al. Changes in radiographic and clinical outcomes with primary treatment adult spinal deformity surgeries from two years to three- to five-years follow-up. Spine (Phila Pa 1976). 2010;35:1849–54.
27. Smith JS, Shaffrey CI, Berven S, et al. Improvement of back pain with operative and nonoperative treatment in adults with scoliosis. Neurosurgery. 2009;65:86–93.
28. Schwab FJ, Blondel B, Bess S, et al. Radiographical spinopelvic parameters and disability in the setting of adult spinal deformity: a prospective multicenter analysis. Spine (Phila Pa 1976). 2013;38:E803–12.

8

The role of the paravertebral muscles in adolescent idiopathic scoliosis evaluated by temporary paralysis

Christian Wong[1]* ⓘ, Kasper Gosvig[2] and Stig Sonne-Holm[1]

Abstract

Background: Muscle imbalance has been suggested as implicated in the pathology of adolescent idiopathic scoliosis (AIS). The specific "pathomechanic" role of the paravertebral muscles as being scoliogenic (inducing scoliosis) or counteracting scoliosis in the initial development and maintenance of this spinal deformity has yet to be clarified in humans. In the present study, we investigated the radiographic changes of temporal paralysis using botulinum toxin A as localized injection therapy (ITB) in the psoas major muscle in AIS patients.

Methods: Nine patients with AIS were injected one time with ITB using ultrasonic and EMG guidance in the selected spine muscles. Radiographic and clinical examinations were performed before and 6 weeks after the injection. Primary outcome parameters of radiological changes were analyzed using Wilcoxon signed-rank test and binomial test, and secondary outcome parameters of short- and long-term clinical effects were obtained.

Results: Significant radiological corrective changes were seen in the frontal plane in the thoracic and lumbar spine as well as significant derotational corrective change in the lumbar spine according to Cobb's angle measurements and to Nash and Moe's classification, respectively. No serious adverse events were detected at follow-up.

Conclusions: In conclusion, this study demonstrated that the psoas major muscle do play a role into the pathology in adolescent idiopathic scoliosis by maintaining the curvature of the lumbar spine and thoracic spine.

Keywords: Injection therapy, Botulinum toxin A, Idiopathic scoliosis, Prospective study, Radiological Cobb's angle

Background

The Greek physician Hippocrates was the first to describe adolescent idiopathic scoliosis (AIS) as early as 400 BC [1]. Today, the etiology of AIS is still considered multifactorial, even though over time many researchers have tried to explain the pathology by one single etiology, ranging from a broad variety of causes of either biomechanical or genetic nature [2–6]. One relative recent observation by Modi et al. is that the spinal deformity in mild AIS tries to return to the neutral midline position, thereby displaying a "wavy" curve pattern with fluctuations in a lateral curve shape when followed closely [4]. They suggested that the paravertebral muscles would have a "tuning/balancing

mechanism" that tries to correct the spinal deformity of mild scoliosis into apparent spontaneous regression or to prevent further progression of curve, and if failing, this would result in further progression [4]. The natural history of AIS, where the majority spontaneously remains stable while the rest either regresses or progresses, may be seen as suggestive for this hypothesis [7], and the paravertebral muscles or rather a misbalance of the paravertebral muscles has been suggested as causative for progression or regression of AIS [3, 4, 6, 8, 9]. Differences in morphology examined by MRI, behavioral response to exercise, and electromyographic response of the paravertebral muscle have indicated that muscle imbalance may play a role in the pathologic pathway that leads to progression or regression of AIS. This important question of the "pathomechanic role" of paravertebral muscles is still debated [10], but the evidence for the specific role as scoliogenic

* Correspondence: chwo123@gmail.com
[1]Department of Orthopaedics, University Hospital of Hvidovre, Kettegaard Allé 30, 2650 Hvidovre, Denmark
Full list of author information is available at the end of the article

(inducing scoliosis) or counteracting scoliosis in human is still circumstantial [2, 3, 9–13]. Recently, Grivas et al. examined this for the quadratus lumborum muscle by comparing the length of the 12th rib in a group of children with right lumbar idiopathic scoliosis and straight spines; he suggested that stimulation of the paravertebral muscles should be performed to determine the "pathomechanic role" in future studies [10]. In this study, we examined if the hypnotized "pathomechanic role" of the psoas major (PM) of the iliopsoas muscle is scoliogenic—not by stimulation but by paralysis. The PM muscle is interesting for examining the "pathomechanic role" for AIS; Bruggi et al. found an interrelationship between the paravertebral muscle iliopsoas and AIS, where the muscle in isometric contraction had a corrective effect of the scoliotic curve [14]. In addition, a volumetric asymmetry of the PM has also been demonstrated in patients with degenerative AIS, where hypertrophy of 6.3% on the convex side was concluded to be associated with the scoliosis [12]. Yet, another study was unable to demonstrate that this difference had a significant effect in either the maximal voluntary isometric contraction force between healthy girls (161.4 N) and girls with scoliosis (144.3 N) or in the strength of the paravertebral muscle on either side of the scoliosis [15]. This interest in the PM in regard to AIS stems from the anatomy of the PM; it is a long fusiform muscle that is distributed on the lateral side of the lumbar spine from Th12 to L5, where it inserts on the transverse processes,

the two adjacent vertebral bodies and their intervertebral discs. Moreover, it inserts from a series of tendinous arches extending across the bodies of the lumbar vertebrae. The PM then descends through the pelvic brim and passes beneath the ligamentum inguinale. It is finally attached to the trochanter minor of the femur. The function of PM is that of having an antigravity compensation, which also acts as a stabilizer of the lumbar lordosis in an upright posture [16]. The hypnotized scoliogenic role of the PM muscle would be that of initiating or maintaining a lumbar scoliotic curvature by muscle contraction. The PM would act by performing a lateral pull in the upper part of the lumbar spine into a concave scoliotic curvature, thus creating a convex thoracic curve in the thoracic and thoracolumbar scoliosis. This is illustrated in Fig. 1. The PM muscle would seem an ideal case in which to examine and clarify this specific scoliogenic effect, since it is of such a strength/magnitude/size that temporary paralysis would affect the scoliotic curves when recorded radiographically and at the same time would be attainable for safe percutaneous injection treatment.

Botulinum toxin A as a localized injection therapy (ITB) has been utilized to reduce spasticity and improve the motor dysfunction in cerebral palsy. ITB has already been examined for neuromuscular scoliosis by injection in the back muscles for treatment, where the corrective and clinical efficacy was examined [17, 18]. However, to our knowledge, ITB for AIS has not been investigated

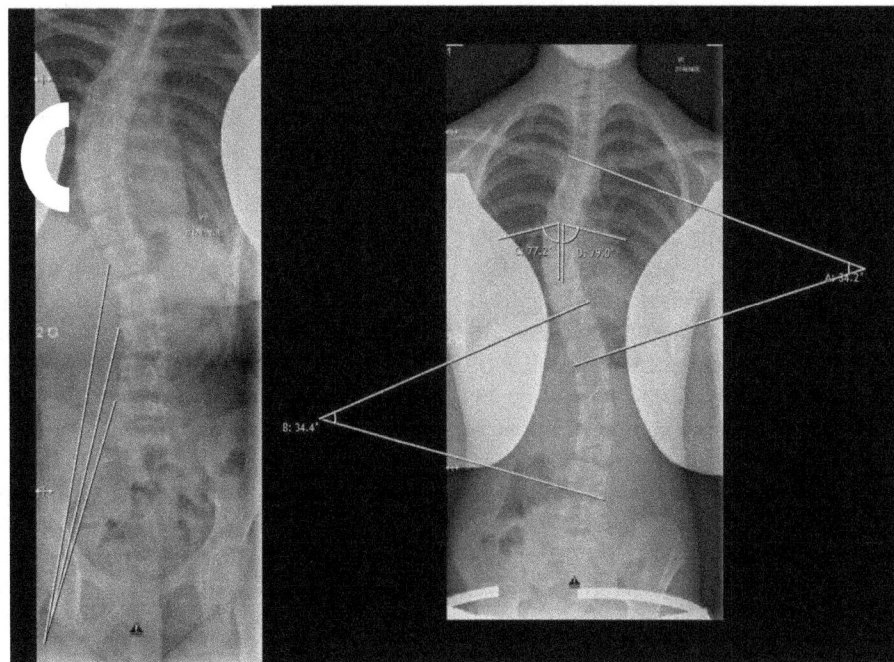

Fig. 1 Schematic representation of the psoas major on the concave side of a thoracic scoliosis; C marks the stronger muscles on the thoracic convex side scoliosis in accordance with the literature (left). Measurements of thoracic and lumbar Cobb's angle and concave and convex rib vertebra angle (right)

and would seem to be ideal for examining the role of the muscles in AIS, since it provides temporary muscle paralysis without long-term side effects or complications in therapeutic doses in otherwise healthy humans [19]. In this study, we conducted a small longitudinal prospective series using ITB for AIS, examining the radiological changes when treatment would have maximal paralytic effects (after 6 weeks). The purpose was to examine if ITB would induce a change in curvature in AIS. This could clarify if the spinal muscles play in the pathological process of the AIS, whether the spinal muscles would in fact induce the spinal deformity of AIS by the muscle forces/pull of the PM, thus having a scoliogenic effect, where regression of the AIS after paralysis would happen.

Methods

In the present study, the patients were recruited patients from those already being treated for AIS at our hospital from the out-patient clinic. We carried out inclusion after oral and written informed consent. Inclusion criteria included a history of AIS, an age between 10 and 14 years, and a Cobb's angle of at least 10°. Exclusion criteria were hypersensitivity or allergy to botulinum toxin A, ongoing infection at the injection sites, or prior ITB within the last 6 months. The patients are characterized clinically in Table 1.

The injection treatment was given as a standard dose with three injections on the concave side of the lumbar scoliosis in the PM part of the iliopsoas muscle, so that the maximum dose in the single muscle did not exceed 100 units as in the earlier studies [17, 18]. After placement of the injection needle in the target muscle, we confirmed the correct placement by an ultrasound and by electric simulation through the needle for correct identification of the target muscle, since correct targeting of the deep back muscles otherwise seemed unreliable [20]. An experienced

anesthesiologist and pediatric orthopedic surgeon performed the injections under general anesthesia using propofol infusion and spontaneous breathing, when lying in lateral position. We performed the radiographic examinations before and 6 weeks after injection treatment with standing radiographs, when botulinum toxin A would have the maximum effect on the muscles (visit window of 2 weeks). The same staff performed the radiographic acquisitions in a uniform, systematic manner, where patients omitted the brace for 24 h before the acquisition [21]. The primary outcome measures were the measurements of Cobb's angle for primary and secondary curves, and the secondary parameters were the level of measurements for primary and secondary curves, rib vertebra angles for the thoracic apex vertebra, rib vertebrae angle difference, Nash and Moe's classification at the apex vertebrae of the primary and secondary curves, and level of the apex vertebra for primary and secondary curves. Three experienced doctors performed all measurements similarly, separately and blinded, and we used the average results for further analyses. See Fig. 1 for a schematic representation of the radiographic evaluation.

Tertiary outcome measures were clinical, where patients and/or their parents were questioned openly at follow-up after treatment and specifically about their/the patient's general well-being, about the effect of treatment in regard to brace tolerance if any, about respiratory problems, and about pain, endurance, and weight change. The statistical analyses performed on the study data were Wilcoxon signed-rank test (significance level 0.05) using SPSS (IBM Corp. released in 2013. IBM SPSS Statistics for Windows, Version 22.0. Armonk, NY: IBM Corp.) for measurements before and after ITB of Cobb's angle (primary parameter), rib vertebra angle, and rib vertebrae angle difference and one sample binomial test for change in the levels of apex vertebrae and levels of curve measurements and Nash and Moe's classification

Table 1 Patient characteristics

Pt[a]	1	2	3	4	5	6	7	8	9
Age[b]	14.5 (13.3)	14.0 (2.8)	13.5 (13)	11.9 (19)	10.4 (11)	8.44 (1)	12.5 (51)	11.7 (5.9)	14.6 (10.7)
Sex[c]	fem	fem	fem	fem	fem	male	fem	fem	fem
Risser	0	4	0	0	1	2	4	4	4
Mena[d]	0[f]	13.6	14.2	0[e]	11.6	0[e]	16	12.3	14.2
Type of scoliosis[g]	Right TLS	Right TS	Right TLS	Right TS	Left TLS	Right TLS	Right TLS	Right TLS	Right TLS
Med. C[d]	BP + ED[h]	SPH + CM[h]	–	–	–	BP	–	–	BP

[a]Patient ID
[b]Age when diagnosed in years (time of injection after diagnosed in month)
[c]Gender (*fem* female, *male* male)
[d]Age of menarche (years)
[e]Before menarche
[f]No menarche due to hormonal imbalance
[g]Type of scoliosis (*right* right-handed, *left* left-handed, *TLS* S-shaped convex thoracolumbar scoliosis, *TS* thoracic scoliosis)
[h]Medical condition before injection (*BP* back pain, *SPH* physiological disorder of schizophrenia, *ED* eating disorder of anorexia, *CM* cyst in medulla)

Table 2 Radiological effects

Pt ID[a]	1	2	3	4	5	6	7	8	9	P value[b]
cobb t pre[c]	23.5(6.1)	38.7(8.1)	29.5(2.3)	12(19.6)	11.7(15.2)	18.6(14.0)	23(10.0)	31.1(17.0)	43.5(3.0)	
cobb t post[c]	16.2(12.2)	33.3(8.1)	33.1(3.3)	3.8(6.4)	7.1(4.5)	7.3(11.7)	24.4(16.4)	33.3(15.5)	28.4(3.0)	0.015**
cobb l pre[d]	40.9(7.3)	21(9.8)	11.6(13.8)	3.6(16.3)	22.7(9.6)	14.5(12.1)	16.5(12.0)	31.5(14.0)	41.8(10.4)	
cobb l post[d]	37.3(5.4)	20.4(0.1)	12(1.4)	1(2.6)	26(6.8)	6.5(3.6)	18.8(1.7)	28.2(18.3)	39.1(3.2)	0.038**
RA conc pre[e]	46.6	60.6	75.8	62.5	78.6	55.1	65.5	72.2	73.6	
RA conc post[e]	73	64	65.8	58.6	64.4	56.4	78.5	68.6	75	0.953
RA conv pre[f]	72.6	80.3	58.5	62.7	76.9	55.4	63.9	73.5	70.5	
RA conv post[f]	69.7	69.4	54.5	69.6	83.2	63.4	58.6	61.1	69.1	0.594
RVAD pre[g]	− 26	− 19.7	17.3	− 0.2	1.7	− 0.3	1.6	− 1.3	3.1	
RVAD post[g]	3.3	− 5.4	11.3	− 11	− 18.8	− 7	19.9	7.5	5.9	0.594

Pt ID[h]	Pre Pt1	Post Pt1	Pre Pt2	Post Pt2	Pre Pt3	Post Pt3	Pre Pt4	Post Pt4	Pre Pt5	Post Pt5
TuppV[i]	Th3	Th5	Th6	Th6	Th5	Th4	Th5	Th6	Th4	Th4
TlowV	Th11	Th11	Th12	Th12	L1	L1	Th11	L3	Th11	Th11
ThoNM[j]	2	1	3	1	2	1	1	2	1	1
T apex[k]	Th7	Th7	Th9	Th9	Th10	Th10	Th9	Th10	Th7	Th8
LuppV	Th9	Th10	Th12	Th12	Th12	Th12	Th10	Th12	Th10	Th10
LlowV	L4	L4	L4	L4	L4	L5	L4	L4	L4	L4
LumNM	3	2	3	1	2	1	1	1	3	1
L apex	L1	L1	L2	L2	L2	L2	L1	L2	L2	L1

Pt ID[h]	Pre Pt6	Post Pt6	Pre Pt7	Post Pt7	Pre Pt8	Post Pt8	Pre Pt9	Post Pt9		P value[l]
TuppV	Th1	Th1	Th7	Th4	Th4	Th5	Th5	Th5		
TlowV	L3	L4	Th12	Th12	Th12	Th12	Th11	Th12		0.508
ThoNM	1	1	2	2	2	1	2	1		0.201
T apex	Th9	Th10	Th9	Th9	Th7	Th8	Th8	Th8		1.00
LuppV	Th11	Th12	Th12	Th12	Th11	Th11	Th11	Th11		
LlowV	L4	L5	L4	L4	L4	L5	L4	L4		0.180
LumNM	1	1	1	1	2	1	3	2		0.023***
L apex	L2	L3	L2	L2	L2	L2	L1	L2		1.00

[a]Pre- and post-injection values for patient ID
[b]Significance level after Wilcoxon signed-rank test (**significant at a level < 0.05)
[c]Pre- and post-injection thoracic Cobb's angle
[d]Pre- and post-injection lumbar Cobb's angle
[e]Pre- and post-injection rib vertebrae angle on the concave side
[f]Pre- and post-injection rib vertebrae angle on the convex side
[g]Pre- and post-injection rib vertebrae angle difference
[h]Pre- and post-injection values for patient ID
[i]Upper and lower levels for measurement of Cobbs angle (T thoracic, L lumbar)
[j]Measurements of Nash and Moe's classification (Tho thoracic, Lum lumbar)
[k]Apex vertebra (T thoracic, L lumbar)
[l]Significance level after Wilcoxon signed-rank test or binomial test (***significant at a level < 0.05)

(significance level 0.05); if, in the Nash and Moe's classification, the level of measurement of Cobb's angle or apex vertebrae changed with one, we considered this as a change (+ 1), otherwise as no effect (0).

In this study, an *off label* medicine was used in children and adolescents. We obtained appropriate permissions from the Danish local ethical committee and the Danish Health and Medicine Authority (EudraCT number 2008-004584-19). The good clinical practice unit of Copenhagen monitored this study, and we screened the patients continuously for events, adverse events, and serious adverse events throughout the study period according to national guidelines, the European GCP guidelines, and the Helsinki II Declaration for biomedical research involving humans. We received no commercial or public financial support during the study.

Results

Nine patients with AIS met the inclusion criteria. The patients maintained prior treatment of physiotherapy, bracing and otherwise throughout the study period. No patients were excluded, lost at follow-up, or withdrew from the study.

The primary outcome parameters with their subsequent statistical analyses are shown in Table 2. Figures 2 and 3 illustrate the changes of radiographic parameters graphically and schematically.

Table 3 shows the clinical history of using brace treatment and subsequent surgery, the ITB and the clinical feedback throughout the study, where we noted remarks from patients and parents after ITB by open questioning. Two patients reported temporary soreness at the injection site, which regressed within days, and no other serious adverse events occurred during the study, except for one patient who was injected in the erector spine and quadratus lumborum as well as in the PM. No other major medical or orthopedic surgical events at the time of and after termination of the study; the subsequent spinal surgeries took placed years after injection treatment.

Discussion

The temporary muscular paralysis of the PM leads to radiological changes in the spinal deformity of thoracolumbar AIS. These radiographic changes were a significant improvement (lesser curve) in thoracic and lumbar Cobb's angle and a non-significant thoracic and significant lumbar derotation (changes in Nash and Moe's classification), and a non-significant small average change in rib vertebra angles with an improvement on the convex side and a deterioration on the concave side. These changes were as expected better in the lumbar region, since the primary effect is in the lumbar region, thus having subsequent less change in the thoracic region as seen in Fig. 2. This implies that the spine muscles do play a role in maintaining the human adolescent idiopathic scoliosis by the muscle contraction or pull by the PM, which was to be expected if the muscle pull by contraction was released in the lumbar area with subsequent effect in the thoracic area as hypnotized earlier. We prescribed the radiological changes to the induced muscular paralysis due to the short follow-up of 6 weeks, since all prior treatments were maintained and no other clinical events occurred in the patient's life.

A methodological obstacle of this study was to find an adequate way of evaluating our radiographic results. In clinical practice, a Cobb's angle of at least in between 5° and 10° would be a cutoff value of clinical radiographic change [21]. The diurnal variation in Cobb's angle for AIS is 5° and the inter- and intra-observer variations are 7.2° and 4.9°, respectively [22]. In this study, we would expect subtle smaller radiographic changes, due to ITB which induces only partial reduction of muscle function [23, 24], and seen in this perspective, we would not

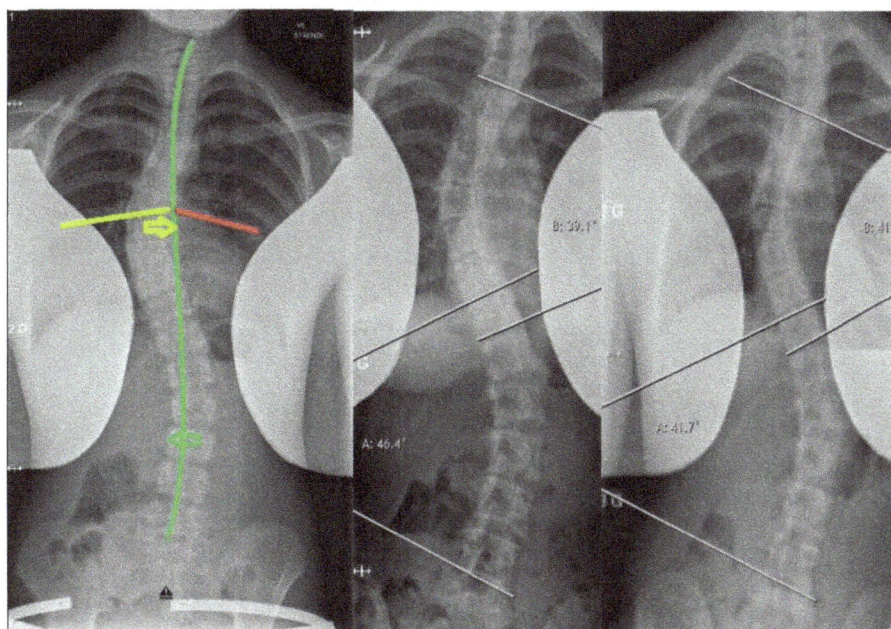

Fig. 2 Changes in radiographic parameters. To the left: dark green, significant improvement in Cobb's angle (curves) and Nash and Moe's classification (error); light green, insignificant improvement in Nash and Moe's classification (error) and in rib vertebra angle (line); red, insignificant deterioration in rib vertebra angle (line). To the middle and right: an example of pre- (middle) and post-injection (right) radiographs for patient number 9, where there is a smaller lumbar Cobb's angle and larger thoracic Cobb's angle after injection of botulinum toxin A

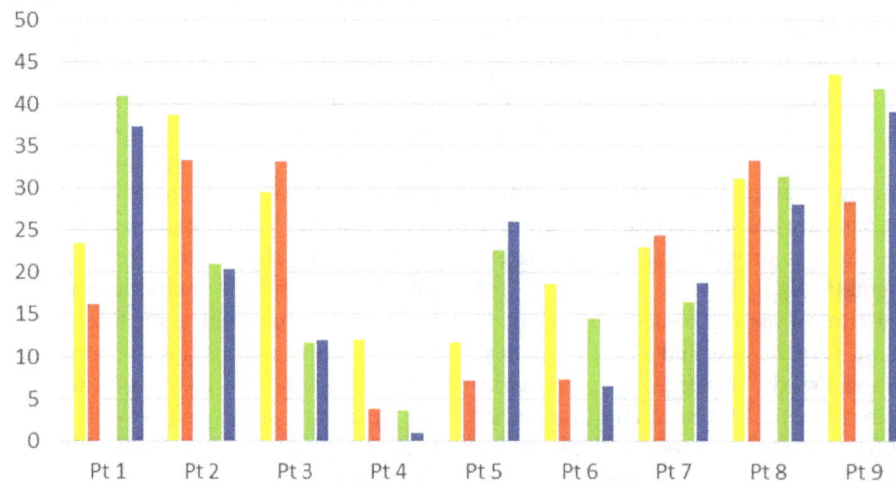

Fig. 3 Changes in radiographic parameters: patient number on the ordinal axis (x) and Cobb's angle on the vertical axis (y): yellow = Cobb's angle pre-injection in the thoracic spine, red = Cobb's angle post-injection in the thoracic spine, green = Cobb's angle pre-injection in the lumbar spine, and blue = Cobb's angle post-injection in the lumbar spine

expect to detect radiological changes as high as clinical cutoff values [18]. Moreover, three patients had main thoracic curves (patients 3, 4, and 7), and we would expect lesser effect (as in fact seen) than if all patients had main lumbar curves. Additionally, our intra-observer variation for Cobb's angle was high (average SD of 9.1°) in spite of trying to minimize measuring error by using three blinded experienced doctors and achieve higher accuracy in our radiological recordings by a standardized standing radiographic protocol. For these reasons, we used nonparametric statistical analyses of Wilcoxon signed-rank and one sample binomial test, in which the clinical cutoff value was not included.

In this study, the role of the PM muscle in humans would be scoliogenic, which maintains AIS, but this conclusion can probably not be extrapolated to all of the paravertebral muscles in general. However, to our knowledge, this is the first study in the paravertebral muscles that are influenced directly by the immediate temporary paralysis in humans in order to examine the role in AIS, which in our view is being an important step for the further exploration and understanding of the etiology of AIS. We would recommend to examine this by stimulation instead of paralysis for future studies as suggested by Grivas et al. [10]. Our above-described radiographic changes may be seen as mimicking a "wavy pattern" as described earlier [4], where slight changes in level and size occurred as a response to the almost immediate paralysis of the PM muscle. However, if bilateral paralyses were performed instead of unilateral, this might have resulted in larger changes and have shed light on the role of the paravertebral muscles even further, but bilateral paralysis was omitted for safety reasons to minimize botulinum toxin dosage for the patients to prevent

Table 3 Clinical treatment and Experimental injections

Pt. [*1]	1	2	3	4	5	6	7	8	9
Brace[*2]	Prov	Prov	Prov	0	Prov	0	Prov	Prov	Prov
IniBra[*3]	7.6	6.3	3.0		6		26.5	16.4	9.3
TermBra[*4]	52.4	21.7[*5]	51.8		28[*6]		67.9	42.7	31.7
TInj[*7]	10.7	2.87	13.45	11.94	1	10.4	51.2	5.9	13.37
IDose[*8]	100	100	100	100	100	100	100	100	420
TMusc[*9]	IP dex	IP dex	IP dex	IP dex	IP dex	IP dex	IP dex	IP dex	IPQE
Med. E[*10]	S, TBP	–	–	–	–	NBP	–	–	S, NBP
Surg. E	–	SU [*13]	SU [*13]	SU [*13]	cancelled SU[*12]	SU [*14]	–	–	–

*1 Patient ID *2 Type of Brace (Prov = Providence brace, 0 = no brace) *3 treated with Brace from time of diagnosis - initiation (months) *4 treated with brace from time of diagnosis - termination (months) *5 Brace abandoned due to physiological disorder of schizophrenia *6 omit brace treatment due to discomfort and psychological reasons *7 treated with injection from time of diagnosis (months) *8 Injection dose (Allergan units) *9 Injection in target muscles (IP = Iliopsoas, IPQE = Iliopsoas, quadratus lumborum and erector spinae, dex = right side, sin = left side) *10 clinical effects or adverse events after injection (S = soreness, NBP = no effect on back pain, TBP = temporary effect on back pain) * 11 surgical history at a later stage (SU = Spinal corrective surgery) *12 Su cancelled due to eating disorder and hormone treatment *13 correction at level Th4-L1 ad modem K2 M *14 correction at level Th3-L2 ad modem MESA Range + removal of cyst in medulla systemic spread, and ethical approval was only for unilateral treatment. Moreover, studies using electromyography and/or magnetic resonance imaging for muscle volume and muscle quality (fatty infiltration) indicate that the spinal muscles are significantly stronger and larger on the convex side at the apex of the curve of the scoliosis [9, 11, 25, 26]; this would indicate that ITB of the paravertebral muscles would have a correcting effect, when injected on the convex side. At the initiation of this study, we evaluated that the muscle contraction/pull of PM on the concave side of the lumbar curve of the thoracolumbar scoliosis in fact brought about the deformity as seen in Fig. 1. In retrospect, the ITB should have been performed either on the convex side or bilaterally, and this could be undertaken in a future study, if another study using ITB in humans was to be undertaken. Our suggestion would be to focus on primary lumbar curves, since the radiological effects were more pronounced in this region. Also, the multifidi and quadratus lumborum muscles have been examined as potential scoliogenic muscles and could be of interest for future studies [10, 27].

The ethical motivation to perform such a study in humans should be discussed. Firstly, our primary ethical motivation for initiating this experimental study was to discover a potential effective corrective or clinical beneficial treatment for AIS. This should be performed strenuously protocolled experimental and monitored study as in this study. The window for effective ITB treatment for AIS would be in the small curve AIS as a supplement for our current conservative treatment of bracing. This might have been able to alleviate humans with brace-treated AIS, since it currently is strenuous and with low compliance to follow [28–30]. From this point of view, it would seem inappropriate not to look for alternate treatment strategies and it certainly would be attractive to find an alternative treatment or to supplement the current conservative treatment. This was our motivation for initiating this study, namely, to investigate if using ITB to treat AIS would lead to improvement of curve and stop curve progression for affected humans. This radiological corrective effect was plausible since we supposedly addressed the culprit of the potential pathology, namely, the PM muscle of the back. However, we did not find radiological corrective effect or patient-reported benefits to a convincing clinical level in our population of patients with AIS—even though radiological correction of significant magnitudes was achieved. We expected that it would be less stressful for the patients when wearing a corrective brace, but we did not find such an effect. In the aftermath of the study, five patients were candidates for surgery, which would suggest that the long-term effect of ITB was not seen. The ITB was in our evaluation unrelated to surgery, since these were performed several years later and ITB have an expected effect of

3 months and severe deterioration after ITB was not seen. However, since we were unable to detect a coherent clinical or corrective treatment for short-term effects, we decided not to perform a second injection in any of the patients in an "interim" analysis after inclusion after the ninth patient.

Conclusions

In conclusion, this study demonstrated that the paravertebral muscle psoas major do play a role in the pathology in maintaining adolescent idiopathic scoliosis, and this role is maintaining the curvature of the lumbar spine primarily and affecting the curvature of the thoracic spine secondarily.

Abbreviations

AIS: Adolescent idiopathic scoliosis; ITB: Botulinum toxin A as localized injection therapy

Acknowledgements

We acknowledge Billy B. Kristensen and Lene Larsen from the Department of Anesthesiology, University Hospital of Hvidovre, Denmark, for their participation in this study.

Funding

No funding was received during the study. All authors have no financial relationships relevant to this article to disclose. All authors have no conflicts of interest to disclose in relation to this study. No commercial or public financial support was received during the study.

Authors' contributions

All authors consented for the publication. All authors contributed equally in all the parts of this article. All authors read and approved the final manuscript.

Authors' information

None

Competing interests

The authors declare that they have no competing interests.

Author details

[1]Department of Orthopaedics, University Hospital of Hvidovre, Kettegaard Allé 30, 2650 Hvidovre, Denmark. [2]Department of Radiology, University Hospital of Hvidovre, Kettegaard Allé 30, 2650 Hvidovre, Denmark.

References

1. Vasiliadis ES, Grivas TB, Kaspiris A. Historical overview of spinal deformities in ancient Greece. Scoliosis. 2009;4(6):1–13.

2. Weinstein SL, Dolan LA, Cheng JC, Danielsson A, Morcuende JA. Adolescent idiopathic scoliosis. Lancet 3. 2008;371(9623):1527–37.

3. Kouwenhoven JW, Castelein RM. The pathogenesis of adolescent idiopathic scoliosis: review of the literature. Spine (Phila Pa 1976) 15. 2008;33(26):2898–908.

4. Modi HN, Suh SW, Yang JH, Hong JY, Venkatesh K, Muzaffar N. Spontaneous regression of curve in immature idiopathic scoliosis—does spinal column play a role to balance? An observation with literature review. J Orthop Surg Res 4. 2010;5(80):1–8.

5. Archer IA, Dickson RA. Stature and idiopathic scoliosis. A prospective study J Bone Joint Surg Br. 1985;67(2):185–8.

6. Wong C. Mechanism of right thoracic adolescent idiopathic scoliosis at risk for progression; a unifying pathway of development by normal growth and imbalance. Scoliosis. 2015;

7. Soucacos PN, Zacharis K, Gelalis J, et al. Assessment of curve progression in idiopathic scoliosis. Eur Spine J. 1998;7(4):270–7.

8. Machida M, Saito M, Dubousset J, Yamada T, Kimura J, Shibasaki K. Pathological mechanism of idiopathic scoliosis: experimental scoliosis in pinealectomized rats. Eur Spine J. 2005;14(9):843–8.

9. Riddle HF, Roaf R. Muscle imbalance in the causation of scoliosis. Lancet. 1955;18;268(6877):1245–7.

10. Grivas TB, Burwell RG, Kechagias V, et al. Idiopathic and normal lateral lumbar curves: muscle effects interpreted by 12th rib length asymmetry with pathomechanic implications for lumbar idiopathic scoliosis. Scoliosis and Spinal Disorders. 2016;11(Suppl 2):35.

11. Cheung J, Veldhuizen AG, Halberts JP, Sluiter WJ, Van Horn JR. Geometric and electromyographic assessments in the evaluation of curve progression in idiopathic scoliosis. Spine (Phila Pa 1976). 2006;1;31(3):322–9.

12. Kim H, Lee CK, Yeom JS, Lee JH, Cho JH, Shin SI, Lee HJ, Chang BS. Asymmetry of the cross-sectional area of paravertebral and psoas muscle in patients with degenerative scoliosis. Eur Spine J. 2013;22(6):1332–8.

13. Smidt GL, Blanpied PR, White RW. Exploration of mechanical and electromyographic responses of trunk muscles to high-intensity resistive exercise. Spine (Phila Pa 1976). 1989;14(8):815–30.

14. Bruggi M, Lisi C, Rodigari A, Nava M, Carlisi E, Dalla TE. Monitoring iliopsoas muscle contraction in idiopathic lumbar scoliosis patients. G Ital Med Lav Ergon. 2014;36(3):186–91.

15. Starcević-Klasan G, Cvijanović O, Peharec S, Zulle M, Arbanas J, Ivancić Jokić N, Bakarcić D, Malnar-Dragojević D, Bobinac D. Anthropometric parameters as predictors for iliopsoas muscle strength in healthy girls and in girls with adolescent idiopathic scoliosis. Coll Antropol. 2008;32(2):461–6.

16. Hansen L, de Zee M, Rasmussen J, Andersen TB, Wong C, Simonsen EB. Anatomy and biomechanics of the back muscles in the lumbar spine with reference to biomechanical modeling. Spine (Phila Pa 1976). 2006;1;31(17):1888–99.

17. Nuzzo RM, Walsh S, Boucherit T, et al. Counterparalysis for treatment of paralytic scoliosis with botulinum toxin type A. AmJOrthop. 1997;26:201–7.

18. Wong C, Pedersen SA, Gosvig K, Kristensen BB, Sonne-Holm S. The effect of botulinum toxin A injections in the spine muscles for cerebral palsy scoliosis. Spine (Phila Pa 1976). 2015 Dec;40(23):E1205–11.

19. Graham HR. Botulinum toxin: the first 25 years. A critical assessment of the role of Botox in CP: the first 25 years. 7th annual International Pediatric Orthopaedic Symposium. Florida, USA: Wolters Kluwer Health, Inc. 2010;2:605–610.

20. Schroeder AS, Berweck S, Lee SH, Heinen F. Botulinum toxin treatment of children with cerebral palsy—a short review of different injection techniques. Neurotox Res. 2006 Apr;9(2–3):189–96.

21. V.N. Cassar-PullicinoS.M. Eisenstein. (2002) Imaging in scoliosis: what, why and how? Clinical radiology. Vol57(7):543–562.

22. Carman DL, Browne RH, Birch JG. Measurement of scoliosis and kyphosis radiographs. Intraobserver and interobserver variation. J Bone Joint Surg Am. 1990;72(3):328–33.

23. Herzog W, Longino D, Clark A. The role of muscles in joint adaptation and degeneration. Langenbeck's Arch Surg. 2003 Oct;388(5):305–15.

24. Stone AV, Ma J, Whitlock PW, Koman LA, Smith TL, Smith BP, Callahan MF. Effects of Botox and Neuronox on muscle force generation in mice. J Orthop Res. 2007 Dec;25(12):1658–64.

25. Jiang J, Meng Y, Jin X, Zhang C, Zhao J, Wang C, Gao R, Zhou X. Volumetric and fatty infiltration imbalance of deep paravertebral muscles in adolescent idiopathic scoliosis. Med Sci Monit. 2017 May 2;23:2089–95.

26. Zoabli G, Mathieu PA, Aubin CE. Back muscles biometry in adolescent idiopathic scoliosis. Spine J. 2007 May-Jun;7(3):338–44.

27. Fidler MW, Jowett RL. Muscle imbalance in the aetiology of scoliosis. J Bone Joint Surg Br. 1976 May;58(2):200–1.

28. Reichel D, Schanz J. Developmental psychological aspects of scoliosis treatment. Pediatr Rehabil. 2003;6(3–4):221–5.

29. Bunnell WP. Nonoperative treatment of spinal deformity: the case for observation. Instr Course Lect. 1985;34:106–9.

30. Chan SL, Cheung KM, Luk KD, Wong KW, Wong MS. A correlation study between in-brace correction, compliance to spinal orthosis and health-related quality of life of patients with adolescent idiopathic scoliosis. Scoliosis. 2014;22;9(1):1.

9

Do the SRS-22 self-image and mental health domain scores reflect the degree of asymmetry of the back in adolescent idiopathic scoliosis?

James Cheshire[1]* ⓘD, Adrian Gardner[2,3], Fiona Berryman[2] and Paul Pynsent[3]

Abstract

Background: Patient-reported outcomes are becoming increasingly recognised in the management of patients with adolescent idiopathic scoliosis (AIS). Integrated Shape Imaging System 2 (ISIS2) surface topography is a validated tool to assess AIS. Previous studies have failed to demonstrate strong correlations between AIS and patient-reported outcomes highlighting the need for additional objective surface parameters to define the deformities associated with AIS. The aim of this study was to examine whether the Scoliosis Research Society-22 (SRS-22) outcome questionnaire reflects the degree of measurable external asymmetry of the back in AIS and thus is a measure of patient outcome for external appearance.

Methods: A total of 102 pre-operative AIS patients were identified retrospectively. Objective parameters were measured using ISIS2 surface topography. The associations between these parameters and the self-image and mental health domains of the SRS-22 questionnaire were investigated using correlation coefficients.

Results: All correlations between the parameters of asymmetry and SRS-22 self-image score were of weak strength. Similarly, all correlations between the parameters of asymmetry and SRS-22 mental health score were of weak strength.

Conclusion: The SRS-22 mental health and self-image domains correlate poorly with external measures of deformity. This demonstrates that the assessment of mental health and self-image by the SRS-22 has little to do with external torso shape. Whilst the SRS-22 assesses the patient as a whole, it provides little information about objective measures of deformity over which a surgeon has control.

Keywords: Adolescent idiopathic scoliosis (AIS), Surface topography, Scoliosis Research Society-22 (SRS-22), Patient-reported outcomes, Health-related quality of life (HRQOL), ISIS2

Background

Adolescent idiopathic scoliosis (AIS) is a three-dimensional deformity of the spine typically associated with a range of torso abnormalities including rib and scapula prominences, asymmetry of the shoulders, chest wall deformity and waist asymmetry [1].

Correction of visible deformity is increasingly becoming recognised as an important indication for surgical intervention [2] with one of the goals of surgery being to improve both physical health and health-related quality of life (HRQOL) [3]. Both AIS patients and their parents have associated aesthetic concerns [4, 5], with reduction of visible deformity found to be the second most common reason for patients requesting surgical intervention [5].

In light of the increasing recognition and importance of patient-reported outcomes, attempts have been made to develop objective measures to address patient's HRQOL. One questionnaire by the Scoliosis Research Society (SRS), the SRS-22 [6], has been validated in pre-operative AIS and adult scoliosis patients and has been shown to have excellent internal consistency and reliability [7–9].

* Correspondence: james.cheshire@nhs.net
[1]Institute of Metabolism and Systems Research (IMSR), University of Birmingham, Birmingham, UK
Full list of author information is available at the end of the article

It is established that patients with AIS suffer from reduced HRQOL, often experiencing more pain, impaired function, lower self-esteem and increased rates of depression than their contemporaries [10–13]. A review by Rushton and Grevitt found that, compared to unaffected peers, patients with AIS had statistically worse pain and poorer self-image [14]. Of these SRS domains, self-image was the only one found to be consistently worse clinically.

The traditional measurement for quantifying spinal deformity is the Cobb angle [15], which is a measurement of the size of the curve in the spine in the coronal plane measured on a posterior-anterior radiograph. This measurement assesses spinal deformity in a two-dimensional uni-planar manner. Due to the three-dimensional nature of the deformity in AIS, the use of the Cobb angle has drawbacks and fails to take into account patients' perceptions of their deformity. Furthermore, several studies have demonstrated that radiological parameters do not correlate well with patients' subjective perception of body image [1, 16–18]. For this reason, it is increasingly recognised that in addition to radiological measurements, supplementary outcome measures are required to better quantify the deformity [16].

Over the years, new modes of assessing deformity have been developed. Surface topography is one such method allowing a non-invasive, three-dimensional assessment of the surface of the back or torso to be performed, and it has been well validated for assessing spinal deformity in scoliosis [19–23]. Several studies have demonstrated moderate correlation between surface topography and the SRS-22 scores specifically in the self-image and mental health domains [8, 23, 24]. Despite demonstrating these correlations, Brewer et al. [24] concluded that the patients' view of deformity may be related to other factors that were not fully assessed by their current methodology, highlighting a need to determine additional objective parameters that would better correlate with the patients' perceptions of their condition.

When attempting to define these additional parameters, reference was made to previous work demonstrating that the shoulder balance, scapula prominence and waistline asymmetry are the most important factors that contribute to overall trunk deformity in AIS patients [25–27].

The purpose of the study was to analyse how well the SRS-22 domains of mental health and self-image reflect the objective parameters of asymmetry measured using the Integrated Shape Imaging System 2 (ISIS2) surface topography system. The overriding aim was to assess whether the SRS-22 questionnaire reflects the measured trunk deformity in areas known to be of concern in AIS and that the surgeon has the opportunity to influence during surgery.

Methods

This study retrospectively identified 102 pre-operative patients with previously untreated AIS. Patients between 10 and 18 years of age were included. Patients undergoing conservative management with bracing were excluded from the study. The patient cohort was a consecutive series of patients presenting to the spinal clinic at our institution that met the inclusion/exclusion criteria. Each patient had undergone clinical assessment and surface topography using ISIS2 within 6 weeks of completing the SRS-22 questionnaire (mean difference 1 day, SD 6 days, range 0–41 days). Available spinal radiographs were only considered to be appropriate for assessment if taken within 6 weeks of the ISIS2 scan. All patients had undergone a whole spine MRI confirming a diagnosis of idiopathic scoliosis, as is standard practice at our institution. Prior ethical approval was gained (15/EM/0283) through the national ethical approval process.

A perfectly symmetrical back is one without difference between the right and left side of the body. Noting the importance of shoulder balance, scapula prominence and waistline asymmetry [24–26], the following parameters were chosen for use in our study.

The parameters 'AxDiffOff' for the axilla and 'WaistDiffOff' for the waist describe the difference (right minus left) in the distances from the midline for points marking the proximal end of the posterior axillary fold and the most medial part of the flank for the waist as shown in Fig. 1. A positive number indicates that the right side had a larger offset than the left. The parameters 'ShDiffHt', AxDiffHt and WaistDiffHt describe the difference (right minus left) in the relative heights of the shoulders, axillae and waist in a similar fashion. A positive number indicates that the right side was higher than the left. The parameters AxDiffOff, WaistDiffOff, ShDiffHt, AxDiffHt and WaistDiffHt were all measured from a two-dimensional photograph. The point used for the shoulder in ShDiffHt is marked from a vertical line from the axillary point as that line crosses over the edge of the shoulder girdle.

The three-dimensional aspect of ISIS2 is defined using volumetric asymmetry. The methodology for this parameter is as follows. Markers are placed on the bony landmarks of the spine and lumbar dimples so that the three-dimensional surface of the back can be related to body axes. A zero plane is defined through the sacrum and the vertebra prominens, parallel to the line running between the markers on the lumbar dimples. A curve is fitted through the markers on the spinous processes on the measured surface and is then used as the axis of symmetry. The difference between the areas of the back surface above the zero plane on each side of the symmetry line is then calculated for each transverse (horizontal) section and allocated to the higher side. The left

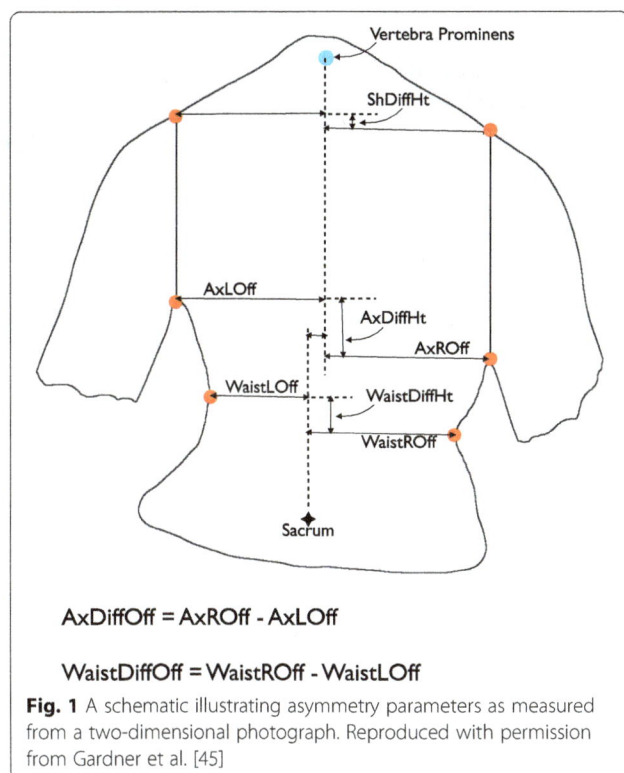

AxDiffOff = AxROff - AxLOff

WaistDiffOff = WaistROff - WaistLOff

Fig. 1 A schematic illustrating asymmetry parameters as measured from a two-dimensional photograph. Reproduced with permission from Gardner et al. [45]

and right volumetric asymmetry parameters are then calculated by summing the area differences on each side and normalising for back length, as shown in Fig. 2. The parameters 'VolL' and 'VolR' give objective values for the size (volume) of any rib or lumbar humps seen on the back. A new parameter 'VolSum' is defined as the sum of VolL and VolR. 'VolDiff' is defined as the difference of VolR minus VolL. These parameters give a measure of the total amount of asymmetry (right and left together) and the difference in the asymmetry between the two sides. An additional parameter 'ZScapDiff' is defined as the difference in magnitude between the maximum point (maximum height away from the zero plane) in the left and right scapular areas. These parameters give a measure of the three-dimensional asymmetry of the back.

Modifications were coded adding to the standard ISIS2 user interface to allow the user to locate the positions of the waist creases, axillae and shoulders by identifying these points with the mouse. The remaining parameters based on the standard ISIS2 parameters were calculated automatically as normal [21]. The analysis was carried out by a single researcher (AG) on the new two-dimensional parameters based on the manual identification of the waist, axilla and shoulder locations. The magnitudes of the radiographic spinal curves were measured using the Cobb angle method by the treating surgeon using Picture Archiving and Communication System software (GE Systems, New York, NY, USA).

The relationships between the scores for the SRS-22 self-image and mental health domains and the surface topography parameters were investigated using either the Pearson correlation coefficient (r) or Spearman's rank correlation coefficient depending on distribution of data type. R software was used for all data analysis [28]. The strength of correlation is defined as 0–0.29 is weak, 0.3–0.69 is moderate and 0.7–1.0 is strong [29]. Statistical significance was set at $p < 0.05$.

Results

Of the 102 patients included in the study, six (5.9%) were males and 96 (94.1%) females. The mean age of the patients at time of assessment was 14.3 years (standard deviation 1.29 years, range 11.32–17.6 years). Of the 102 patients, only 54 had an appropriate accompanying radiograph. There were 39 patients with Lenke type 1 curves, 13 with Lenke type 3 curves and two with Lenke type 5 curves.

Median total SRS score was 3.30 (interquartile range 2.91–3.82); median self-image score was 2.65 (interquartile range 2.20–3.15) and median mental health score was 3.38 (interquartile range 2.80–4.00). Median Cobb angle was 66.0° (interquartile range 54.0–74.8°).

Table 1 shows the statistics for the parameters of asymmetry and the SRS-22 questionnaire. All correlations between the parameters of asymmetry and SRS-22 self-image score were of weak strength. Similarly, all correlations between parameters of asymmetry and SRS-22 mental health score were of weak strength. Scatterplots of the SRS-22 self-image and mental health domain scores against parameters of asymmetry were drawn, but none showed a strong relationship. A sample scatterplot for WaistDiffOff and SRS-22 self-image is shown in Fig. 3.

Correlation analysis was also carried out on the Lenke 1 subgroup. The results were similar to the whole group, with all measured correlations being of weak strength. Analysis was not done on the Lenke 3 and 5 subgroups because of the low numbers.

Discussion

It is well established that patients with untreated AIS tend to suffer a reduced HRQOL often experiencing increased pain, impaired day to day function, lower self-image and self-esteem and increased rates of depression than their contemporaries [10–13]. The need to consider HRQOL when deciding treatment strategy is becoming increasingly recognised among clinicians [2] with one of the main goals of surgery now to improve both physical health and HRQOL.

There has been an increasing use of disease-specific, patient-reported questionnaires such as the SRS-22, the Spinal Appearance Questionnaire (SAQ) [30] and the Trunk Appearance Perception Scale (TAPS) [31], to help

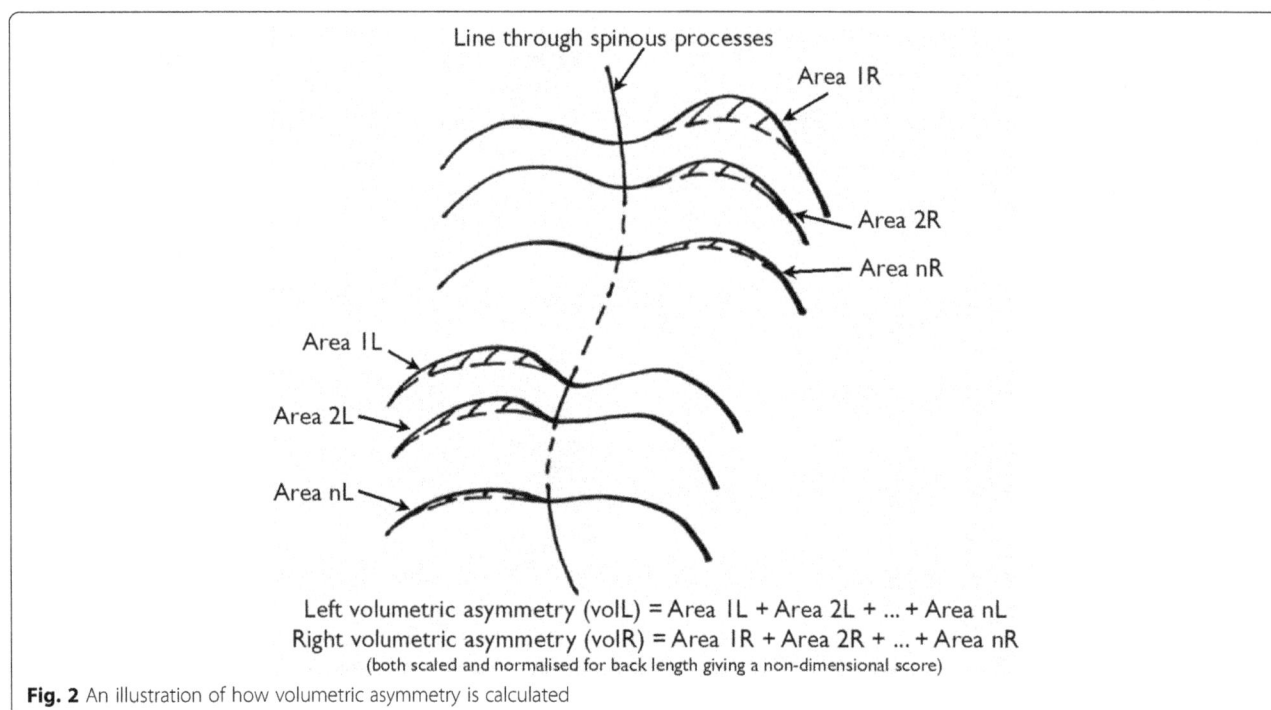

Left volumetric asymmetry (volL) = Area 1L + Area 2L + ... + Area nL
Right volumetric asymmetry (volR) = Area 1R + Area 2R + ... + Area nR
(both scaled and normalised for back length giving a non-dimensional score)

Fig. 2 An illustration of how volumetric asymmetry is calculated

clinicians assess a patient's HRQOL and decide on the most suitable management. Furthermore, questionnaires also allow clinicians to assess the impact of a specific management strategy.

Despite Cobb angle being the traditionally accepted standard for measuring the size of a scoliotic curve [15], Brewer et al. [24] demonstrated that volumetric asymmetry correlated better than the Cobb angle with the self-image and mental health domains of the SRS-22 questionnaire. This is not unexpected. Goldberg et al. in their paper of 2001 stated "it is the rib hump that the patient is unhappy with, not the value of the Cobb angle" [20]. The measurement of volumetric asymmetry enables clinicians to better address patient perceptions of their own deformity and in turn goes some way in understanding the psychological impact the resultant deformity has in AIS [11, 13].

Whilst the Brewer et al. study [24] demonstrated better correlation of the SRS-22 self-image and mental health domains with a volumetric asymmetry parameter from surface topography than with Cobb angle, the correlations were only of a moderate level. The authors concluded that volumetric asymmetry alone, as calculated by surface topography, was insufficient to completely explain a patient's own perception of self-image and mental health in AIS and that additional objective parameters were needed. This led to the development of the anatomical points for the shoulder, axilla and waist as used in this paper as it has been previously demonstrated that shoulder balance, scapula prominence and

waistline asymmetry are the most important factors that contribute to overall trunk deformity in AIS patients [25–27]. Using photographic measures to evaluate waistline asymmetry in patients with idiopathic scoliosis, Matamalas et al. [32] demonstrated significant correlation between anatomic landmarks of waistline asymmetry and

Table 1 A table of correlation coefficients and p values from parameters of asymmetry compared with Scoliosis Research Society–22 self-image and mental health domains

	Self-image	Mental health
ShDiffHt	$r = 0.06$	$r = 0.01$
	$p = 0.58$	$p = 0.94$
AxDiffHt	$r = -0.16$	$r = -0.21$
	$p = 0.10$	$p = 0.033$
WaistDiffHt	$r = 0.24$	$r = 0.10$
	$p = 0.014$	$p = 0.31$
AxDiffOff	$r = -0.17$	$r = -0.23$
	$p = 0.084$	$p = 0.02$
WaistDiffOff	$r = -0.28$	$r = -0.22$
	$p < 0.01$	$p = 0.027$
VolDiff	$r = -0.26$	$r = -0.13$
	$p < 0.01$	$p = 0.19$
VolSum	$r = -0.22$	$r = -0.09$
	$p = 0.024$	$p = 0.30$
ZScapDiff	$r = -0.21$	$r = -0.15$
	$p = 0.035$	$p = 0.13$

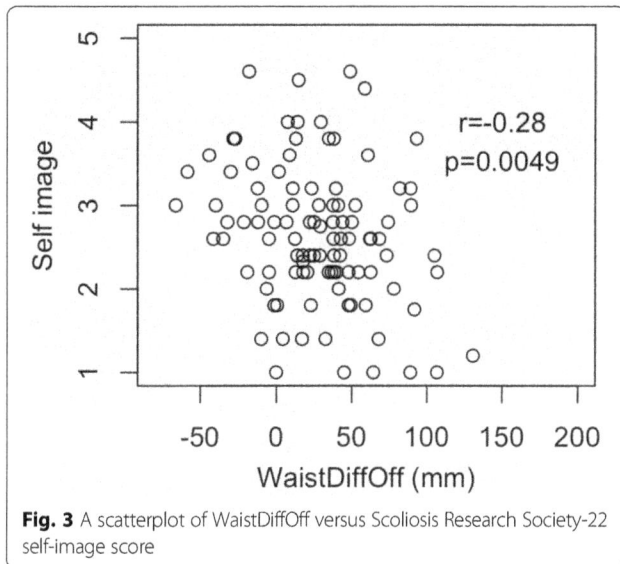

Fig. 3 A scatterplot of WaistDiffOff versus Scoliosis Research Society-22 self-image score

Cobb angle. Furthermore, a significant, yet weak, correlation between clinical measures of waistline asymmetry and the patients' perception of their deformity was demonstrated. Whilst considered a key factor in the perception of trunk deformity in scoliotic patients [25, 27], it has recently been suggested that patients' perceptions of their shoulder deformity do not correspond with clinical measures of shoulder balance. Using clinical photography, Matamalas et al. [33] demonstrated no correlation between clinical measures of shoulder balance and patients' perceptions of their deformity in non-operated scoliotic patients, calling into question the value of shoulder balance in the overall assessment of trunk deformity. Interestingly in a normal study population, Akel et al. [34] found that 28% had a shoulder imbalance greater than 10 mm. However, all of these people perceived themselves as having balanced shoulders. These findings suggest that in the absence of other aspects of trunk deformity shoulder balance goes unnoticed. In the scoliotic population it is possible that the presence of other aspects of trunk deformity may negatively impact their perception of their own shoulder balance.

This paper adds to the literature by demonstrating that the assessment of external deformity in AIS is not well performed when using the SRS-22 scores. Despite the extensive number of parameters of asymmetry used, our study was only able to identify weak correlations with the SRS-22 self-image and mental health domains. This demonstrates that the assessment of mental health and self-image by the SRS-22 seems to have little to do with measurable external torso shape. Whilst the SRS-22 assesses the patient as a whole, it provides little information about objective measures of deformity over which a surgeon has control during a scoliosis operation, one aim of which is to change torso shape.

It was interesting to note that WaistDiffHt and ShDiffHt demonstrated a positive correlation with SRS-22 self-image and mental health domains, although only WaistDiffHt with self-image was statistically significant. One would expect that as the difference in relative heights between the shoulder and waist points increases, the self-image and mental health domain scores would decrease, demonstrating a negative correlation. The significant unexpected positive correlation for WaistDiffHt could possibly be explained by the difficulty encountered whilst identifying the waist in some patients with scoliosis. The waist crease on the concave side is often clear while the waist on the convex side is not. The ability of surgeons to reliably determine waist and shoulder asymmetry in scoliotic patients has been shown to be poor [26]. It should be noted that all correlations measured here were of weak strength whether in the positive or negative directions.

The SAQ [30, 35], TAPS [31] and SRS-22 [7–9] have all been validated in AIS, with the SAQ validated for use with surface topography [23]. Despite the robustness of the SRS-22, it has been shown to have weak to moderate correlation with scoliosis magnitude measured using the Cobb angle [36]. Bago et al. demonstrated that this problem could be overcome by adding dimensions from a pictorial scale to improve correlation with scoliosis curve magnitude [37]. Both the SAQ and TAPS are pictorial questionnaires with their designs previously described [30, 31, 35]. Whilst both the SRS-22 and SAQ have been identified as having significant floor and ceiling effects limiting their ability to detect change [38, 39], the TAPS questionnaire offers an alternative and has been shown to have lower floor and ceiling effects [31].

No studies are known to have used surface topography to directly compare which questionnaires correlate better with HRQOL in AIS. Several studies have, however, used Cobb angle to do this [40, 41]. Matamalas et al. compared three questionnaires; SRS-22, SAQ and TAPS in idiopathic scoliosis [41]. The study found that all questionnaires demonstrated good internal consistency and correlation with scoliosis magnitude. SAQ and TAPS demonstrated the strongest correlation with each other ($r = -0.8$) whilst SRS-22 demonstrated medium strength correlation with SAQ ($r = -0.67$) and TAPS ($r = 0.46$). This finding suggests that pictorial scales such as the SAQ and TAPS might assess different constructs within body image. Both SAQ and TAPS correlated better with Cobb angle compared to SRS-22 self-image ($r = 0.61$, $r = 0.62$ vs. $r = -0.41$ respectively). Specifically, in younger age groups, there was a lack of correlation between the SRS-22 and Cobb angle, thus questioning the ability of textual scales to address self-image issues effectively in the young, a finding previously highlighted by Parent et al. [38]. Whilst pictorial scales clearly demonstrated a superior ability to address body image, they also correlated lower with the other HRQOL domains than textual scales. This led the authors to conclude that the concurrent use of both pictorial and textual scales would be best to address patient-reported outcome measures in AIS, a view supported in other reviews [40, 42].

There are several limitations to this study. Firstly, both its retrospective nature and method of patient sample selection have inherent shortcomings in terms of study design. Our cohort was a consecutive series of patients presenting to our institution's spinal clinic. We acknowledge that obtaining a random sample of patients would have been preferential and would have reduced any associated sampling bias. In our cohort, the ratio of females to males (16:1) is greater than the quoted sex ratio for AIS in the literature, where a ratio of 10:1 for curves greater than 30° is reported [43]. This bias towards a greater number of females may have caused a distortion of the results as females and males may react differently to the perceived aesthetic effects of their scoliosis [44]. Secondly, study patients may well have had concomitant mental health issues that were not necessarily a result of their scoliosis meaning that we may have been measuring the psychological consequences of other unrelated issues.

Future work should look to repeat the methodology described in this study but employing the concurrent use of the SAQ, TAPS and SRS-22 questionnaires to assess which questionnaire best addresses different facets of patient HRQOL in AIS. Future development of a combined pictorial and textual questionnaire to assess outcome measures in AIS should be considered.

Conclusion
Despite extensive use of surface topography parameters known to be important to patients, only weak correlations to the SRS-22 mental health and self-image domains could be demonstrated. Whilst the SRS-22 assesses the patient as a whole, it provides little information about objective measures of deformity over which a surgeon has control.

Abbreviations
AIS: Adolescent idiopathic scoliosis; HRQOL: Health-related quality of life; ISIS2: Integrated Shape Imaging System 2; SAQ: Spinal Appearance Questionnaire; SRS: Scoliosis Research Society; SRS-22: Scoliosis Research Society-22; TAPS: Trunk Appearance Perception Scale

Acknowledgements
We would like to acknowledge Professor Joanne Wilton of the Department of Anatomy, Institute of Clinical Science, University of Birmingham for her continued support.

Funding
None.

Authors' contributions
AG, FB and PP made substantial contributions to conception and design of the study. JC, AG and FB were involved in the acquisition of data, its analysis and interpretation of the data. All authors were involved in drafting the manuscript and revising it critically for important intellectual content. All authors read and approved the final manuscript.

Competing interests
The authors declare that they have no competing interests.

Author details
[1]Institute of Metabolism and Systems Research (IMSR), University of Birmingham, Birmingham, UK. [2]The Royal Orthopaedic Hospital NHS Foundation Trust, Birmingham, UK. [3]Department of Anatomy, Institute of Clinical Science, University of Birmingham, Birmingham, UK.

References
1. Smith PL, Donaldson S, Hedden D, Alman B, Howard A, Stephens D, et al. Parents' and patients' perceptions of postoperative appearance in adolescent idiopathic scoliosis. Spine. 2006;31(20):2367–74.
2. Negrini S, Grivas TB, Kotwicki T, Maruyama T, Rigo M, Weiss HR, et al. Why do we treat adolescent idiopathic scoliosis? What we want to obtain and to avoid for our patients. SOSORT 2005 Consensus paper. Scoliosis. 2006;1(1):4.
3. Kreder HJ, Wright JG, McLeod R. Outcome studies in surgical research. Surgery. 1997;121(2):223–5.
4. Koch KD, Buchanan R, Birch JG, Morton AA, Gatchel RJ, Browne RH. Adolescents undergoing surgery for idiopathic scoliosis: how physical and psychological characteristics relate to patient satisfaction with the cosmetic result. Spine. 2001;26(19):2119–24.
5. Bridwell KH, Shufflebarger HL, Lenke LG, Lowe TG, Betz RR, Bassett GS. Parents' and patients' preferences and concerns in idiopathic adolescent scoliosis: a cross-sectional preoperative analysis. Spine. 2000;25(18):2392–9.
6. Haher TR, Gorup JM, Shin TM, Homel P, Merola AA, Grogan DP, et al. Results of the Scoliosis Research Society instrument for evaluation of surgical outcome in adolescent idiopathic scoliosis. A multicenter study of 244 patients. Spine. 1999;24(14):1435–40.
7. Asher M, Min Lai S, Burton D, Manna B. The reliability and concurrent validity of the Scoliosis Research Society-22 patient questionnaire for idiopathic scoliosis. Spine. 2003;28(1):63–9.
8. Asher M, Lai SM, Burton D, Manna B. The influence of spine and trunk deformity on preoperative idiopathic scoliosis patients' health-related quality of life questionnaire responses. Spine. 2004;29(8):861–8.
9. Bridwell KH, Cats-Baril W, Harrast J, Berven S, Glassman S, Farcy J-P, et al. The validity of the SRS-22 instrument in an adult spinal deformity population compared with the Oswestry and SF-12: a study of response distribution, concurrent validity, internal consistency, and reliability. Spine. 2005;30(4):455–61.
10. Han J, Xu Q, Yang Y, Yao Z, Zhang C. Evaluation of quality of life and risk factors affecting quality of life in adolescent idiopathic scoliosis. Intractable rare Dis Res. 2015;4(1):12–6.
11. Freidel K, Petermann F, Reichel D, Steiner A, Warschburger P, Weiss HR. Quality of life in women with idiopathic scoliosis. Spine. 2002;27(4):E87–91.
12. Akazawa T, Minami S, Kotani T, Nemoto T, Koshi T, Takahashi K. Health-related quality of life and low back pain of patients surgically treated for scoliosis after 21 years or more of follow-up: comparison among nonidiopathic scoliosis, idiopathic scoliosis, and healthy subjects. Spine. 2012;37(22):1899–903.
13. Payne WK, Ogilvie JW, Resnick MD, Kane RL, Transfeldt EE, Blum RW. Does scoliosis have a psychological impact and does gender make a difference? Spine. 1997;22(12):1380–4.
14. Rushton PRP, Grevitt MP. Comparison of untreated adolescent idiopathic scoliosis with normal controls: a review and statistical analysis of the literature. Spine. 2013;38(9):778–85.
15. Cobb J. Outline for the study of scoliosis. Am Acad Orthop Surg Instr Course Lect. 1948;5:261–75.
16. Qiu X, Ma W, Li W, Wang B, Yu Y, Zhu Z, et al. Discrepancy between

radiographic shoulder balance and cosmetic shoulder balance in adolescent idiopathic scoliosis patients with double thoracic curve. Eur Spine J. 2009; 18(1):45–51.

17. Kuklo TR, Lenke LG, Graham EJ, Won DS, Sweet FA, Blanke KM, et al. Correlation of radiographic, clinical, and patient assessment of shoulder balance following fusion versus nonfusion of the proximal thoracic curve in adolescent idiopathic scoliosis. Spine. 2002;27(18):2013–20.

18. D'Andrea LP, Betz RR, Lenke LG, Clements DH, Lowe TG, Merola A, et al. Do radiographic parameters correlate with clinical outcomes in adolescent idiopathic scoliosis? Spine. 2000;25(14):1795–802.

19. Berryman F, Pynsent P, Fairbank J, Disney S. A new system for measuring three-dimensional back shape in scoliosis. Eur Spine J. 2008;17(5):663–72.

20. Goldberg CJ, Kaliszer M, Moore DP, Fogarty EE, Dowling FE. Surface topography, Cobb angles, and cosmetic change in scoliosis. Spine. 2001; 26(4):E55–63.

21. Sangole AP, Aubin C-E, Labelle H, IAF S, Lenke LG, Jackson R, et al. Three-dimensional classification of thoracic scoliotic curves. Spine. 2009;34(1):91–9.

22. Patias P, Grivas TB, Kaspiris A, Aggouris C, Drakoutos E. A review of the trunk surface metrics used as scoliosis and other deformities evaluation indices. Scoliosis. 2010;5(1):12.

23. Gorton GE, Young ML, Masso PD. Accuracy, reliability, and validity of a 3-dimensional scanner for assessing torso shape in idiopathic scoliosis. Spine. 2012;37(11):957–65.

24. Brewer P, Berryman F, Baker D, Pynsent P, Gardner A. Influence of Cobb angle and ISIS2 surface topography volumetric asymmetry on Scoliosis Research Society-22 outcome scores in scoliosis. Spine Deform. 2013;1(6):452–7.

25. Raso VJ, Lou E, Hill DL, Mahood JK, Moreau MJ, Durdle NG. Trunk distortion in adolescent idiopathic scoliosis. J Pediatr Orthop. 1998;18(2):222–6.

26. Donaldson S, Hedden D, Stephens D, Alman B, Howard A, Narayanan U, et al. Surgeon reliability in rating physical deformity in adolescent idiopathic scoliosis. Spine. 2007;32(3):363–7.

27. Kotwicki T, Negrini S, Grivas TB, Rigo M, Maruyama T, Durmala J, et al. Methodology of evaluation of morphology of the spine and the trunk in idiopathic scoliosis and other spinal deformities––6th SOSORT consensus paper. Scoliosis. 2009;4:26.

28. R Core Team. R: a language and environment for statistical computing. Vienna, Austria: R Foundation for Statistical Computing; 2013.

29. Jackson SL. Research methods and statistics: a critical thinking approach. 4th ed. Belmont CW. 2011. 69 p.

30. Sanders JO, Harrast JJ, Kuklo TR, Polly DW, Bridwell KH, Diab M, et al. The spinal appearance questionnaire: results of reliability, validity, and responsiveness testing in patients with idiopathic scoliosis. Spine. 2007; 32(24):2719–22.

31. Bago J, Sanchez-Raya J, Perez-Grueso FJS, Climent JM. The Trunk Appearance Perception Scale (TAPS): a new tool to evaluate subjective impression of trunk deformity in patients with idiopathic scoliosis. Scoliosis. 2010;5(1):6.

32. Matamalas A, Bago J, D'Agata E, Pellise F. Validity and reliability of photographic measures to evaluate waistline asymmetry in idiopathic scoliosis. Eur Spine J. 2016;25(10):3170–9.

33. Matamalas A, Bagó J, D'Agata E, Pellisé F. Does patient perception of shoulder balance correlate with clinical balance? Eur Spine J. 2016;25(11):3560–7.

34. Akel I, Pekmezci M, Hayran M, Genc Y, Kocak O, Derman O, et al. Evaluation of shoulder balance in the normal adolescent population and its correlation with radiological parameters. Eur Spine J. 2008;17(3):348–54.

35. Sanders JO, Polly DW, Cats-Baril W, Jones J, Lenke LG, O'Brien MF, et al. Analysis of patient and parent assessment of deformity in idiopathic scoliosis using the Walter Reed Visual Assessment Scale. Spine. 2003; 28(18):2158–63.

36. Asher M, Min Lai S, Burton D, Manna B. Discrimination validity of the Scoliosis Research Society-22 patient questionnaire: relationship to idiopathic scoliosis curve pattern and curve size. Spine. 2003;28(1):74–8.

37. Bago J, Climent JM, Pineda S. Adding a domain to the SRS-22 questionnaire may improve its metric characteristics. EurSpine J. 2008;17:151.

38. Parent EC, Dang R, Hill D, Mahood J, Moreau M, Raso J, et al. Score distribution of the Scoliosis Research Society-22 questionnaire in subgroups of patients of all ages with idiopathic scoliosis. Spine. 2010 Mar 1;35(5):568–77.

39. Roy-Beaudry M, Beauséjour M, Joncas J, Forcier M, Bekhiche S, Labelle H, et al. Validation and clinical relevance of a French-Canadian version of the Spinal Appearance Questionnaire in adolescent patients. Spine. 2011;36(9):746–51.

40. Bagó J, Climent JM, FJS P-G, Pellisé F. Outcome instruments to assess scoliosis surgery. Eur Spine J. 2013;22:S195–202.

41. Matamalas A, Bagó J, D'Agata E, Pellisé F. Body image in idiopathic scoliosis: a comparison study of psychometric properties between four patient-reported outcome instruments. Health Qual Life Outcomes. 2014;12:81.

42. Carrasco MIB, Ruiz MCS. Perceived self-image in adolescent idiopathic scoliosis: an integrative review of the literature. Rev Esc Enferm USP. 2014; 48(4):748–58.

43. Weinstein SL. Natural history. Spine. 1999;24(24):2592–600.

44. Brennan MA, Lalonde CE, Bain JL. Body image perceptions: do gender differences exist? Psy Chi J Undergrad Res. 2010;15(3):130–8.

45. Gardner A, Berryman F, Pynsent P. What is the variability in shoulder, axillae and waist position in a group of adolescents? J Anat. 2017;231(2):221–8.

10

Appraisal of the DIERS method for calculating postural measurements: an observational study

Brian Degenhardt[*], Zane Starks, Shalini Bhatia and Geoffroey-Allen Franklin

Abstract

Background: Surface topography is increasingly used with postural analysis. One system, DIERS formetric 4D, measures 40 defined spine shape parameters from a 6-s scan. Through system algorithms, a set of spine shape parameter values from 1 of 12 recorded images obtained during a scan becomes the DIERS-reported value (DRV) for postural assessment. The purpose of the current study was to compare DRV with a standard average value (SAV) calculated from all 12 images to determine which method is more appropriate for assessing postural change.

Methods: One mannequin and 30 human participants were scanned over 5 days. Values from each image and the DRV for 40 defined spine shape parameters were exported, and mean DRV, mean SAV, mean DRV, and within-scan variance were calculated. Absolute difference and percent change between mean DRV and mean SAV were calculated for the mannequin and humans. Inter-method reliability was calculated for humans. Within-scan variance for each parameter was tested for significant variability.

Results: For all spine shape parameters on the mannequin, absolute difference (< 0.6 mm, 0.1°, or 0.1%) and percent change (< 2.90%) between mean DRV and mean SAV for each parameter were small. Nine parameters on human participants had a large percent change (> 7%). Absolute difference between mean DRV and mean SAV for those nine parameters was small ($\leq$ 0.87 mm or 0.61°). Absolute difference for all other parameters ranged from 0.02 to 6.98 mm for distance measurements, from 0.01 to 1.21° for angle measurements, and from 0.15 to 0.22% for percentage measurements. Inter-method reliability between DRV and SAV was excellent (0.94–1.00). For the mannequin, within-scan variance was small (< 1.62) for all parameters. For humans, within-scan variance ranged from 0.05 to 36.04 and was different from zero for all parameters (all $P < 0.001$).

Conclusions: The minimal variability observed in the mannequin suggested the DIERS formetric 4D instrument had high within-scan reliability. The DRV and SAV provided comparable spine shape parameter values. Because within-scan variability is not reported with the DRV, the clinical usefulness of current DRV values is limited. Establishing an estimate of variance with the SAV will allow clinicians to better identify a clinically meaningful change.

Keywords: DIERS formetric 4D, Postural sway, Posture, Rasterstereography, Spine shape, Surface topography

* Correspondence: bdegenhardt@atsu.edu
A.T. Still University, 800 W. Jefferson St, Kirksville 63501, Missouri, USA

Background

Surface topography has recently gained popularity for the assessment of postural deformities. One method of surface topography, called rasterstereography, was developed by Drerup and Hierholzer in the 1980s [1]. This radiation-free technique projects horizontal stripes of light onto the surface of the participant's back, and static images of the lines are recorded and digitized. Based on the distortion of the projected horizontal lines, a three-dimensional image of the surface of the back can be produced, measured, and correlated with underlying spinal curve deformities [2–5]. Because of its non-invasive, non-contact, and radiation-free ability to observe posture and spinal deformities, one surface topography instrument, the DIERS formetric 4D (DIERS Medical Systems, Chicago, IL), allows researchers to observe a full profile of posture changes without the hazards associated with radiography. As such, it has increasingly been used in clinical practice.

Using the DIERS formetric 4D, a typical scan of the back for static standing posture analysis takes 6 s. During a scan, 12 images are collected of the posterior trunk. With each scan, the surface topography instrument calculates 40 defined shape parameters based on angles, distances, rotations, and deviations of the spine and pelvis. To determine the individual shape parameters reported from the series of images, an algorithm calculates average values from the entire scan for specific parameters. As a means of data reduction, the algorithm selects 1 of the 12 images closest to the average values and reports the spine shape parameter values for that image.

In general, there are two potential factors that contribute to variability in any instrument's output: the equipment and the patient being observed. For the DIERS formetric 4D, postural sway and body movement caused by respiration are sources of variability and are observed even when a person is standing still. While data reduction is a common practice with big datasets, it is unclear whether the above data reduction process, which prioritizes presenting data consistent with a graphical image, creates limitations when using the instrument longitudinally in the clinical and research arenas. By calculating the reported spine shape parameters from only one image, the data from each of the remaining images are ignored. Without this additional data, it is impossible to assess the precision or variability within a scan. Further, this data may influence the degree of change that is needed to identify real postural change when comparing studies over time. Studies involving patients with adolescent idiopathic scoliosis [2, 6] and without spinal deformities [7–10] have reported the reliability of the DIERS formetric 4D, but it is unclear whether reported values were the DIERS-reported value (DRV) from a single image or whether the values from each image

were exported and averaged to a standard average value (SAV) for each of the spine shape parameters.

The purpose of the current study was to compare the algorithm-selected DRV with the SAV calculated from the 12 images recorded during a single scan to determine which method is more appropriate for evaluating data. To our knowledge, no other study has evaluated a standard averaging method for the defined spine shape parameters available to the clinician. Rather than presenting the results from the image that most closely represents the average values of the images, we believe a true average of all values with an assessment of variability will be more clinically meaningful. As such, we hypothesized that, when scanning a human-shaped mannequin, minimal variability would be inherent within the instrument. Further, variability from postural sway and respiration in human participants would affect the spine shape parameter values. Therefore, representing the spine shape parameters as SAV with an indication of within-scan variability would be a more effective method for observation of postural changes in longitudinal and interventional studies.

Methods

For the current observational study, 30 male and female participants aged 18 to 65 years were recruited through campus email, posters, and word-of-mouth. Potential participants were excluded if they had a history of surgery to the spine or back tattoos, were unable to stand without assistance, or had a body mass index (BMI) above 35 or below 20. All participants reported to a university research laboratory and completed an approved informed consent form before participating. The local institutional review board approved all aspects of the study.

As a control, an adult-sized female mannequin was scanned daily for 7 days. The mannequin eliminated the human factor of postural sway and breathing and allowed for evaluation of the variability inherent to DIERS formetric 4D instrument. Any observed variability in those scans would indicate variability from the instrument rather than the more variable human form. To more appropriately approximate the human form, the two sacral dimples near the posterior superior anterior spines were modified on the mannequin using modeling clay (Fig. 1).

Before being scanned, human participants completed a short medical history and a demographic questionnaire. They then removed all clothing except for a pair of shorts so that the entire surface of the back was exposed from the top of the gluteal cleft to the base of the hairline. Participants were positioned on a platform 2 m from the DIERS formetric 4D projection unit. The heels of their bare feet were placed on the platform, so they were touching a plastic tube reference line. The plastic tube was secured perpendicular to the surface of the

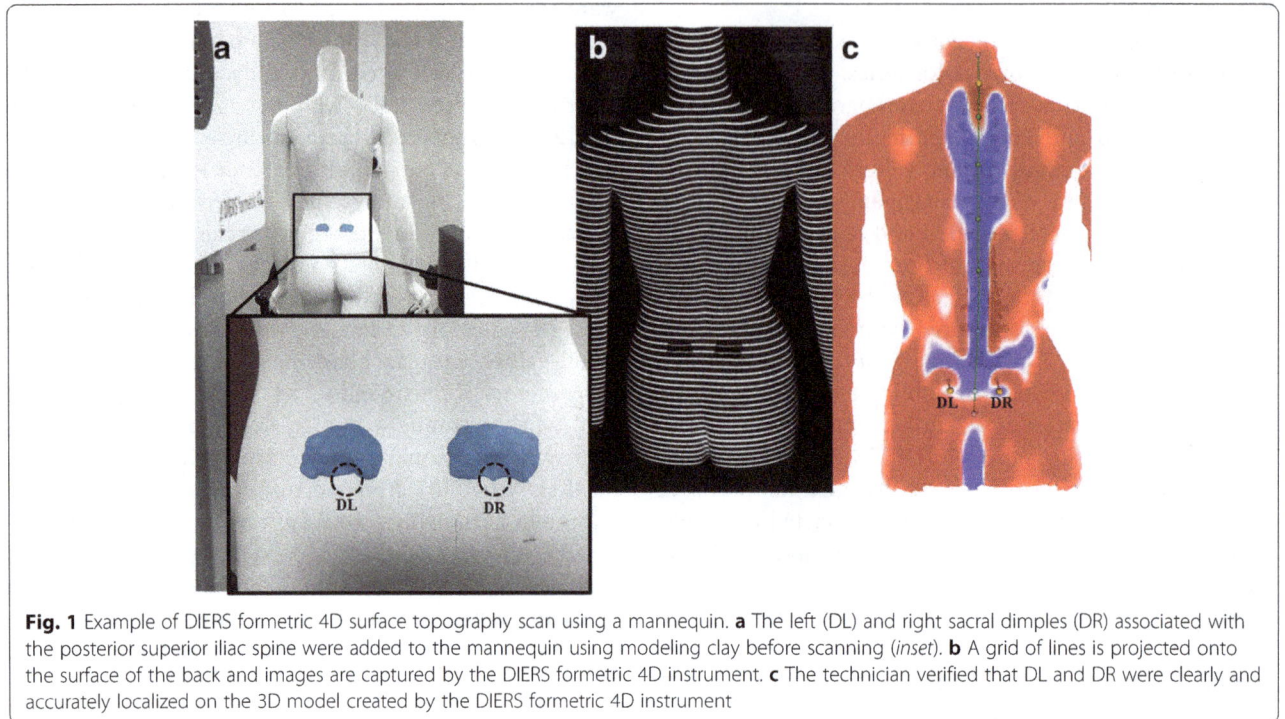

Fig. 1 Example of DIERS formetric 4D surface topography scan using a mannequin. **a** The left (DL) and right sacral dimples (DR) associated with the posterior superior iliac spine were added to the mannequin using modeling clay before scanning (*inset*). **b** A grid of lines is projected onto the surface of the back and images are captured by the DIERS formetric 4D instrument. **c** The technician verified that DL and DR were clearly and accurately localized on the 3D model created by the DIERS formetric 4D instrument

platform to ensure consistent anterior and posterior foot placement at a standardized distance from the camera, but it did not inhibit any natural hip internal or external rotation. After foot placement, the participants were asked to stand in a relaxed, natural position. In front of the participants, an adjustable fixed point was provided as a visual reference and was based on the shoulder height of the participants. Participants were instructed to focus their gaze on this fixed point during the scans to control head position. Thirty scans were completed for each participant over 5 days. Participants were scanned six times consecutively before moving from the platform. During each 6-s scan, participants were asked to stand naturally. Between scans, participants were asked not to move from the original position on the platform. The time to complete six scans was less than 6 min.

Each scan was completed in the DIERS data collection and processing software, DiCAM III, in the 4D average module. During each scan, 12 images were recorded over the 6 s (2 Hz). For each image, up to 50,000 points were captured, digitized, and analyzed automatically by the DIERS formetric 4D instrument. From each of the images, 40 spine shape parameters were exported for evaluation. These parameters were sorted into five subgroups based on the clinical relatedness of the parameter. These subgroup parameters included localization and distance, trunk and pelvis imbalances, spinal reference points, spinal curve measurements, and spinal deviation (Table 1). Spine shape parameters are reported in millimeters, percentage, or degrees depending on the specific parameter.

Each scan was processed as per the manufacturer's instructions. On each of the collected images, the software automatically indicated the location of the left (DL) and right (DR) sacral dimples associated with the posterior superior iliac spine [1] and the location of the vertebral prominens (VP), which is typically located at C7 [11]. The middle point between the dimples (DM) was determined from the location of DL and DR. Since accurate localization of these reference landmarks is vital for accurate spinal reconstruction, the location of these points was confirmed by the technician. The positions of DL and DR were represented by round, blue areas and indicated by a concave dimple on both sides of the spine near the posterior superior iliac spine (Fig. 2). For some scans, the DIERS formetric 4D improperly localized DL and DR markers on the participant's shorts or within concave areas outside of the actual dimple area. This problem was addressed by cropping at the lower edge of the image. The system then reprocessed the image and relocated the landmarks. If this method still failed to locate the dimples, the markers representing those dimples were manually moved within the DIERS processing program to their proper relative position, and the image was reprocessed so the marker was at the deepest point of the dimple. The VP was represented by a convex region at the base of the neck (Fig. 2). In a similar fashion, if the VP marker fell outside of this area, it was moved to the proper position at the most prominent portion of the convex region. Although the cropping tool is also available at the top of the image, cropping was not used

Table 1 Spine shape parameters output by the DIERS formetric 4D instrument and their definitions

Spine shape parameters by subgroup	Definition
Localization and distance	
Trunk length VP-DM, mm	The distance from VP to DM
Trunk length VP-SP, mm	The distance from VP to the SP
Trunk length VP-SP, %	The distance of VP-SP expressed as a percentage of VP-DM
Dimple distance, mm	The distance from DL to DR
Dimple distance, %	The distance of DL to DR expressed as a percentage of VP-DM
Trunk and pelvis imbalances	
Trunk inclination VP-DM, °	The angle between the line connecting VP-DM and an external vertical line
Trunk inclination VP-DM, mm	The distance between VP and the connecting external vertical line
Trunk imbalance VP-DM, °	The angle between the line connecting VP-DM and a vertical line through VP
Trunk imbalance VP-DM, mm	The lateral distance between VP and DM
Pelvic tilt DL-DR, °	The angle between the line connecting DL and DR and an external horizontal line
Pelvic tilt DL-DR, mm	The difference in height between DL and DR
Pelvic torsion DL-DR, °	The torsion of the surface normals of DL and DR
Pelvic inclination dimples, °	The mean vertical components of the surface normals at DL and DR
Rotation correction pelvis, °	In the frontal plane the angle of rotation of DR in the frontal plane in relation to DL
Spinal reference points	
Inflection point ICT, mm	The point of maximum positive surface inclination above the KA
Kyphotic apex, mm	The location of the posterior apex of the sagittal profile
Inflection point ITL, mm	The point of maximum negative surface inclination between the KA and the LA
Lordotic apex, mm	The location of the frontal apex of the sagittal profile in the lower region
Inflection point ILS, mm	The point of maximum positive surface inclination in the region between the LA and the sacrum
Fleche cervicale, mm	The horizontal distance between the cervical apex and the tangent through the KA
Fleche lombaire, mm	The horizontal distance between the LA and the tangent through the KA
Fleche cervicale VP, mm	The horizontal distance between the VP and the KA
Spinal curve measurements	
Kyphotic angle ICT-ITL, °	The angle between the surface tangents from the ICT and ITL
Kyphotic angle VP-ITL, °	The angle between the surface tangents from VP and ITL
Kyphotic angle VP-T12, °	The angle between the surface tangents on VP and the location of the calculated T12
Lordotic angle ITL-ILS, °	The angle between the surface tangents from ITL and ILS
Lordotic angle ITL-DM, °	The angle between the surface tangents from ITL and DM
Lordotic angle T12-DM, °	The angle between the surface tangents from T12 and DM
Pelvic inclination, °	The angle of the vertical surface normals from the horizontal of DM
Spinal deviation	
Surface rotation RMS, °	The RMS of the horizontal components of the surface normals on the symmetry line
Surface rotation, °	The maximum value of the horizontal components of the surface normals on the symmetry line
Surface rotation right °	The maximum value of the horizontal components of the surface normals on the symmetry line to the right
Surface rotation left, °	The maximum value of the horizontal components of the surface normals on the symmetry line to the left
Surface rotation amplitude, °	The maximal spinal torsion calculated from the maximal rotation to the right and the left
Trunk torsion, °	The maximal value of the horizontal components on VP compared to the horizontal components of the symmetry line on DM
Lateral deviation RMS, mm	The RMS deviation of the midline of the spine from the direct connection of VP-DM in the frontal plane
Lateral deviation, mm	The maximum deviation of the midline of the spine from the direct connection of VP-DM in the frontal plane

Table 1 Spine shape parameters output by the DIERS formetric 4D instrument and their definitions *(Continued)*

Lateral deviation right, mm	The maximum deviation of the midline of the spine from the VP-DM line to the right
Lateral deviation left, mm	The maximum deviation of the midline of the spine from the VP-DM line to the left
Lateral deviation amplitude, mm	The sum of the maximum deviation of the right and the left lateral deviation values

Spine shape parameter definitions adapted from DIERS formetric III 4D Manual (Created 21.06.2010, Revision grade 5) and DIERS Optical Measurement of the Spine Information for the Assessment (Version 1, Created 04.08.2009)
DL left sacral dimple, *DM* middle point between the left and right sacral dimples, *DR* right sacral dimple, *ICT* cervical-thoracic inflection point, *ILS* lumbar-sacral inflection point, *ITL* thoracic-lumbar inflection point, *KA* kyphotic apex, *LA* lordotic apex, *RMS* root mean square, *SP* sacral point, *VP* vertebral prominens

to relocate VP. Once it was confirmed by the technician that the points representing DL, DR, and VP were localized within the concave area of the dimples and on the convex area at the base of the neck on each image, no further changes were made to the scan.

To evaluate the SAV, a nested random effects model was built in SAS version 9.4 (SAS Institute, Inc., Cary, NC) for the 40 spine shape parameters (Table 1) using data from the mannequin that was collected on all 5 days and included the six scans from each day and the 12 images produced during each scan. Mean SAV and within-scan variance for each spine shape parameter were calculated from this model. Another nested random effects model was built for the mannequin using only the DRV for each scan rather than the values from each of the 12 images. Mean DRV for each parameter was calculated from this model.

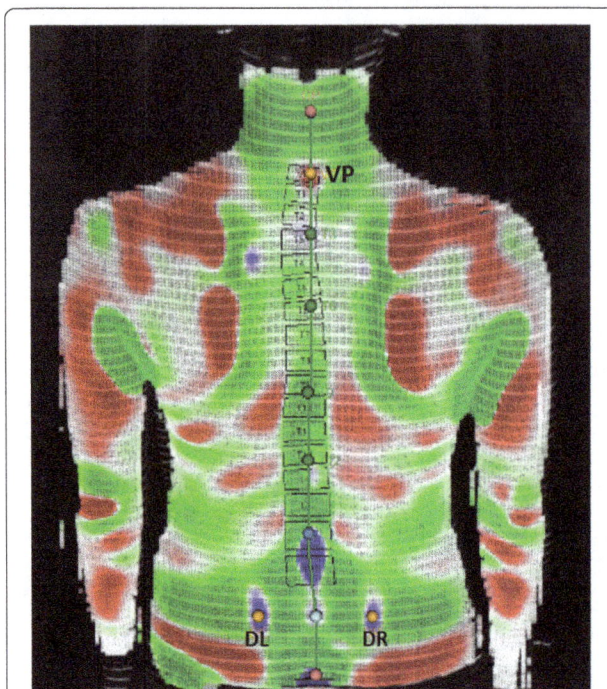

Fig. 2 Example of correct landmark localization by DIERS formetric 4D scan on a human participant. The technician verified that the automatically localized points of the left sacral dimple (DL) and right sacral dimple (DR) were within the concave dimples of the lower back (*blue*), and the vertebral prominens (VP) was within the convex region just below the neck (*red*) on each image from each scan

Percent change in mean was calculated between the mean SAV and the mean DRV for each parameter using the following formula: $\left| \frac{\text{mean of SAV} - \text{mean of DRV}}{\text{mean of SAV}} \right| \times 100$. Percent change was represented as an absolute value, so values of percent change are all positive.

Similar nested models were built using pooled data from the 30 human participants. Like the mannequin, two different models were built for human participants: one that contained the SAV and one that contained the DRV from each scan. Mean SAV for each parameter, mean SAV for each participant, and within-scan variance were calculated from the first model, and mean DRV for each parameter and mean DRV for each participant were calculated from the second model. Mixed effects analysis of variance models were built using mean SAV and mean DRV for each participant, treating method (SAV or DRV) as a fixed effect, and inter-method reliability was calculated for each of the 40 spine shape parameters using intraclass correlation coefficients (ICC). Percent change for human participants was also calculated between the mean SAV and the mean DRV for each spine shape parameter with the same formula described above. Using data from the human participants, we tested whether the within-scan variance from the 12 images within a scan was significantly different from zero. A significant variance would indicate that respiration and postural sway affected measurements within a scan, so evaluating parameters based on SAV would be more appropriate than using DRV. A *P* value less than 0.05 was considered statistically significant.

Results

The mannequin was scanned 42 times over 7 days. After the first 2 days, the landmarks were adjusted to ensure that the location of DL and DR were clearly defined. Thirty human participants (age 30.2 ± 9.8 years, BMI 27.3 ± 4.4) completed the current study: 15 males (age 31.9 ± 11.5 years, BMI 27.5 ± 4.1) and 15 females (age 28.6 ± 7.3 years, BMI 27.1 ± 4.8). Each participant completed 30 scans in 5 days for a total of 900 processed and analyzed scans. The location of at least 1 of the landmarks had to be manually adjusted for at least 1 image for 399 (43.33%) of the scans (Table 2).

On the mannequin, the mean DRV and mean SAV for each of the 40 spine shape parameters were similar

Table 2 Number of scans with landmarks adjusted

Scans	Landmarks adjusted, no. (%)
Total (n = 900)	399 (44.33)
Male (n = 450)	201 (44.67)
Female (n = 450)	198 (44.00)

(Table 3). The absolute difference between the mean DRV and mean SAV for each parameter ranged from 0.01 to 0.55 mm for all distance parameters and from 0.00 to 0.08° for all angle parameters. The percent change ranged from 0 to 2.90%.

For human participants, inter-method reliability between mean DRV and mean SAV was excellent for each of the 40 spine shape parameters (ICC = 0.94–1.00) (Table 4). The absolute difference between the mean DRV and mean SAV for localization and distance subgroup parameters ranged from 1.40 to 3.37 mm for distance parameters and from 0.15 to 0.22% for percentage parameters; the percent change ranged from 0.14 to 1.44% (Table 3). The absolute difference in the trunk and pelvis imbalances subgroup parameters ranged from 0.17 to 0.50 mm for distance parameters and from 0.04 to 1.18° for angle parameters; the percent change ranged from 1.55 to 719.76%. The absolute difference for the spinal reference points subgroup parameters ranged from 0.62 to 6.98 mm, and the percent change ranged from 0.56 to 20.32%. The absolute difference for spinal curve measurements subgroup parameters ranged from 0.67 to 1.21°, and the percent change ranged from 1.81 to 6.11%. The absolute difference for spinal deviation subgroup parameters ranged from 0.02 to 0.29 mm for distance parameters and from 0.01 to 0.61° for angle parameters; the percent change ranged from 0.23 to 31.68%.

For the mannequin, the largest absolute difference observed between the mean DRV and mean SAV was for kyphotic apex (0.55 mm) followed by trunk length from VP to the sacral point (0.13 mm) (Table 3). For human participants, the largest absolute difference observed between the mean DRV and mean SAV was for kyphotic apex (6.98 mm) followed by lordotic apex (3.75 mm), inflection point between the kyphotic apex and lordotic apex (3.64 mm), and trunk length from VP to the sacral point (3.37 mm). For the mannequin, the maximum lateral deviation of the spine to the left of VP-DM (2.90%) and the maximum surface rotation to the left (1.78%) had the greatest percent change between means. For human participants, pelvic tilt angle had the highest percent change (719.76%) followed by pelvic torsion (195.92%), rotation correction (123.16%), and pelvic tilt height difference (100.61%).

Within-scan variance for measurements on the mannequin was small (Table 5). For the mannequin, variance ranged from 0.0000 for rotation correction of the pelvis

to 1.6175 for the kyphotic apex. For human participants, within-scan variance ranged from 0.05 for the angle of trunk inclination between VP-DM to 36.04 for the inflection point between the kyphotic apex and lordotic apex. A significant within-scan variance was found for each of the 40 spine shape parameters for human participants (all P < 0.001).

Discussion

The current study was conducted to evaluate the difference between DRV and SAV for calculating spine shape parameters collected from the DIERS formetric 4D. Our results suggested that significant variability occurred within a scan and should be considered when evaluating the parameters of the DIERS formetric 4D. To optimally use the DIERS formetric 4D for longitudinal within-subject comparisons in research and clinical settings, investigators need to understand what the spine shape parameter values represent and the level of variability that occurs within a scan. This information will help researchers and clinicians to determine the level of change in spine shape parameters that can be attributed to an actual change rather than inherent variability that occurs within the human participant and instrument. To our knowledge, no previous studies have investigated the DIERS formetric 4D parameters with this level of critical within-scan analysis.

In the current study, completing scans on a mannequin allowed us to use a model of the human body to evaluate the instrument's algorithms for DRV in comparison with the calculated SAV while eliminating the influence of postural sway and breathing on within-scan variability. The absolute difference between the mean DRV and mean SAV was very small for all of the spine shape parameters. The largest percent change observed between the mean DRV and mean SAV was for the maximum lateral deviation of VP-DM to the left, which had an absolute difference of only 0.03 mm. The extremely small within-scan variance observed throughout each of the spine shape parameters was an indication of the ability of the DIERS formetric 4D instrument to evaluate the static human shape with a high level of consistency. In this circumstance, the DRV provides an adequate estimation of the SAV.

Larger differences between the mean DRV and mean SAV for each parameter were observed for our human participants because of the added variability from postural sway and breathing. Nine of the 40 spine shape parameters had a large percent change (> 7%). Parameters in the localization and distance subgroup and the spinal curve measurements subgroup did not have a large percent change when comparing mean DRV and mean SAV.

The parameters with the largest percent change were from the trunk and pelvis imbalances subgroup. Six of the nine trunk and pelvis imbalances parameters had an

Table 3 Comparison of means for DIERS-reported values (DRV) and standard average values (SAV) for each parameter

Spine shape parameter by subgroup	Mannequin				Human participants			
	Mean DRV	Mean SAV	Absolute difference	Change (%)	Mean DRV	Mean SAV	Absolute difference	Change (%)
Localization and distance								
Trunk length VP-DM, mm	426.95 (1.23)	426.98 (1.09)	0.03	0.01	463.35 (33.38)	465.83 (33.06)	2.48	0.53
Trunk length VP-SP, mm	462.34 (4.92)	462.47 (2.28)	0.13	0.03	511.31 (35.03)	514.68 (33.69)	3.37	0.65
Trunk length VP-SP, %	108.30 (1.12)	108.32 (1.11)	0.02	0.02	110.34 (1.81)	110.49 (1.77)	0.15	0.14
Dimple distance, mm	74.80 (2.94)	74.88 (1.58)	0.08	0.10	95.64 (11.95)	97.03 (11.06)	1.40	1.44
Dimple distance, %	17.47 (0.69)	17.49 (0.77)	0.02	0.12	20.68 (2.99)	20.90 (2.98)	0.22	1.03
Trunk and pelvis imbalances								
Trunk inclination VP-DM, °	2.41 (0.36)	2.42 (0.64)	0.01	0.37	3.09 (2.25)	3.14 (2.31)	0.05	1.55
Trunk inclination VP-DM, mm	18.26 (2.68)	18.32 (1.74)	0.06	0.33	25.49 (18.32)	25.99 (18.72)	0.50	1.92
Trunk imbalance VP-DM, °	0.78 (1.21)	0.78 (1.20)	0.00	0.62	0.16 (0.85)	0.11 (0.83)	0.04	37.28
Trunk imbalance VP-DM, mm	5.94 (9.16)	5.99 (3.29)	0.05	0.75	1.32 (7.16)	1.00 (7.15)	0.32	31.49
Pelvic tilt DL-DR, °	−2.25 (2.21)	−2.26 (1.67)	0.01	0.50	−0.11 (3.39)	0.02 (3.46)	0.13	719.76
Pelvic tilt DL-DR, mm	−2.98 (2.90)	−3.00 (1.91)	0.02	0.61	0.00 (5.78)	0.17 (5.91)	0.17	100.61
Pelvic torsion DL-DR, °	4.93 (0.71)	4.93 (0.89)	0.00	0.01	0.16 (2.70)	−0.17 (2.51)	0.33	195.92
Pelvic inclination dimples, °	36.47 (1.02)	36.40 (0.91)	0.07	0.18	19.06 (7.38)	17.88 (5.97)	1.18	6.59
Rotation correction pelvis, °	6.18 (1.47)	6.21 (0.91)	0.03	0.47	0.07 (3.14)	−0.32 (2.75)	0.40	123.16
Spinal reference points								
Inflection point ICT, mm	17.95 (2.25)	17.92 (1.68)	0.03	0.16	5.13 (10.40)	4.27 (10.15)	0.87	20.32
Kyphotic apex, mm	−81.19 (21.17)	−80.64 (4.64)	0.55	0.68	−183.81 (36.58)	−190.79 (24.53)	6.98	3.66
Inflection point ITL, mm	−257.38 (2.20)	−257.29 (1.46)	0.09	0.03	−307.74 (36.01)	−311.38 (34.68)	3.64	1.17
Lordotic apex, mm	−326.82 (4.25)	−326.74 (2.23)	0.08	0.02	−384.56 (35.82)	−388.31 (33.38)	3.75	0.97
Inflection point ILS, mm	−420.35 (3.59)	−420.23 (2.13)	0.12	0.03	−460.46 (42.03)	−463.06 (42.21)	2.60	0.56
Fleche cervicale, mm	33.11 (1.58)	33.09 (1.28)	0.02	0.06	71.08 (19.67)	73.69 (17.61)	2.61	3.54
Fleche lombaire, mm	27.14 (1.77)	27.16 (1.40)	0.02	0.06	36.62 (12.62)	37.24 (12.73)	0.62	1.67
Fleche cervicale VP, mm	9.25 (0.93)	9.31 (0.99)	0.07	0.70	45.32 (16.71)	47.71 (14.29)	2.40	5.03
Spinal curve measurements								
Kyphotic angle ICT-ITL, °	35.13 (0.72)	35.13 (0.84)	0.00	0.00	47.23 (9.35)	48.10 (9.05)	0.87	1.81
Kyphotic angle VP-ITL, °	31.53 (0.78)	31.55 (0.87)	0.02	0.08	45.33 (8.95)	46.27 (8.61)	0.94	2.03
Kyphotic angle VP-T12, °	31.47 (0.76)	31.50 (0.88)	0.03	0.08	41.87 (8.44)	42.54 (8.44)	0.68	1.59
Lordotic angle ITL-ILS, °	46.11 (0.63)	46.15 (0.78)	0.04	0.09	36.26 (8.53)	35.59 (8.35)	0.67	1.88
Lordotic angle ITL-DM, °	45.27 (1.08)	45.29 (1.05)	0.03	0.06	34.32 (8.77)	33.57 (8.53)	0.75	2.24
Lordotic angle T12-DM, °	45.24 (1.10)	45.26 (1.06)	0.02	0.05	30.86 (9.27)	29.84 (8.74)	1.02	3.41
Pelvic inclination, °	39.36 (0.50)	39.34 (0.68)	0.03	0.07	21.05 (8.74)	19.84 (7.49)	1.21	6.11
Spinal deviation								
Surface rotation RMS, °	4.56 (0.24)	4.56 (0.44)	0.00	0.02	3.74 (1.24)	3.75 (1.37)	0.01	0.23
Surface rotation, °	11.26 (0.49)	11.28 (0.70)	0.02	0.15	2.35 (7.23)	1.79 (7.20)	0.57	31.68
Surface rotation right, °	11.26 (0.49)	11.28 (0.70)	0.02	0.15	5.97 (3.51)	5.61 (3.43)	0.36	6.41
Surface rotation left, °	−2.20 (0.80)	−2.23 (0.89)	0.04	1.78	−4.38 (2.71)	−4.55 (2.93)	0.18	3.85
Surface rotation amplitude, °	13.49 (0.80)	13.57 (0.99)	0.08	0.60	10.38 (3.05)	10.20 (3.04)	0.18	1.78
Trunk torsion, °	12.08 (0.96)	12.06 (1.41)	0.02	0.18	3.96 (4.35)	3.35 (3.89)	0.61	18.11
Lateral deviation RMS, mm	4.51 (2.11)	4.50 (1.10)	0.01	0.23	5.53 (2.92)	5.59 (2.97)	0.06	0.99
Lateral deviation, mm	7.39 (1.33)	7.36 (1.36)	0.02	0.33	3.87 (10.05)	3.63 (10.28)	0.25	6.79

Table 3 Comparison of means for DIERS-reported values (DRV) and standard average values (SAV) for each parameter *(Continued)*

Lateral deviation right, mm	7.39 (2.08)	7.36 (1.36)	0.02	0.33	7.86 (5.60)	7.88 (5.76) 0.02	0.25
Lateral deviation left, mm	−1.16 (0.43)	−1.19 (0.57)	0.03	2.90	−4.73 (4.11)	−5.01 (4.13) 0.27	5.45
Lateral deviation amplitude, mm	8.59 (1.81)	8.60 (1.27)	0.01	0.15	12.64 (5.34)	12.93 (5.43) 0.29	2.27

DRV and SAV are reported as mean (SD)
DL left sacral dimple, *DM* middle point between the left and right sacral dimples, *DR* right sacral dimple, *ICT* cervical-thoracic inflection point, *ILS* lumbar-sacral inflection point, *ITL* thoracic-lumbar inflection point, *RMS* root mean square, *SP* sacral point, *VP* vertebral prominens

extremely large percent change between the mean DRV and mean SAV: angle of trunk imbalance between VP-DM, trunk imbalance distance between VP-DM, pelvic tilt angle, pelvic tilt height difference, pelvic torsion, and rotation correction. The high percent change for these parameters may be attributed to their small mean DRV and mean SAV values. Parameters from the trunk and pelvis imbalances subgroup, such as pelvic tilt angle, pelvic tilt height difference, and pelvic torsion, have been reported as less reliable [7, 10] and more variable [8, 10]. Further, studies have attributed the increased variability and the decreased reliability of these parameters to outside influence from inconsistent patient positioning between scans [7, 8]. Although these studies [7, 8, 10] focused on between-scan variability and reliability, positioning seems to have influenced their results. In the current study, only a single scan was considered, and the participants remained in the same position during the entire scan, as recommended by the manufacturer. The mannequin we scanned lacked postural sway and breathing, and we found very low variability for pelvic tilt angle, pelvic tilt height difference, and pelvic torsion. This variability increased with the human participants even though the magnitude of the means were very small. Taken together, these results suggest that postural sway and breathing should be considered as a component of within-scan variability and are likely a meaningful contributor to the reported between-scan variability due to patient positioning [7, 8].

Previous studies support this approach. Schroeder et al. [10] suggested that measurement error may be influenced by individual variation in the soft tissue structure. Although BMI has not been found to influence the reliability of the DIERS formetric 4D in calculating spine shape parameters [9, 12], parameters related to the pelvis are calculated and represented based on the localization or a derivative of the localization of DL and DR. Since the location of DL and DR are correlated to but not necessarily representative of the underlying structures of the pelvis [13] and because the position of these landmarks is used to create the Cartesian coordinate plane for back shape reconstruction [14, 15], postural sway may manipulate the contour of the soft tissue that makes up either dimple. The change in soft tissue contour could influence the consistency at which the DIERS formetric 4D localizes DL and DR and increase variability in the

evaluation of any parameter directly related to the pelvis. Although the current study did not investigate the effect of variability within the localization of DL and DR, clinicians and researchers should be aware that that observable changes within those landmarks may add to the within-scan variability and influence the ability to generate meaningful and comparable results.

Two of the nine spine shape parameters with a large percent change between the mean DRV and mean SAV were in the spinal deviation subgroup: trunk torsion and maximum surface rotation. The high percent change in trunk torsion is likely related to soft tissue changes. The maximum surface rotation evaluates the maximum rotation of the vertebra in either direction. Because this parameter accounts for the greatest rotation in either direction, a small change in posture because of normal postural sway during a scan has the potential to change the rotational characteristics of each vertebral segment and the location of the maximum rotation along the spine. Within the maximum surface rotation parameter, a change of direction or location could cause the value to flip from positive to negative, creating a large amount of variability. Therefore, the results of the current study show a larger percent change and variance for maximum surface rotation (percent change = 31.68%, variance = 6.30) than for maximum surface rotation to the right (percent change = 6.41%, variance = 1.36) and maximum surface rotation to the left (percent change = 3.85%, variance = 0.98). Without knowing the segment of maximum rotation, any observable change in maximum surface rotation which takes into account two directions along the entire length of the spine should be interpreted with caution.

One of the nine spine shape parameters with a large percent change between the mean DRV and mean SAV was in the spinal reference points subgroup: cervical-thoracic inflection point. To our knowledge, the reliability and variability of this spine shape parameter has not been previously reported. In the current study, a large increase in within-scan variance from the mannequin to the human participant was observed. Since the inflection point above the kyphotic apex is dependent on the change in surface curvature of the neck, any change in the head position because of postural sway or other reasons would be expected to influence the variability of this parameter. If the inflection point is a spine shape parameter of interest,

Table 4 Inter-method reliability for human participants between DIERS-reported value (DRV) and standard average value (SAV)

Spine shape parameter by subgroup	ICC
Localization and distance	
Trunk length VP-DM, mm	0.94
Trunk length VP-SP, mm	0.94
Trunk length VP-SP, %	0.99
Dimple distance, mm	0.99
Dimple distance, %	1.00
Trunk and pelvis imbalances	
Trunk inclination VP-DM, °	1.00
Trunk inclination VP-DM, mm	0.99
Trunk imbalance VP-DM, °	1.00
Trunk imbalance VP-DM, mm	1.00
Pelvic tilt DL-DR, °	0.99
Pelvic tilt DL-DR, mm	0.99
Pelvic torsion DL-DR, °	1.00
Pelvic inclination dimples, °	1.00
Rotation correction pelvis, °	0.99
Spinal reference points	
Inflection point ICT, mm	0.99
Kyphotic apex, mm	0.98
Inflection point ITL, mm	0.97
Lordotic apex, mm	0.97
Inflection point ILS, mm	0.95
Fleche cervicale, mm	1.00
Fleche lombaire, mm	0.98
Fleche cervicale VP, mm	0.99
Spinal curve measurements	
Kyphotic angle ICT-ITL, °	0.99
Kyphotic angle VP-ITL, °	0.96
Kyphotic angle VP-T12, °	0.97
Lordotic angle ITL-ILS, °	0.98
Lordotic angle ITL-DM, °	0.99
Lordotic angle T12-DM, °	0.99
Pelvic inclination, °	1.00
Spinal deviation	
Surface rotation RMS, °	1.00
Surface rotation max, °	0.98
Surface rotation right, °	0.97
Surface rotation left, °	1.00
Surface rotation amplitude, °	0.97
Trunk torsion, °	0.98
Lateral deviation RMS, mm	1.00
Lateral deviation, mm	0.96
Lateral deviation right, mm	0.98

Table 4 Inter-method reliability for human participants between DIERS-reported value (DRV) and standard average value (SAV) *(Continued)*

Lateral deviation left, mm	0.95
Lateral deviation amplitude, mm	1.00

DL left sacral dimple, *DM* middle point between the left and right sacral dimples, *DR* right sacral dimple, *ICC* intraclass correlation coefficient, *ICT* cervical-thoracic inflection point, *ILS* lumbar-sacral inflection point, *ITL* thoracic-lumbar inflection point, *RMS* root mean square, *SP* sacral point, *VP* vertebral prominens

because of the amount of mobility within the neck, more focus should be placed on finding a consistent stable position of the head.

Based on results of the current study and even though we observed large percent changes between DRV and SAV, the absolute differences between the mean DRV and mean SAV for each parameter in our human participants were small and likely not clinically meaningful. In addition, the inter-method reliability between DRV and SAV was excellent, indicating little difference between the two methods. Therefore, using either the DRV or the SAV is an acceptable method for evaluating spine shape parameters. The greatest determinant of which method to use may lie in the intention of the user. For instance, the DRV may currently be more useful for clinicians who want to quickly access parameter values, such as when looking at a pictorial representation of the posture. On the other hand, researchers may find the SAV is more meaningful when they want to observe the variability associated with each parameter. As found in the current study, when postural sway occurs, each of these parameters varies. Although no clinically relevant differences between DRV and SAV were observed, a significant within-scan variance was observed for all 40 of the human spine shape parameters, indicating that for an individual scan each parameter contained significant information not accounted for in the DRV. As such, we recommend that an indication of variability be reported to adequately represent the change that occurs from normal postural sway and breathing. Currently, to evaluate within-scan variability, data files from each image collected must be parsed, compiled, and analyzed. A representation of the within-scan variability inside the DIERS data collection and processing software would provide clinicians and researchers with immediate information to determine meaningful change whether they are evaluating the natural change of posture longitudinally or change from an intervention. Further, reporting variability will allow researchers to explore the normal range of changes that occur in the spine and pelvis during quiet stance and to determine normative ranges that can be used to understand meaningful change in future studies.

The current study had several limitations. One limitation is that the influence of head positioning on the spine shape parameters is unknown, but it is possible that variation in

Table 5 Within-scan variance for the mannequin and human participants calculated using the standard average value (SAV)

Spine shape parameter by subgroup	Mannequin	Human participants
Localization and distance		
Trunk length VP-DM, mm	0.0006 (0.02)	2.79 (1.67)
Trunk length VP-SP, mm	0.0010 (0.03)	7.21 (2.69)
Trunk length VP-SP, %	0.0001 (0.01)	0.22 (0.47)
Dimple distance, mm	0.0006 (0.02)	3.22 (1.79)
Dimple distance, %	0.0001 (0.01)	0.15 (0.39)
Trunk and pelvis imbalances		
Trunk inclination VP-DM, °	0.0001 (0.01)	0.05 (0.22)
Trunk inclination VP-DM, mm	0.0005 (0.02)	3.69 (1.92)
Trunk imbalance VP-DM, °	0.0001 (0.01)	0.06 (0.24)
Trunk imbalance VP-DM, mm	0.0007 (0.03)	4.13 (2.03)
Pelvic tilt DL-DR, °	0.0006 (0.02)	0.90 (0.95)
Pelvic tilt DL-DR, mm	0.0010 (0.03)	2.28 (1.51)
Pelvic torsion DL-DR, °	0.0007 (0.03)	0.62 (0.79)
Pelvic inclination dimples, °	0.0190 (0.14)	1.01 (1.00)
Rotation correction pelvis, °	0.0000 (0.00)	0.35 (0.59)
Spinal reference points		
Inflection point ICT, mm	0.0043 (0.07)	6.10 (2.47)
Kyphotic apex, mm	1.6175 (1.27)	8.04 (2.84)
Inflection point ITL, mm	0.0321 (0.18)	36.04 (6.00)
Lordotic apex, mm	0.0320 (0.18)	10.72 (3.27)
Inflection point ILS, mm	0.0112 (0.11)	15.90 (3.99)
Fleche cervicale, mm	0.0011 (0.03)	2.32 (1.52)
Fleche lombaire, mm	0.0010 (0.03)	2.07 (1.44)
Fleche cervicale VP, mm	0.0011 (0.03)	2.88 (1.70)
Spinal curve measurements		
Kyphotic angle ICT-ITL, °	0.0007 (0.03)	1.02 (1.01)
Kyphotic angle VP-ITL, °	0.0006 (0.02)	1.54 (1.24)
Kyphotic angle VP-T12, °	0.0004 (0.02)	1.18 (1.09)
Lordotic angle ITL-ILS, °	0.0004 (0.02)	2.29 (1.51)
Lordotic angle ITL-DM, °	0.0002 (0.01)	1.92 (1.39)
Lordotic angle T12-DM, °	0.0005 (0.02)	1.75 (1.32)
Pelvic inclination, °	0.0094 (0.10)	0.73 (0.85)
Spinal deviation		
Surface rotation RMS, °	0.0003 (0.02)	0.29 (0.54)
Surface rotation max, °	0.0013 (0.04)	6.30 (2.51)
Surface rotation right, °	0.0013 (0.04)	1.36 (1.17)
Surface rotation left, °	0.0015 (0.04)	0.98 (0.99)
Surface rotation amplitude, °	0.0026 (0.05)	0.92 (0.96)
Trunk torsion, °	0.1244 (0.35)	2.66 (1.63)
Lateral deviation RMS, mm	0.0003 (0.02)	0.53 (0.73)
Lateral deviation, mm	0.0008 (0.03)	6.29 (2.51)
Lateral deviation right, mm	0.0008 (0.03)	1.79 (1.34)

Table 5 Within-scan variance for the mannequin and human participants calculated using the standard average value (SAV) *(Continued)*

Lateral deviation left, mm	0.0010 (0.03)	1.22 (1.10)
Lateral deviation amplitude, mm	0.0017 (0.04)	2.50 (1.58)

Data are reported as variance (within-scan SD). Variance for all human spine shape parameters was significant ($P < 0.001$)
DL left sacral dimple, *DM* middle point between the left and right sacral dimples, *DR* right sacral dimple, *ICT* cervical-thoracic inflection point, *ILS* lumbar-sacral inflection point, *ITL* thoracic-lumbar inflection point, *RMS* root mean square, *SP* sacral point, *VP* vertebral prominens

head placement may affect results. In anticipation of this limitation, a fixed point was provided as a visual reference in front of each participant near shoulder height in an attempt to establish a consistent head position. Future studies should investigate the effect of changing head positions on the spine shape parameters. Another limitation is that the landmarks (DL, DR, and VP) that the instrumentation automatically identifies may require repositioning. In nearly 45% of scans (399), at least 1 landmark had to be adjusted in 1 or more images because of improper localization by the DIERS system. The possibility of this adjustment is reported in the instrument's operations manual, and the user is instructed to reposition the landmark to the correct location. Within our dataset of 900 scans, a total of 32,400 landmarks/data points could be adjusted. In nearly all of the 399 scans where marker location was adjusted, only 1–2 of the markers were adjusted for 1 of the 3 landmarks. So estimating for the entire dataset, only 798 of the 32,400 data points were adjusted, resulting in a conservative correction rate of 3%. While adjusting landmarks is not ideal and could be a cause of variability, such infrequently required modification better represents the true parameter value than if the landmark was left in its original position. Finally, the current study included participants with a BMI range from 25 to 35, which is a wider range than previously reported studies [9, 12]. We have no reason to believe our BMI range would influence our results. The variability and reliability for the wider BMI range are currently being investigated.

Current studies in progress are focusing on the influence of within-scan, within-day, between-day, and between-participant variability on the measured variability of the DIERS formetric 4D over time. Understanding these components will allow for the establishment of population-based normative spinal parameter ranges that could improve our understanding of what outcomes can be determined as meaningful change. Although previous studies [9, 12] have evaluated the influence of BMI on the reliability of the spine shape parameters, more definitive analysis of the influence of BMI and other measures, such as sex and body fat percent, should be evaluated as well. Future studies should also investigate how changes in the location of DL and DR influence the stability of parameters from postural sway or modifications in land-mark localization by a technician during processing.

Conclusions

In the current study, the minimal variability observed in the mannequin suggested the DIERS formetric 4D instrument had high within-scan reliability. The absolute difference between the mean DRV and mean SAV for human participants was small, and the inter-method reliability was excellent. Both the DRV and SAV provided comparable spine shape parameter values. Because significant within-scan variability was identified, reporting the SAV along with the within-scan variability will increase the clinical usefulness of each spine shape parameter, especially when researchers and clinicians are trying to determine when a clinically meaningful change has occurred.

Abbreviations

BMI: body mass index; DL: left sacral dimple; DM: middle point between the left and right sacral dimples; DR: right sacral dimple; DRV: DIERS-reported value; ICC: intraclass correlation coefficient; SAV: standard average value; VP: vertebral prominens

Acknowledgments

The authors would like to acknowledge Steve Webb for his assistance in study development, Jane Johnson for her contributions in data analysis, and Deborah Goggin for editing the manuscript.

Funding

This research was supported by the Osteopathic Heritage Foundation, grant no. 509-305. The Osteopathic Heritage Foundation had no role in the design of the study; collection, analysis, and interpretation of the data; or writing of the manuscript.

Authors' contributions

BD, ZS, and SB designed the study. ZS completed all of the data collection. ZS, SB, and GF completed the data analysis and interpretation. ZS drafted the article. All authors were responsible for critical revision of the article and approved the final manuscript to be published.

Competing interests

The authors declare that they have no competing interests.

References

1. Drerup B, Hierholzer E. Automatic localization of anatomical landmarks on the back surface and construction of a body-fixed coordinate system. J Biomech. 1987;20:961–70.
2. Frerich JM, Hertzler K, Knott P, Mardjetko S. Comparison of radiographic and surface topography measurements in adolescents with idiopathic scoliosis. Open Orthop J. 2012;6:261–5.
3. Hackenberg L, Hierholzer E, Pötzl W, Götze C, Liljenqvist U. Rasterstereographic back shape analysis in idiopathic scoliosis after anterior correction and fusion. Clin Biomech (Bristol, Avon). 2003;18:1–8.
4. Hackenberg L, Hierholzer E, Pötzl W, Götze C, Liljenqvist U. Rasterstereographic back shape analysis in idiopathic scoliosis after posterior correction and fusion. Clin Biomech (Bristol, Avon). 2003;18:883–9.
5. Knott P, Sturm P, Lonner B, Cahill P, Betsch M, McCarthy R, et al. Multicenter comparison of 3D spinal measurements using surface topography with those from conventional radiography. Spine Deform. 2016;4:98–103.
6. Tabard-Fougere A, Bonnefoy-Mazure A, Hanquinet S, Lascombes P, Armand S, Dayer R. Validity and reliability of spine rasterstereography in patients with adolescent idiopathic scoliosis. Spine (Phila Pa 1976). 2017;42:98–105.
7. Guidetti L, Bonavolonta V, Tito A, Reis VM, Gallotta MC, Baldari C. Intra- and interday reliability of spine rasterstereography. Biomed Res Int. 2013;2013:745480.
8. Lason G, Peeters L, Vandenberghe K, Byttebier G, Comhaire F. Reassessing the accuracy and reproducibility of Diers formetric measurements in healthy volunteers. Int J Osteopath Med. 2015;18:247–54.
9. Mohokum M, Mendoza S, Udo W, Sitter H, Paletta JR, Skwara A. Reproducibility of rasterstereography for kyphotic and lordotic angles, trunk length, and trunk inclination: a reliability study. Spine (Phila Pa 1976). 2010;35:1353–8.
10. Schroeder J, Reer R, Braumann KM. Video raster stereography back shape reconstruction: a reliability study for sagittal, frontal, and transversal plane parameters. Eur Spine J. 2015;24:262–9.
11. Drerup B, Hierholzer E. Objective determination of anatomical landmarks on the body surface: measurement of the vertebra prominens from surface curvature. J Biomech. 1985;18:467–74.
12. Goh S, Price RI, Leedman PJ, Singer KP. Rasterstereographic analysis of the thoracic sagittal curvature: a reliability study. J Musculoskelet Res. 1999;03:137–42.
13. Drerup B, Hierholzer E. Movement of the human pelvis and displacement of related anatomical landmarks on the body surface. J Biomech. 1987;20:971–7.
14. Drerup B, Ellger B, Meyer zu Bentrup F, Hierholzer E. Functional rasterstereographic images. A new method for biomechanical analysis of skeletal geometry [in German]. Orthopade. 2001;30:242–50.
15. Drerup B, Hierholzer E. Back shape measurement using video rasterstereography and three-dimensional reconstruction of spinal shape. Clin Biomech (Bristol, Avon). 1994;9:28–36.

11

Effectiveness of the Rigo Chêneau versus Boston-style orthoses for adolescent idiopathic scoliosis

Miriam K. Minsk[1], Kristen D. Venuti[1], Gail L. Daumit[2,3,4,5] and Paul D. Sponseller[1,6*]

Abstract

Background: Bracing can effectively treat adolescent idiopathic scoliosis (AIS), but patient outcomes have not been compared by brace type. We compared outcomes of AIS patients treated with Rigo Chêneau orthoses (RCOs) or custom-molded Boston-style thoracolumbosacral orthoses (TLSOs).

Methods: We retrospectively reviewed patient records from one scoliosis center from 1999 through 2014. Patients were studied from initial treatment until skeletal maturity or surgery. Inclusion criteria were a diagnosis of AIS, initial major curve between 25° and 40°, use of an RCO or TLSO, and no previous scoliosis treatment.

Results: The study included 108 patients (93 girls) with a mean (±standard deviation) age at brace initiation of 12.5 ± 1.3 years. Thirteen patients wore an RCO, and 95 wore a TLSO. Mean pre-bracing major curves were 32.7° ± 4.8° in the RCO group and 31.4° ± 4.4° in the TLSO group ($p = 0.387$). Mean brace wear time was similar between groups. Mean differences in major curve from baseline to follow-up were −0.4° ± 9.9° in the RCO group and 6.9° ± 12.1° in the TLSO group ($p = 0.028$). Percent changes in major curve from baseline to follow-up were 0.0% ± 30.5% for the RCO group and 21.3% ± 38.8% for the TLSO group ($p = 0.030$). No RCO patients and 34% of TLSO patients progressed to spinal surgery ($p = 0.019$). At follow-up, major curves improved by 6° or more in 31% of the RCO group and 13% of the TLSO group ($p = 0.100$).

Conclusions: Patients treated with RCOs compared with Boston-style TLSOs had similar baseline characteristics and brace wear time yet significantly lower rates of spinal surgery. Patients with RCOs also had lower mean and percent major curve progression versus those with TLSOs.

Keywords: Adolescent, Bracing, Major curve, Orthosis, Outcomes, Scoliosis

Background

Adolescent idiopathic scoliosis (AIS) affects 2 to 3% of adolescents between the ages of 10 and 18 years [1, 2]. Brace treatment is commonly offered when the spinal curve has reached 25° [3]. Since the Bracing in Adolescent Idiopathic Scoliosis Trial study in 2013 [4], bracing has been increasingly recognized as an effective nonsurgical means of scoliosis treatment. However, the comparative effectiveness of most types of braces for AIS has not been definitively established [5].

A rigid thoracolumbosacral orthosis (TLSO) is a brace worn to minimize progression of AIS. There are various TLSO designs (e.g., Boston, Milwaukee, Wilmington) [6]. Rigo Chêneau orthoses (RCOs) were developed approximately two decades ago, with the intent to combine biomechanical forces in three dimensions, including curve derotation. They use an open pelvis design with anterior opening. However, studies of the RCO are limited, and we know little about its effectiveness, particularly in relation to other braces [5, 7, 8].

In the current study, we reviewed records of patients treated at one large academic medical center's pediatric orthopedic scoliosis practice who were prescribed full-time bracing for AIS. Our objective was to determine if brace type, specifically the RCO compared with a

* Correspondence: psponse@jhmi.edu
[1]Department of Orthopaedic Surgery, The Johns Hopkins University, Baltimore, MD, USA
[6]Bloomberg Children's Center, 1800 Orleans Street, 7359A, Baltimore, MD 21287, USA
Full list of author information is available at the end of the article

Boston-style TLSO, affected outcomes. Our hypothesis was that different brace designs would lead to different patient outcomes.

Methods

Study population

We retrospectively reviewed medical records of patients treated at an academic scoliosis center from 1999 through 2014. The study population consisted of adolescents aged 10 years or older at presentation who met the following criteria: (1) diagnosis of AIS; (2) Risser stage between 0 and 2; (3) major curve between 25° and 40°; (3) no previous treatment for scoliosis; (4) if female, premenarchal or less than 1 year postmenarchal; (5) prescribed full-time brace treatment; and (6) follow-up until skeletal maturity or surgery.

Measurements

Outcome variables followed the recommendations of the Scoliosis Research Society (SRS) Committee on Bracing and Nonoperative Management and the Society on Scoliosis Orthopaedic and Rehabilitation Treatment (SOSORT) and incorporated other relevant clinical outcomes [9, 10]. Outcomes included the following: major curve exceeding 30° and major curve exceeding 50°, difference in major curve from baseline to follow-up, percent change in major curve, progression to spinal surgery, progression of curve to 45° or more after bracing, progression to spinal surgery or curve of at least 45° after bracing, major curve progression of 6° or more, major curve improvement of 6° or more, and major curve unchanged (within 5°). For the outcomes that included progression to curvature of 45° or more, we measured the patients whose major curve progressed to at least 45°.

Our primary independent variable was the type of brace. We compared an RCO with a custom Boston-style TLSO. Patients self-selected their orthotists and brace type. Follow-up orthopedist recommendations were the same for all patients: in-brace radiography and clinic visit 4 weeks after treatment initiation, then out-of-brace radiography and clinic visits every 4 months before menarche and every 6 months after menarche. We abstracted information on age, sex, race, curve location, pre-bracing initial major curve magnitude, pre-bracing Risser stage, initial in-brace major curve, time in brace, and mean patient-reported number of hours the brace was worn in Risser stages 0 and 1 and overall. We recorded information for the total course of treatment for each patient and calculated the mean brace wear time for the course of treatment.

We performed univariate and bivariate descriptive analyses, including Student t tests, Fisher exact tests, and χ^2 tests, comparing baseline characteristics and

outcomes. A two-sided alpha with $p < 0.05$ was considered statistically significant.

Results

Baseline characteristics

Of the 108 patients (93 girls) who met the inclusion criteria, the mean age at treatment initiation was 12.5 ± 1.3 years (Table 1). Ninety-five patients were treated with a TLSO, and 13 patients were treated with an RCO. Of the study population, 72% were Caucasian and 15% were African American. Major curves were mainly thoracic (47%), lumbar (22%), or thoracic and thoracolumbar (18%). The mean pre-brace major curves were $31.6° \pm 4.4°$ overall, $32.7° \pm 4.8°$ in the RCO group, and $31.4° \pm 4.4°$ in the TLSO group, corresponding to 52% of patients having an initial pre-brace major curve of more than 30°. Sixty-three percent of patients began bracing at Risser stage 0, 22% at Risser stage 1, and 15% at Risser stage 2. Demographic and clinical characteristics at baseline were similar for patients in both groups.

Treatment and outcomes

We followed all patients until skeletal maturity or progression to surgery, whichever came first. Mean initial in-brace major curves were $22.6° \pm 6.4°$ in the RCO group and $22.6° \pm 7.2°$ in the TLSO group ($p = 0.924$) (Table 2). In-brace correction of major curve from baseline of at least 35% was achieved in 42% of the RCO group and 36% of the TLSO group ($p = 0.943$, data not shown). Patients in the RCO group wore the brace for a mean 17.0 ± 6.1 h per day, and patients in the TLSO group wore the brace for a mean 16.1 ± 5.2 h per day ($p = 0.641$).

After bracing was complete, the mean final measurements for major curves were $32.3° \pm 10.4°$ (RCO group) and $38.3° \pm 13.5°$ (TLSO group) ($p = 0.077$) (Table 2). Forty-six percent of RCO patients had a major curve at follow-up of greater than 30°, compared with 67% of TLSO patients ($p = 0.133$). The mean difference in major curves from baseline to follow-up was $-0.4° \pm 9.9°$ for the RCO group versus $6.9° \pm 12.1°$ for the TLSO group ($p = 0.028$). Figure 1 shows each patient's change in major curve magnitude from baseline to follow-up. The percent changes in major curves from baseline to follow-up were $0.0\% \pm 30.5\%$ for the RCO group and $21.3\% \pm 38.8\%$ for the TLSO group ($p = 0.030$) (Table 2). No patients in the RCO group progressed to surgery, compared with 32 patients in the TLSO group ($p = 0.019$). Fifteen percent of patients in the RCO group had a final major curve of 45° or greater or progressed to spinal surgery, compared with 38% of patients in the TLSO group ($p = 0.133$). At follow-up, major curves improved by 6° or more in 31% of the RCO group and 13% of the TLSO group ($p = 0.100$).

Table 1 Demographic and clinical characteristics at baseline for 108 patients with adolescent idiopathic scoliosis

Characteristics	Patients						P
	All (n = 108)		RCO group (n = 13)		Boston-style TLSO group (n = 95)		
	Mean (SD)	n (%)	Mean (SD)	n (%)	Mean (SD)	n (%)	
Age (years)	12.5 (1.3)		12.5 (1.3)		12.5 (1.3)		0.762
Female sex		93 (86)		11 (85)		82 (86)	1.00
Race							0.282
Caucasian		78 (72)		10 (77)		68 (72)	
African American		16 (15)		0 (0)		16 (17)	
Hispanic		1 (1)		0 (0)		1 (1)	
Asian/Pacific Islander		2 (2)		0 (0)		2 (2)	
Other		11 (10)		3 (23)		8 (8)	
Major curve location							
Thoracic		51 (47)		5 (38)		46 (48)	0.500
Thoracolumbar		3 (3)		0 (0)		3 (3)	1.00
Lumbar		24 (22)		1 (7.7)		23 (24)	0.290
Double major		0 (0)		0 (0)		0 (0)	
Double thoracic		9 (8)		3 (23)		6 (6)	0.075
Thoracic and thoracolumbar		19 (18)		4 (31)		15 (16)	0.238
Triple		2 (2)		0 (0)		2 (2)	1.00
Major curve (°)	31.6 (4.4)		32.7 (4.8)		31.4 (4.4)		0.387
Major curve >30°		56 (52)		7 (54)		49 (51)	0.878
Risser stage							0.710
0		68 (63)		7 (54)		61 (64)	
1		24 (22)		4 (31)		20 (21)	
2		16 (15)		2 (15)		14 (15)	

RCO Rigo Chêneau orthosis, TLSO thoracolumbosacral orthosis, SD standard deviation

Discussion

In this retrospective review of a large academic medical center's patients with AIS and their experience with full-time brace treatment, we found that patients treated with RCOs were substantially less likely to progress to spinal surgery and had smaller mean change and smaller percent increase in major curves from treatment initiation through follow-up than patients treated with a TLSO, despite similar baseline characteristics and brace wear time. The outcomes of curve progression less than 45° or progression to surgery and major curve improvement of at least 6° were not statistically different; however, they appeared to favor RCOs. Although previous studies have shown the benefits of bracing [4, 11–13] and the benefits of the RCO for treatment of AIS [7, 8], none has compared efficacy of the RCO with other orthoses. For this study, we incorporated guidelines from the SRS Bracing Committee and SOSORT to establish our inclusion criteria [10] and tracked patients from early Risser stages until maturity or surgery to understand the effects of brace type, specifically RCO versus TLSO, on outcomes.

We consider our outcomes for brace treatment in relation to previous studies' findings. In the Bracing in Adolescent Idiopathic Scoliosis Trial study, 72% of those with TLSO bracing had curve progression to less than 50° [4]. Similarly, our study showed that 68% of patients with TLSO bracing had major curve progression to less than 45° [4]. Previous studies, mostly using Milwaukee TLSO braces, have shown a large spectrum of success rates for a range of curve outcomes, likely because of dissimilarity in brace quality, patient characteristics, and decision thresholds for spinal surgery [14–18]. Most of these studies took place before SRS and SOSORT guidelines on reporting; thus, standards of outcome measurement and participant selection varied [10].

Little research has been published on outcomes for RCOs. Zaborowska-Sapeta et al. [8] reported on 79 patients with RCOs in Poland. In their study, 12.9% of patients progressed to a major curve greater than 50° at final follow-up, with a mean major curve increase of 9.2° for the overall study population [8]. Although we used the SRS-recommended outcome of 45°, our results are comparable to those of Zaborowska-Sapeta et al. [8].

Table 2 Bracing treatment and outcomes for 108 patients with adolescent idiopathic scoliosis

Parameter	Patients						P
	All (n = 108)		RCO group (n = 13)		Boston-style TLSO group (n = 95)		
	Mean (SD)	n (%)	Mean (SD)	n (%)	Mean (SD)	n (%)	
Initial in-brace major curve[a] (°)	22.8 (7.2)		22.6 (6.4)		22.6 (7.2)		0.924
Percent initial in-brace major curve correction[a]	28.4 (20.1)		31.5 (15.2)		27.8 (20.1)		0.538
Time in brace (year)	2.4 (1.4)		2.8 (0.9)		2.4 (1.4)		0.193
Brace wear time per day (h)							
All patients[b]	16.2 (5.3)		17.0 (6.1)		16.1 (5.2)		0.641
Patients with Risser stage 0 or 1[c]	17.0 (5.8)		18.9 (5.8)		16.8 (5.8)		0.296
Final major curve (°)	37.6 (13.3)		32.3 (10.4)		38.3 (13.5)		0.077
Final major curve							
>30°		70 (65)		6 (46)		64 (67)	0.133
>50°		18 (17)		1 (8)		17 (18)	0.464
Change in major curve from baseline[d] (°)	6.0 (12.1)		−0.4 (9.9)		6.9 (12.1)		0.028
Percent change in major curve from baseline	18.6 (38.9)		0.0 (30.5)		21.3 (38.8)		0.030
Progression to surgery		32 (30)		0 (0)		32 (34)	0.019
At skeletal maturity							
Major curve ≥45°		32 (30)		2 (15)		30 (32)	0.337
Progression to surgery or major curve ≥45°		38 (35)		2 (15)		36 (38)	0.133
Major curve change							
Progression ≥6°		52 (48)		5 (38)		47 (49)	0.556
Decrease ≥6°		16 (15)		4 (31)		12 (13)	0.100
Unchanged (±5°)		40 (37)		4 (31)		36 (38)	0.764

SD standard deviation, *RCO* Rigo Chêneau orthosis, *TLSO* thoracolumbosacral orthosis
[a]n = 83 (RCO, n = 12; TLSO, n = 70)
[b]n = 107 (RCO, n = 13; TLSO, n = 94)
[c]RCO, n = 10; TLSO, n = 71
[d]n = 95 (RCO, n = 11; TLSO, n = 84)

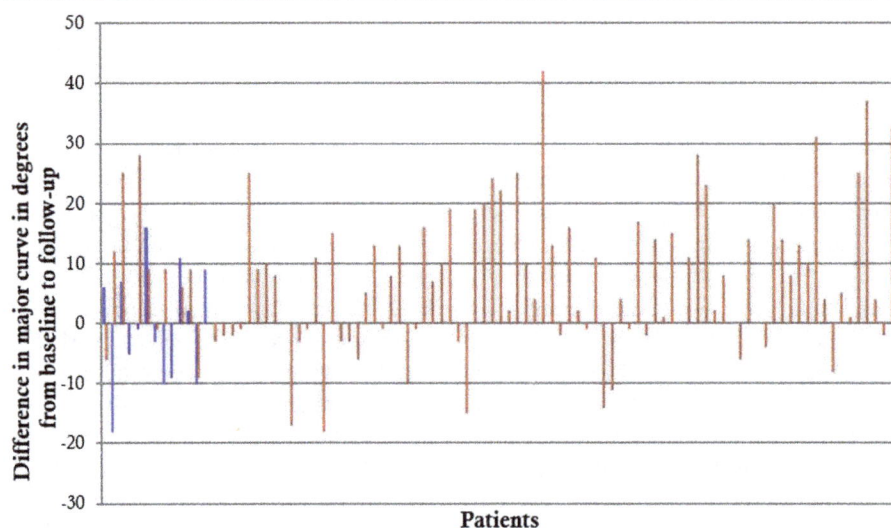

Fig. 1 Difference in major curve after treatment with Rigo Chêneau orthoses (*blue lines*) compared with Boston-style thoracolumbosacral orthoses (*red lines*) in 108 patients with adolescent idiopathic scoliosis

However, our population had a lower mean change in major curve from baseline to follow-up with the RCO. Ovadia et al. [7] published the results of 93 patients in Israel treated with RCOs and found that 84% of patients' curves progressed by less than 5°. Although we studied a smaller number of patients with RCOs than these two international reports, our study is an important addition to the research because it is one of the first to compare outcomes after RCO use versus general Boston-style TLSO bracing.

Several factors could have contributed to the favorable outcomes for RCOs compared with TLSOs in our study. First, the RCO construction with three-dimensional corrective forces may have a better effect on scoliosis curves compared with the TLSO. Second, the lighter weight of the RCO and more open design may have made it more desirable and comfortable for patients to wear, leading to increased compliance. However, we did not observe a difference in patient-reported mean wear time between brace types during the course of follow-up. Third, because this was an observational study of clinical practice, families had a choice of orthotists and orthoses. Although we did not measure how families made these decisions, we believe variation in geographical distance to orthotists and heterogeneity of insurance coverage for orthoses could have influenced the type of brace adolescents received. In addition, families who chose the RCOs could have had other factors that made their adolescents more likely to have successful bracing outcomes.

This study has limitations. Despite the large number of records encompassing 15 years of a busy, academic scoliosis clinical practice, we had a relatively small sample of patients using RCOs compared with the two international reports, and this may have limited our ability to detect statistically significant differences in some measures [7, 8]. RCO braces were principally made by one skilled orthotist in the region, which contributed to their lower frequency. Despite this, the relative comparability of our outcomes with previous TLSO and RCO studies provides face validity. In addition, this was a retrospective review of an outpatient clinical practice, and we did not have quality-of-life measures, objective monitoring of time wearing the brace, or blinded, independent outcome assessment. Although self-reports tend to overestimate brace wear time [19], it is unlikely that reported wear time would differ systematically between patients with TLSOs and RCOs in this review of a real-world clinical practice.

Another potential limitation was that although the percent initial in-brace major curve correction appeared to be better in RCOs compared with TLSOs, the difference was not statistically significant, as we may have expected given the positive RCO outcomes at the end of treatment. This could have been caused in part by the smaller number of RCOs and by the fact that if the initial correction was not clinically acceptable to the orthopedist, he would recommend the patient return for brace adjustments to achieve optimal correction. Further, in-brace radiography was generally not performed. Thus, the 1-month in-brace measurements presented here may underestimate actual in-brace correction, particularly for RCOs. In addition, the in-brace measured curve correction reflects coronal changes only, not rotational changes, which could not be studied. However, on clinical assessment such as out-of-brace examination of forward bending, the orthopedist noticed that rotational prominence often diminished in RCO-treated patients. The RCO's influence on curve derotation may be particularly important for its effectiveness in treating scoliosis; however, future research is needed to elucidate how this mechanism contributes to bracing success [7].

There are several strengths of our report. We followed guidelines for patient inclusion and choice of clinical outcome variables [9, 10]. Our results provide a real-world comparison of patient experience with brace types in a large outpatient scoliosis practice. This use of SRS and SOSORT criteria to compare outcomes by brace type is rare in prior studies. Moreover, the similar clinical characteristics at baseline allow an assessment of differences between brace types, despite a relatively small sample size for the RCO group.

Conclusions

In this large retrospective review of an academic outpatient scoliosis practice, patients treated with RCOs were substantially less likely to progress to spinal surgery than those treated with Boston-style TLSOs. Patients treated with RCOs also had smaller mean change and smaller percent increase in major curves from treatment initiation through follow-up. Future studies should examine differences in outcomes by brace type in other settings and in larger samples, and they should investigate the impact of the rotational dimension of correction with RCOs. Clinicians may consider increasing use of RCOs for AIS.

Abbreviations
AIS: Adolescent idiopathic scoliosis; RCO: Rigo Chêneau orthosis; SOSORT: Society on Scoliosis Orthopaedic and Rehabilitation Treatment; SRS: Scoliosis Research Society; TLSO: Thoracolumbosacral orthosis

Acknowledgements
Not applicable.

Funding
Not applicable. There was no funding for this study.

Authors' contributions

MKM designed the data abstraction, abstracted the data from the records, performed the analyses, and drafted the manuscript. KDV was a major contributor in the data abstraction design and participated in writing the manuscript. GLD contributed to the analyses, interpretation of the data, and editing the manuscript. PDS designed the study and was a major contributor to the interpretation of the data and editing the manuscript. All authors provided approval of the final manuscript.

Competing interests

The authors declare that they have no competing interests.

Author details

[1]Department of Orthopaedic Surgery, The Johns Hopkins University, Baltimore, MD, USA. [2]Division of General Internal Medicine, The Johns Hopkins University School of Medicine, Baltimore, MD, USA. [3]Welch Center for Prevention, Epidemiology, and Clinical Research, The Johns Hopkins University, Baltimore, MD, USA. [4]Department of Epidemiology, The Johns Hopkins Bloomberg School of Public Health, Baltimore, MD, USA. [5]Department of Health Policy and Management, The Johns Hopkins Bloomberg School of Public Health, Baltimore, MD, USA. [6]Bloomberg Children's Center, 1800 Orleans Street, 7359A, Baltimore, MD 21287, USA.

References

1. Nachemson A, Lonstein J, Weinstein S. Report of the SRS Prevalence and Natural History Committee 1982. Presented at the Scoliosis Research Society 17th Annual Meeting, Denver, CO, September 22-25, 1982.
2. Weinstein SL, Dolan LA, Cheng JCY, Danielsson A, Morcuende JA. Adolescent idiopathic scoliosis. Lancet. 2008;371(9623):1527–37.
3. Parent S, Newton PO, Wenger DR. Adolescent idiopathic scoliosis: etiology, anatomy, natural history, and bracing. Instr Course Lect. 2005;54:529–36.
4. Weinstein SL, Dolan LA, Wright JG, Dobbs MB. Effects of bracing in adolescents with idiopathic scoliosis. N Engl J Med. 2013;369(16):1512–21.
5. Negrini S, Aulisa AG, Aulisa L, Circo AB, de Mauroy JC, Durmala J, Grivas TB, Knott P, Kotwicki T, Maruyama T, Minozzi S, O'Brien JP, Papadopoulos D, Rigo M, Rivard CH, Romano M, Wynne JH, Villagrasa M, Weiss HR, Zaina F. 2011 SOSORT guidelines: orthopaedic and rehabilitation treatment of idiopathic scoliosis during growth. Scoliosis. 2012;7(1):3.
6. Zaina F, De Mauroy JC, Grivas T, Hresko MT, Kotwizki T, Maruyama T, Price N, Rigo M, Stikeleather L, Wynne J, Negrini S. Bracing for scoliosis in 2014: state of the art. Eur J Phys Rehabil Med. 2014;50(1):93–110.
7. Ovadia D, Eylon S, Mashiah A, Wientroub S, Lebel ED. Factors associated with the success of the Rigo System Chêneau brace in treating mild to moderate adolescent idiopathic scoliosis. J Child Orthop. 2012;6(4):327–31.
8. Zaborowska-Sapeta K, Kowalski IM, Kotwicki T, Protasiewicz-Faldowska H, Kiebzak W. Effectiveness of Chêneau brace treatment for idiopathic scoliosis: prospective study in 79 patients followed to skeletal maturity. Scoliosis. 2011;6(1):2.
9. Negrini S, Hresko TM, O'Brien JP, Price N, Boards S, Committee SRSN-O. Recommendations for research studies on treatment of idiopathic scoliosis: consensus 2014 between SOSORT and SRS non-operative management committee. Scoliosis. 2015;10:8.
10. Richards BS, Bernstein RM, D'Amato CR, Thompson GH. Standardization of criteria for adolescent idiopathic scoliosis brace studies. SRS Committee on Bracing and Nonoperative Management. Spine (Phila Pa 1976). 2005;30(18):2068–75.
11. Katz DE, Herring JA, Browne RH, Kelly DM, Birch JG. Brace wear control of curve progression in adolescent idiopathic scoliosis. J Bone Joint Surg Am. 2010;92(6):1343–52.
12. Nachemson AL, Peterson LE, members of The Brace Study Group of the Scoliosis Research Society. Effectiveness of treatment with a brace in girls who have adolescent idiopathic scoliosis. A prospective, controlled study based on data from the Brace Study of the Scoliosis Research Society. J Bone Joint Surg Am. 1995;77(6):815-822.
13. Rowe DE, Bernstein SM, Riddick MF, Adler F, Emans JB, Gardner-Bonneau D. A meta-analysis of the efficacy of non-operative treatments for idiopathic scoliosis. J Bone Joint Surg Am. 1997;79(5):664–74.
14. Danielsson AJ, Hasserius R, Ohlin A, Nachemson AL. A prospective study of brace treatment versus observation alone in adolescent idiopathic scoliosis. A follow-up mean of 16 years after maturity. Spine (Phila Pa 1976). 2007;32(20):2198–207.
15. Fernandez-Feliberti R, Flynn J, Ramirez N, Trautmann M, Alegria M. Effectiveness of TLSO bracing in the conservative treatment of idiopathic scoliosis. J Pediatr Orthop. 1995;15(2):176–81.
16. Goldberg CJ, Moore DP, Fogarty EE, Dowling FE. Adolescent idiopathic scoliosis: the effect of brace treatment on the incidence of surgery. Spine (Phila Pa 1976). 2001;26(1):42–7.
17. Lonstein JE, Winter RB. The Milwaukee brace for the treatment of adolescent idiopathic scoliosis. A review of one thousand and twenty patients. J Bone Joint Surg Am. 1994;76(8):1207–21.
18. Noonan KJ, Weinstein SL, Jacobson WC, Dolan LA. Use of the Milwaukee brace for progressive idiopathic scoliosis. J Bone Joint Surg (Br). 1996;78(4):557–67.
19. Morton A, Riddle R, Buchanan R, Katz D, Birch J. Accuracy in the prediction and estimation of adherence to bracewear before and during treatment of adolescent idiopathic scoliosis. J Pediatr Orthop. 2008;28(3):336–41.

12

Three-dimensional reconstructions of Lenke 1A curves

J-C. Bernard[1][*] (iD), E. Berthonnaud[1,2,3], J. Deceuninck[1], L. Journoud-Rozand[4], G. Notin[4] and E. Chaleat-Valayer[1]

Abstract

Background: Scoliosis is a 3D deformity that can be reconstructed through 2D antero-posterior and lateral radiographs, which provide an upper view of the deformed spine as well as regional planes matching all vertebrae of elective plane for each curve. The objective of this study is to explore whether all idiopathic scoliosis classified Lenke 1A have the same 3D representation made with regional planes.

Methods: All patients treated for idiopathic thoracic scoliosis during the growth period and classified Lenke 1A were included in this study conducted in the pediatric spinal orthopedic department of Centre des Massues. A photogrammetric technique was used to obtain a 3D reconstruction, from regional planes identified on radiographs made with the EOS system. Three regional planes are usually identified in asymptomatic spines: lumbar, dorsal, and cervical—none of them presenting rotation. In the studied group, the number of planes, the rotation, and the limit vertebrae of each plane were looked for.

Results: Sixty-three patients were included (47 girls and 16 boys, mean age 11.3 years). The Cobb angle was meanly 36.5°. The scoliosis was reconstructed with three regional planes (57%) or four ones (43%, with the thoracic plane divided into two planes). Maximal rotation was found in the thoracic plane, especially when scoliosis was represented with four regional planes. The transition between planes 2 and 3 was mainly located between the fourth and sixth dorsal vertebrae.

Conclusion: The use of an arbitrary regional plane representation of a 3D shape leads to conclude that there are two types of Lenke 1A scoliosis, which should be taken into account for designing the brace.

Keywords: Idiopathic scoliosis, Thoracic, 3D reconstruction, Upper view, Lenke classification, Regional planes

Background

Scoliosis is defined as a three-dimensional deformity in frontal, sagittal, and horizontal planes [1–5]. For Berthonnaud et al., the spine is considered as a heterogeneous beam and is modeled as a deformable wire along which vertebrae can be seen as beads turning on this wire [6]. In our modeling, the 3D spinal curve is a compound of plane regions connected together by zones of transition. The 3D spinal curve is uniquely flexed along the plane regions. Biplanar radiographic examination with simultaneous exposures (frontal and sagittal in the EOS system), coupled with photogrammetric reconstructions, may be used for reconstructing the 3D spinal curve [7]. The photogrammetric technique reconstructs points in space from their two images in projection planes.

The photogrammetry applied to radiographic images has been described by Suh [8] and the first presentation of photogrammetric reconstruction of spinal curves from simultaneous biplanar radiography was done by Brown et al. [9]. Biplanar radiography involves the setting of specific devices to get simultaneous exposures, and this has been used for clinical applications. The geometric structure of a 3D spinal curve can be characterized by the size and orientation of regional planes, by the parameters representing flexed regions and by the size and function of zones of transition [6].

Despite the fact that all classifications are only based on 2D like the Scoliosis Research Society (SRS) classification [10] and King classification [11, 12], Lenke introduces with his classification new parameters in radiographic analysis of idiopathic scoliosis, such as lumbar sagittal modifiers (A, B, C) and the difference between structural and non-structural curves [13, 14].

---

* Correspondence: bernard-mpr@cmcr-massues.com
[1]Croix Rouge française – CMCR des Massues, 92, rue Edmond Locard, 69322 Lyon Cedex 05, France
Full list of author information is available at the end of the article

The objective of this study was to show if the use of regional plane analysis could determine if all Lenke 1A curves (main thoracic = thoracic scoliosis without compensation on the lumbar part) would result in the same 3D representation.

Methods

To become familiar with Lenke classification, we classified all the radiographs of patients who consulted for adolescent idiopathic scoliosis and underwent frontal and sagittal radiographs on the EOS system in Centre des Massues in 2015. Although the Lenke classification has already proved its reliability [13], four independent readers (two very familiar with scoliosis and two not) analyzed 223 files, and then we compared results. In order to distinguish Lenke type 1 from type 2, we did not use bending radiographs to determine whether the upper curve was structural or not, because it is difficult in daily practice to multiply radiographs for these patients in the growth period, as they are already very often exposed. We used clinical examination for that, by measuring the upper bump in standing position and comparing it to the one measured in ventral decubitus: if the upper bump disappeared in lying position, it means that the curve was not structural. When we all agreed that the scoliosis could be classified as Lenke 1A, we kept the case and included it in our group for this study.

All patients with Lenke 1A curves who consulted in our institution and underwent frontal and sagittal radiographs on the EOS system in 2015 were recruited. Patient's characteristics were recorded: age, height, weight, and radiographic measures: Cobb angles, pelvic incidence (PI), pelvic tilt (PT).

Median spinal curves were drawn on frontal and sagittal projections. Points of frontal and sagittal curves were then linked together for the photogrammetric reconstruction of the 3D spinal curve. The relation was based on the use of epipolar planes. The 3D spinal curves were projected on fixed plane, and regional planes were detected along this rough spinal curve [6, 7]. Three or four planes were then identified. Figure 1 shows an example of 3D reconstruction of Lenke 1A scoliosis with three planes, whereas Fig. 2 shows an example with four planes.

Statistical analysis

All of the collected information was coded and subsequently captured by computer equipment using SPSS 11.5 software for analysis, which is carried out with the support of the suitable statistical tests (ANOVA and correlation study). The pelvic and spinal parameters have been chosen as dependent variables. Correlation analysis between radiological data and 3D data was performed through the use of Spearman's rank correlation coefficient.

Comparison of the mean values for each of the pelvic and spinal parameters between the groups was carried out through non-parametric analysis of variance (ANOVA). For all the tests, the degree of statistical significance was set at $P < 0.05$.

Results

A total of 63 Lenke 1A patients were included (mean age 11.3 years, with 47 girls and 16 boys). The thoracic Cobb angle in the frontal plane ranged between 14° and 70° (mean 36.5°).

Patient characteristics are presented in Table 1.

Table 2 presents the data for the three planes in our sample. The thoracic plane was the most rotated, but we found also rotation in the lumbar plane and in the upper plane as well.

In our population of Lenke 1A scoliotic patients, the rotation was maximal in the second plane which represents the thoracic plane. The transition from the thoracic plane to the upper plane (between plane 2 and plane 3) occurred mainly between the fourth and the sixth thoracic vertebrae, as shown by Fig. 3.

In 62.3% of cases, the rotation of the third plane was negative (clockwise direction) and positive in 37.7% (counterclockwise direction). We found no correlation between the Cobb angle in the frontal plane and the Cobb angle in the regional plane ($p = 0.298$). We identified three regional planes in 57% of cases and four regional planes in 43% of cases (when the thoracic plane was divided into two parts), and we found a difference between the three-plane group and the four-plane group for the rotation of the thoracic plane, as shown by Table 3 and Fig. 4. This difference was statically not significant, but plane 2 tends to rotate more when the 3D reconstruction identified four planes than when the 3D reconstruction identified three planes.

In the three-plane group, the mean rotation for the thoracic plane (Rot 2) was 67.6° ±29.4 and the transition from plane 2 to plane 3 was mainly located in T5. We found a correlation between the rotation of the plane and the level of transition ($p < 0.0001$).

In the four-plane group, the mean rotation for the thoracic plane (Rot 2) was 77.2° ±16.4 and the transition from plane 2 to plane 3 was mainly located in T6/T7. There was also a correlation between the rotation of the plane and the level of transition ($p = 0.005$).

Discussion

The aim of this work was to study the Lenke 1A thoracic idiopathic scoliosis in 3D using the specific software Optispine® [15] in order to determine if all Lenke 1A curves are similar in 3D analysis.

In daily practice, classifications such as SRS [10], Lenke [13, 14], and King [11, 12] are the most common

Name	Pathology	State	Treatment	Date	Age	Gender	Height	Weight
Patient 1	scoliosis		Brace and Physiotherapy	18/11/2016	13 y.o	F	157	39

THE GEOMETRIC INDEX CARD

The pelvis is modeled as a triangle. The structure of spine is represented by plane regions with homogeneous curvature.

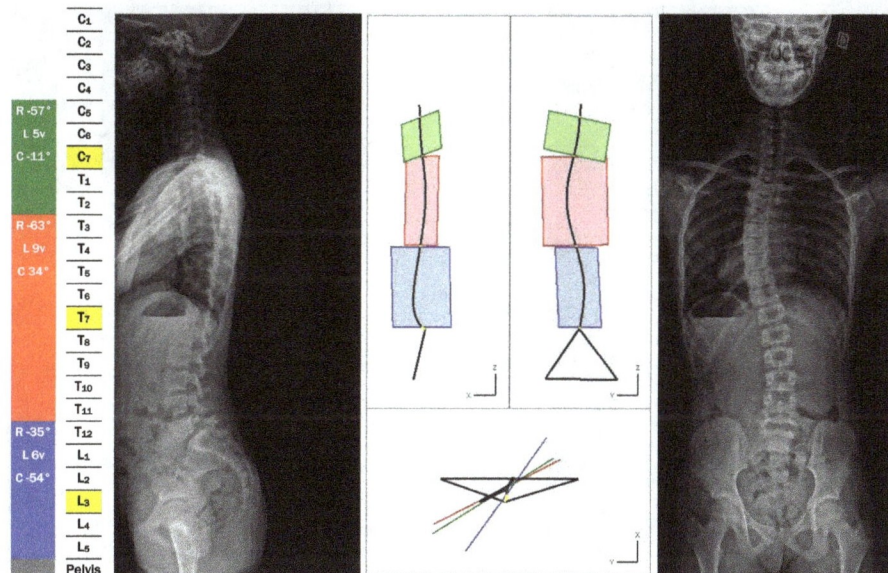

Representative parameters of the pelvis and of plane regions of spine.

	Parameters	Incidence	Pelvic tilt	Frontal tilt	Asymmetry
PELVIS	Values	58.9°	-13.1°	2.2°	7.2 %
	Indices	4	3	2	3

	Nb of regions		Plane regions			Regional curvatures		
	3	Parameters	Rotation	Flexion	Tilting	Length	Curvature	Asymmetry
SPINE	Plane 1	Values	-35.1°	1.0°	-2.9°	6 v	-54.4°	38.2 %
	L5 - T12	Indices	3			4	4	
	Plane 2	Values	-62.6°	-1.5°	-1.2°	9 v	33.8°	50.5 %
	T11 - T3	Indices	4			1	1	
	Plane 3	Values	-57.5°	4.7°	7.8°	5 v	-11.3°	51.8 %
	T2 - C5	Indices	4			3	1	
	Plane 4	Values						
		Indices						

Fig. 1 Example of 3D reconstruction of Lenke 1A scoliosis with three regional planes identified on the lateral, frontal, and horizontal views: the blue plane is for the lumbar region, the red plane for the dorsal region, and the green plane for the cervico-thoracic region

for the surgical or orthopedic treatment of scoliosis. These classifications are based on 2D radiographs of the spine in a standing position: postero-anterior view for SRS and antero-posterior and profile views for Lenke.

The Cobb angle helps in defining the severity of scoliosis by measuring curves in frontal and sagittal planes. The emergence of 3D analysis to evaluate scoliosis [6, 7, 13, 16–21] has allowed a more comprehensive and more correct approach, thanks to the top view.

Among all parameters that have been defined to describe 3D deformation in scoliosis, we retain the plane of major curvature (PMC), the best-fit planes, and the regional planes [6, 14, 22]. This study was conducted with the regional planes, and our results show that there is no correlation between the Cobb angle simply measured on a

front radiograph in standing position and the angle measured on the matching regional plane. This measure on regional plane is done semi-automatically by considering as limits some vertebrae that might not have been identified as such on a frontal radiograph. The Cobb angle on a regional plane is always higher than or equal to the Cobb angle measured on a frontal radiograph. This observation is consistent with the work of Duong and Mac-Thiong [22] who have previously shown how complex it is to classify scoliosis in 3D, specifically for Lenke 1 curves. The earlier works of Stagnara [16, 23] are also in line with our results. He used to measure scoliosis with the Cobb angle on an antero-posterior plane and completed his radiographic assessment for high-range scoliosis with a specific view, characterized by an incidence called "elective plane"

Name	Pathology	State	Treatment	Date	Age	Gender	Height	Weight
Patient 2	scoliosis		Brace and Physiotherapy	08/08/2016	16 y.o	M	173	58

THE GEOMETRIC INDEX CARD

The pelvis is modeled as a triangle. The structure of spine is represented by plane regions with homogeneous curvature.

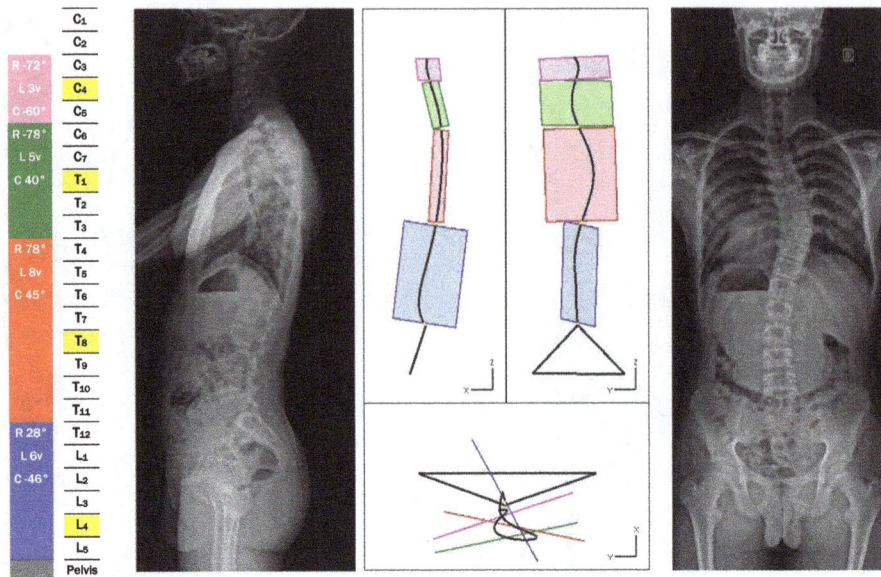

Representative parameters of the pelvis and of plane regions of spine.

PELVIS	Parameters	Incidence	Pelvic tilt	Frontal tilt	Asymmetry
	Values	50.7°	-18.7°	0.2°	3.1 %
	Indices	3	5	3	3

SPINE	Nb of regions		Plane regions			Regional curvatures		
	3	Parameters	Rotation	Flexion	Tilting	Length	Curvature	Asymmetry
	Plane 1	Values	28.2°	-7.0°	1.9°	6 v	-46.4°	31.2 %
	L5 - T12	Indices	2			4	3	
	Plane 2	Values	78.4°	-3.3°	-1.8°	8 v	44.7°	51.3 %
	T11 - T3	Indices	5			1	2	
	Plane 3	Values	-78.3°	13.4°	-2.2°	5 v	39.7°	50.8 %
	T2 - C5	Indices	5			3	5	
	Plane 4	Values	-72.2°	6.8°	-5.8°	3 v	-59.8°	59.7 %
		Indices	5					

Fig. 2 Example of 3D reconstruction of Lenke 1A scoliosis with four planes identified on the lateral, frontal, and horizontal views: the blue plane is for the lumbar region, the red plane for the lower dorsal region, the green plane for the cervico-thoracic region, and the pink plane for the upper cervical region

on the main curve [24]: the spinal deformity is major when projected on a perpendicular plane to this specific incidence. The curve is then measured by the Cobb method and the range of deformity is compared to the one measured in standard conditions, as previously described. The Cobb angle measured on the elective plane

Table 1 Demographic characteristics and radiographic measures for pelvic incidence (PI) and pelvic tilt (PT)

n = 63

	Mean	SD	Min	Max
Age	11.3 (year old)	2.6	7	15
Weight	47.3 (kg)	10.9	20	70
Height	157.4 (cm)	12.1	120	179
PI	50.9 (degree)	9.7	26	78
PT	9.3 (degree)	7.4	-6	29

Table 2 Horizontal rotation of the 3 planes

		Mean	SD	Min	Max
Rot 1	Rotation of the lumbar plane	33.6 (degree)	18.8	-15.7	67.5
Rot 2	Rotation of the thoracic plane	45 (degree)	55.6	-88.8	89
Rot 3	Rotation of the cervical plane	-23.5 (degree)	51.2	-86.7	85.7

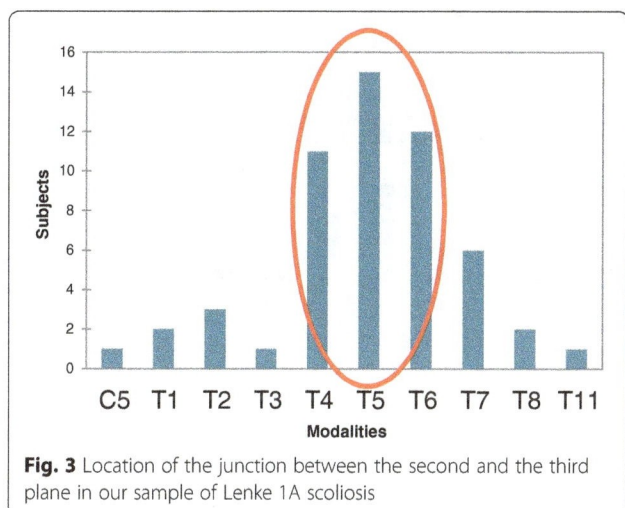

Fig. 3 Location of the junction between the second and the third plane in our sample of Lenke 1A scoliosis

(strict front view of apical vertebrae) was always higher than the Cobb angle measured on the front radiograph.

In asymptomatic subjects, the spinal column is made of three regional planes and three junction points [15]: plane 1 for lumbar level, plane 2 for dorsal level, and plane 3 for cervical level. The results of our study show that in scoliotic patients, plane 3 includes dorsal vertebrae from T4, T5, or T6 in 40% of cases, whereas it includes other dorsal levels in 60% of cases.

Compared to the best fit plane (BFP) with fix limit vertebrae, as described by Duong et al. [22], 3D analysis of scoliosis through regional planes highlights different levels of junction point between plane 2 (thoracic plane) and plane 3, even if the same kind of Lenke curve is considered (i.e., main thoracic). The more rotated the thoracic plane, the lower the junction at the thoracic level. It seems thus interesting to analyze the direction of rotation and to identify the vertebral "breaking point" of this plane 3. Regarding plane rotation, this study reveals that plane 1 (i.e., lumbar plane) mainly presents a direction of rotation similar to the dorsal plane (positive). Plane 1 always rotates less than plane 2, and plane

3 also rotates less than plane 2. Let us specify here again that this work focuses on Lenke 1A scoliosis, which may explain that the rotation of plane 1 is moderate: it would probably have been different if we had considered Lenke 1B or 1C scoliosis, in which thoracic scoliosis is associated with a lumbar non-structural curve destabilized in relation to the center of the sacral plate.

By distinguishing Lenke 1A scoliosis made of three planes from Lenke 1A scoliosis made of four planes after 3D reconstruction, we were able to observe that plane 2 (i.e., thoracic plane) in four-plane scoliosis shows a more important rotation than in three-plane scoliosis. We can thus suppose that the importance of deformity may be responsible for the plane break. Similarly, the junction between plane 2 and plane 3 in four-plane scoliosis is lower when the deformity is more important. In practice, for orthopedic conservative treatment, the first objective with the brace will be to reduce plane rotations, which will lead to a reduction of the Cobb angles and if possible guide this scoliosis from four planes to three planes.

This work also brings to light the fact that the rotation of the cervico-thoracic plane (i.e., plane 3) may either be positive (in counterclockwise direction) or negative (in clockwise direction). Our results show that similar thoracic scoliosis, from a clinical and standard radiographic point of view, may be different from a 3D perspective, with plane 3 presenting either a positive rotation (in the same direction as the dorsal plane) or a negative one (opposite to plane 2)—even if this study does not allow us to come up with an explanation.

We note that Lenke 1A scoliosis could be divided into two classes, depending on the direction of rotation of plane 3 (positive or negative).

The heterogeneity of Lenke 1A has already been demonstrated by Atmaca [25], who added an axial plane analysis to conventional coronal and sagittal evaluations and concluded that it could reveal inherent structural differences that are not apparent in single planar radiographic assessments and may necessitate a different surgical strategy. We also think that this analysis is important to orient treatments, and are convinced that the radiographic evaluation of scoliosis should not be only descriptive in 2D but should also wherever possible be completed by a 3D analysis (upper view), taking into account the regional planes. In daily practice, our evaluation has to consider the Cobb angle on the regional plane and the rotation of the plane. For all that, this analysis is based on a wired reconstruction, which is a limitation for the use of this software, as it does not provide a view of the ribcage (which is important for the conception of the brace) [26]. 3D analysis does not exempt us from a thorough reading of 2D front and profile pictures, in order to have a good radiographic and medical interpretation of issues regarding the spine, ribs, and soft tissues.

Table 3 Pelvic incidence (PI), pelvic tilt (PT), and horizontal rotation of the first three planes for both groups, identified either with three or four planes

	n = 63				
	n = 36 (57%)		n = 27 (43%)		
	3 planes		4 planes		p value
	Mean	SD	Mean	SD	
PI	52.4	9.6	49	9.8	0.209
PT	8.3	7.8	10.5	6.9	0.293
Rot 1	31.9	18.2	35.8	19.7	0.451
Rot 2	67.6	29.4	77.2	16.4	*0.167*
Rot 3	−22.7	52.8	−24.6	50.1	0.89

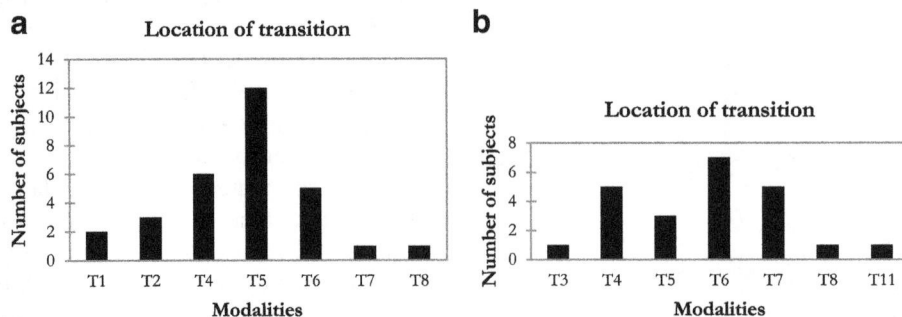

Fig. 4 Location of the junction between the second and the third plane in our sample of Lenke 1A scoliosis, divided into two groups: the three-plane group (**a**) and the four-plane group (**b**)

Conclusion

All scoliotic curves classified 1A from 2D radiographs do not have the same 3D representation. This work underlines the importance of using 3D reconstructions to analyze scoliosis, that is to say including a front view, a profile view, and also a horizontal or top view, in order to assess precisely and understand the deformity. This kind of analysis is particularly useful to identify how scoliosis evolves, by measuring the Cobb angle in regional planes and by quantifying the rotation of the plane, all the while comparing these parameters to clinical data.

Nowadays, the evaluation of scoliotic deformity is based on clinical analysis and morphometric assessment of the trunk, completed by radiographic examination. One needs to go further and use these data to obtain a top view of scoliosis and regional planes, especially when therapeutic options are discussed. To be still more precise, all studied parameters should be connected to their impact on muscular function, and vice versa.

This work can be the starting point for further studies to investigate thoracic scoliosis, depending on the Cobb angle on the plane, number of consecutive planes, and location of breaking point between plane 2 and plane 3, as well as direction of rotation of plane 3. And it will possibly help to develop more adapted therapeutic strategies, especially when considering brace treatment. This has completely changed our daily clinical practice, with a real concern about the orientation and the importance of forces that should be applied through the brace's pads. The top view allows a representation of scoliosis closer to reality and helps to define the ideal brace to correct it.

This regional planes analysis considers each curvature with its rotation, and this is the importance of rotation that helps us to decide and prioritize the to-be-treated curvatures. This is also very helpful to understand why some scoliosis remain stable after brace removal (because the planes rotation is well corrected) whereas others can still become worth, as the plane rotation is not corrected, even if the Cobb angle is corrected on frontal radiographs.

Abbreviations
2D: Two dimensional; 3D: Three dimensional; BFP: Best fit plane; PI: Pelvic incidence; PMC: Plane of major curvature; PT: Pelvic tilt; SRS: Scoliosis Research Society

Acknowledgements
We wish to thank all physiotherapists of the pediatric spine department at the Centre des Massues who kindly gave their time and energy for this work.

Funding
Not applicable.

Authors' contributions
All individuals listed as authors meet the appropriate authorship criteria, and nobody who qualifies for authorship has been omitted from the list. JCB implemented the use of 3D reconstruction in his team's clinical practice and developed the first version of this manuscript. LJ and GN contributed to gathering data. JD collected all study material and gave her substantial contribution to research design, analysis, and interpretation of data, as well as drafting the paper. JD had complete access to the study data that support the publication. EB was in charge of analyzing data and helping interpreting them. He had also complete access to the study data that support the publication. ECV gave substantial contribution to the critical revision, and revised content and accuracy. All authors read and approved the final manuscript.

Authors' information
Jean-Claude Bernard is a physician doctor (in physical and rehabilitation medicine) and a senior clinician at the Centre Médico-Chirurgical de Réadaptation des Massues – Croix Rouge française, in Lyon, France. He received his PhD degree in 1986 and was appointed head of the pediatric department of Physical Medicine and Rehabilitation in Centre des Massues in 1994. He has an extensive experience in working with children with disabilities and has specifically a high daily clinical activity and great interest in spinal deformities in children. This interest has led to research to describe and measure the effects of conservative treatment in children and adolescents with back pain or deformities. Jean-Claude has published a number of journal articles and book chapters relating to his research. He is certified by the European Board of Physical and Rehabilitation Medicine until June 2019 and is also actively involved in medical learned societies, as SOFMER (Société Française de Médecine de Rééducation et Réadaptation Fonctionnelles), GES (Groupe d'Etude sur la Scoliose), SFCR (Société Française de Chirurgie du Rachis), EUROSPINE (Associated member), or SOSORT (Society on Scoliosis Orthopaedic and Rehabilitation Treatment).
Eric Berthonnaud is a biomechanical engineer who has developed a great experience in assessing spinal and pelvic complex. He is working closely with clinicians, medical doctors, and surgeons on these issues at the Centre des Massues, and has published a lot of international papers regarding deformities and spinal balance.

Julie Deceuninck is a physiotherapist and has been working for several years in the pediatric department at the Centre des Massues. She is also actively engaged in research about scoliosis and other spinal issues in children. Lydie Journoud-Rozand and Gregory Notin are orthoprosthesists at Etablissements Lecante, in Lyon, France. Both are particularly involved in orthopedic treatment for scoliosis and work actively with the medical team to develop new options for braces. Emmanuelle Chaleat-Valayer is a doctor in physical and rehabilitation medicine and a senior clinician at the Centre Médico-Chirurgical de Réadaptation des Massues – Croix Rouge française, in Lyon, France. Her extensive experience in spinal disabilities focuses on pain issues, especially in adults with or without deformities. She takes part in a number of research projects about the spine and has published a number of journal articles and book chapters relating to this research. She is also actively involved in medical learned societies, as SOFMER or ANMSR (Association Nationale des Médecins Spécialistes de Rééducation).

Competing interests

The authors declare that they have no competing interests.

Author details

[1]Croix Rouge française – CMCR des Massues, 92, rue Edmond Locard, 69322 Lyon Cedex 05, France. [2]Hôpital Nord Ouest de Villefranche sur Saône, Gleizé 69400, France. [3]Laboratoire de Physiologie de l'Exercice, Saint Etienne, France. [4]Etablissements Lecante, Lyon, France.

References

1. De Smet A, Asher M, Cook L, Goin J, Scheuch H, Orrick J. Three-dimensional analysis of right thoracic idiopathic scoliosis. Spine. 1984;9:377–81.
2. Dubousset J. Three-dimensional analysis of the scoliotic deformity (chapter 22). In: Weinstein SL, editor. The pediatric spine: principles and practice. New York: Raven Press; 1994. p. 479–96.
3. Dubousset J. Scoliose idiopathique: définition, pathologie, classification, étiologie. Bull Acad Natl Med. 1999;183:699–704.
4. Goldstein L, Waugh T. Classification and terminology of scoliosis. Clin Orthop. 1973;93:10–22.
5. Weinstein SL, Dolan LA, Cheng JCY, Danielsson A, Morcuende JA. Adolescent idiopathic scoliosis. Lancet. 2008;371:1527–37.
6. Berthonnaud E, Hilmi R, Dimnet J. Geometric structure of 3D spinal curves: plane regions and connecting zones. ISRN Orthop. 2012;2012:1–11.
7. Berthonnaud E, Papin P, Deceuninck J, Hilmi R, Bernard JC, Dimnet J. The use of a photogrammetric method for the three-dimensional evaluation of spinal correction in scoliosis. Int Orthop. 2016;40:1187–96.
8. Suh C. The fundamentals of computer aided X-ray analysis of the spine. J Biomech. 1974;7:161–9.
9. Brown R, Burstein A, Nash C, Schock C. Spinal analysis using a three-dimensional radiographic technique. J Biomech. 1976;9:355–65.
10. Stokes IA. Three-dimensional terminology of spinal deformity. A report presented to the Scoliosis Research Society by the Scoliosis Research Society working group on 3-D terminology of spinal deformity. Spine. 1994;19:236–48.
11. King H, Moe J, Bradford D, Winter R. The selection of fusion levels in thoracic idiopathic scoliosis. J Bone Joint Surg Am. 1983;65:1302–13.
12. Lenke L, Betz R, Clements D, Merola A, Haher T, Lowe T, et al. Curve prevalence of a new classification of operative adolescent idiopathic scoliosis: does classification correlate with treatment? Spine. 2002;27:604–11.
13. Lenke L, Betz R, Bridwell K, Clements D, Harms J, Lowe T, et al. Intraobserver and interobserver reliability of the classification of thoracic adolescent idiopathic scoliosis. J Bone Joint Surg Am. 1998;80:1097–106.
14. Lenke LG, Betz RR, Harms J, Bridwell KH, Clements DH, Lowe TG, et al. Adolescent idiopathic scoliosis: a new classification to determine extent of spinal arthrodesis. J Bone Joint Surg Am. 2001;83–A:1169–81.
15. Berthonnaud E, Dimnet J, Hilmi R. Classification of pelvic and spinal postural patterns in upright position. Specific cases of scoliotic patients. Comput Med Imaging Graph. 2009;33:634–43.
16. Stagnara P, De Mauroy JC, Dran G, Gonon GP, Costanzo G, Dimnet J, et al. Reciprocal angulation of vertebral bodies in a sagittal plane: approach to references for the evaluation of kyphosis and lordosis. Spine. 1982;7:335–42.
17. Perdriolle R, Le Borgne P, Dansereau J, de Guise J, Labelle H. Idiopathic scoliosis in three dimensions: a succession of two-dimensional deformities? Spine. 2001;26:2719–26.
18. Perdriolle R, Vidal J. A study of scoliotic curve. The importance of extension and vertebral rotation (author's transl). Rev Chir Orthop Reparatrice Appar Mot. 1981;67:25–34.
19. Perdriolle R. La scoliose: son étude tridimensionnelle. Paris: Maloine; 1979.
20. Negrini S, Negrini A, Atanasio S, Santambrogio GC. Three-dimensional easy morphological (3-DEMO) classification of scoliosis, part I. Scoliosis. 2006;1:20.
21. Donzelli S, Zaina F, Lusini M, Minnella S, Respizzi S, Balzarini L, et al. The three dimensional analysis of the Sforzesco brace correction. Scoliosis Spinal Disord. 2016;11(Suppl 2):34.
22. Duong L, Mac-Thiong J, Cheriet F, Labelle H. Three-dimensional subclassification of Lenke type 1 scoliotic curves. J Spinal Disord Tech. 2009;22:135–43.
23. Stagnara P. Les déformations du rachis. Paris: Masson; 1985.
24. Peloux J, Fauchet R, Faucon B, Stagnara P. Le plan d'élection pour l'examen radiologique des cyphoscolioses. Rev Chir Orthop Reparatrice Appar Mot. 1965;51:517–254.
25. Atmaca H, Inanmaz ME, Bal E, Caliskan I, Kose KC. Axial plane analysis of Lenke 1A adolescent idiopathic scoliosis as an aid to identify curve characteristics. Spine J. 2014;14(10):2425–33.
26. Labelle H, Dansereau J, Bellefleur C, Jéquier JC. Variability of geometric measurements from three-dimensional reconstructions of scoliotic spines and rib cages. Eur Spine J. 1995;4:88–94.

13

Non-radiographic methods of measuring global sagittal balance

Larry Cohen*, Sarah Kobayashi, Milena Simic, Sarah Dennis, Kathryn Refshauge and Evangelos Pappas

Abstract

Background: Global sagittal balance, describing the vertical alignment of the spine, is an important factor in the non-operative and operative management of back pain. However, the typical gold standard method of assessment, radiography, requires exposure to radiation and increased cost, making it unsuitable for repeated use. Non-radiologic methods of assessment are available, but their reliability and validity in the current literature have not been systematically assessed. Therefore, the aim of this systematic review was to synthesise and evaluate the reliability and validity of non-radiographic methods of assessing global sagittal balance.

Methods: Five electronic databases were searched and methodology evaluated by two independent reviewers using the 13-item, reliability and validity, Brink and Louw critical appraisal tool.

Results: Fourteen articles describing six methodologies were identified from 3940 records. The six non-radiographic methodologies were biophotogrammetry, plumbline, surface topography, infra-red motion analysis, spinal mouse and ultrasound. Construct validity was evaluated for surface topography ($R = 0.49$ and $R = 0.68$, $p < 0.001$), infra-red motion-analysis (ICC = 0.81) and plumbline testing (ICC = 0.83). Reliability ranged from moderate (ICC = 0.67) for spinal mouse to very high for surface topography (Cronbach $\alpha = 0.985$). Measures of agreement ranged from 0.9 mm (plumbline) to 22.94 mm (infra-red motion-analysis). Variability in study populations, reporting parameters and statistics prevented a meta-analysis.

Conclusions: The reliability and validity of the non-radiographic methods of measuring global sagittal balance was reported within 14 identified articles. Based on this limited evidence, non-radiographic methods appear to have moderate to very high reliability and limited to three methodologies, moderate to high validity. The overall quality and methodological approaches of the included articles were highly variable. Further research should focus on the validity of non-radiographic methods with a greater adherence to reporting actual and clinically relevant measures of agreement.

Keywords: Spine posture, Spine shape, Non-invasive assessment, Sagittal vertical axis, SVA, Measurement, Reliability, Validity

Background

Progressive stooped posture, a common consequence of the ageing process, is associated with poor quality of life [1, 2]. This posture, which can be described according to the vertical alignment of the trunk over the pelvis, is defined as global sagittal balance and is termed anterior sagittal balance when exceeding predetermined threshold values. Anterior sagittal balance is the postural deformity that is most closely correlated with pain, activity limitations and reduced quality of life [2] and affects up to 29% of the population above 60 years of age [3].

The current gold standard for measurement of global sagittal balance is the sagittal vertical axis (SVA) obtained via radiographs. SVA is quantified by measuring, in centimetres, the horizontal distance between the centre of the C7 vertebral body to the postero-superior border of the sacrum on full-length lateral spine radiographs [1]. This requires the use of spine-specific radiographic software [4] which demonstrates excellent intra-rater (ICC = 0.98) and inter-rater (ICC = 0.95) reliability and excellent accuracy between inter-rater tests (ISO reproducibility of 4.02 mm)

* Correspondence: lcoh0894@uni.sydney.edu.au
Faculty of Health Sciences, Discipline of Physiotherapy, The University of Sydney, 75 East Street, Lidcombe, NSW 2141, Australia

[5]. SVA thresholds defining anterior sagittal balance range from 3 to 6 cm [6–10]. Alternate radiographic methods of sagittal spine balance measurement, which do not require spine specific radiographic software, include the angular measurements of T1 spinal inclination (T1Spi) and C7-S1 trunk inclination [11]. T1Spi has been reported to be more closely correlated to clinical outcomes evaluated by the Oswestry Disability Index, Short Form-12 and SRS-23 than SVA [11].

Recent advances in surgical and non-surgical spine management have revealed the importance of identifying, maintaining or restoring sagittal balance to achieve reduction in pain, improvement in function, quality of life and reduction in post-operative complications following spine surgery [11, 12]. Physiotherapy treatment aimed at restoring sagittal balance, primarily by increasing lumbar lordosis, has likewise been demonstrated to improve clinical outcomes in patients with chronic lower back pain [13]. Therefore, the measurement of global sagittal balance is important for the development and monitoring of effective spine therapy interventions.

Although radiographs are the current gold standard, repeated radiographic exposure potentially increases lifetime risk for cancer development [13]. This is compounded when considering that lateral full spine radiographs can deliver an effective radiation dose that is 50–70% higher than standard posterior-anterior (PA) full spine radiographs [14]. Therefore, due to the high cost and radiation exposure, repeated radiographic measurement and monitoring of sagittal balance in the clinical setting have serious limitations [13]. Non-radiographic methods of measuring global sagittal balance are available and may present a viable option for monitoring patient progress. These methods vary with regard to technical complexity and equipment cost. However, the currently available methods and their psychometric properties have not been assessed systematically. Therefore, the aim of this systematic review was to evaluate the reliability and validity of non-radiographic methods of assessing global sagittal balance.

Methods
Protocol and registration
This review protocol was registered in August 2014 with the PROSPERO International prospective register of systematic reviews (ID PROSPERO 2014:CRD42014013071).

Data sources
Electronic database searches of MEDLINE, EMBASE, Web of Science, CINAHL and AMED were conducted from database inception until week 38, September 2016. The search terms were based on three main term groups: sagittal alignment, psychometric properties and physical tests.

The Boolean term "OR" was used within each term group and the Boolean term "AND" was used between each term group. Additional hand searches of relevant bibliographies were completed (Appendix).

Eligibility criteria
Studies were included if they reported reliability and/or validity of non-radiographic methods of measuring standing global sagittal spine parameters in people with or without spine deformity or pain. All studies were considered regardless of publication date, age of participants or language.

Study selection
Two independent reviewers (LC, SK), after trialling a small pilot study, screened the titles and abstracts for eligible studies and reviewed the full texts of those identified. Full texts were retrieved if one reviewer determined that the record could not be excluded by title or abstract. In cases of disagreement, a third reviewer (EP) adjudicated. Bibliographies of included studies were searched for additional references.

Data extraction
In order to extract comprehensive methodological, population and psychometric data two independent reviewers (LC, SK) used a 13-item critical appraisal tool developed by Brink and Louw [15]. The Brink and Louw critical appraisal tool was developed from the Quality Assessment of Diagnostic Accuracy Studies (QUADAS) and Quality Appraisal of Diagnostic Reliability Studies (QUAREL) to test combined or independent reliability and validation studies [16]. The data included a description of the study population and raters, detailed description of blinding, randomisation, between testing time periods, testing procedures, withdrawals and statistics methodology. Disagreement was resolved by consensus and, if necessary, in consultation with a third reviewer (EP). Authors of articles where the results or methodology were unclear were contacted for clarification.

Pearson's r, Cronbach α and intra-class correlation coefficients (ICC) statistics were interpreted as follows: ≤ 0.29 very low correlation, 0.20–0.49 low correlation, 0.50–0.69 moderate correlation, 0.70–0.89 high correlation and ≥ 0.90 very high correlation [17]. Agreement was evaluated by the standard error of measurement (SEM) which, when data were available, was calculated according to the equation: SEM = standard deviation (SD) $\div \sqrt{1}$–reliability coefficient [18].

Quality assessment
Methodological quality of individual studies was evaluated using the Brink and Louw critical appraisal tool and

synthesised within the summary tables. Articles were considered high quality if they scored greater than the accepted 60% threshold on the Brink and Louw critical appraisal tool [16].

Results

Studies included in the review

The database search strategy retrieved a total of 3940 records. After removal of duplicates, 2685 of the remaining citations were excluded as they did not meet the inclusion criteria. Following full text review of 114 articles, 14 articles met the inclusion criteria. The flow of articles through the review process is depicted in the PRISMA flow diagram (Fig. 1). We contacted the lead author of three included studies, a German language article for further information on methodology [19] and the lead authors of two other English language studies, to clarify reported units of measurement [20] and methods of measurement [21].

Global sagittal balance measurement methods

A total of 14 studies describing six global sagittal balance measurement methods were included in the review. Two studies measured construct validity, one by

root mean square deviation [19] and one by ICC [21], two measured both construct validity and reliability [13, 22] and 10 studies [20, 23–31] investigated reliability of the sagittal balance measurement methods.

A description of each non-radiographic measurement method is provided in Table 1. Of the four studies reporting validity, three studies compared surface topography to radiographically measured angular trunk inclination [13, 22] and radiographic SVA [19]. The fourth validity study compared plumbline and infrared (IR) motion analysis to radiographic SVA [21]. Nine studies examined inter- and intra-rater reliability [13, 19, 20, 22–25, 29, 31], and three studies examined test-retest time interval reliability [26–28]. Five studies evaluated the reliability for surface topography and two studies each for spinal mouse, plumbline testing and biophotogrammetry with one study for ultrasonic testing.

In terms of the outcome variables, trunk inclination was measured in four studies; two using spinal mouse [23, 24] and two using surface topography [13, 22] methodology. The distance from a plumbline reference line to the cervical or lumbar lordosis apex and the S1 landmark point was measured in four studies

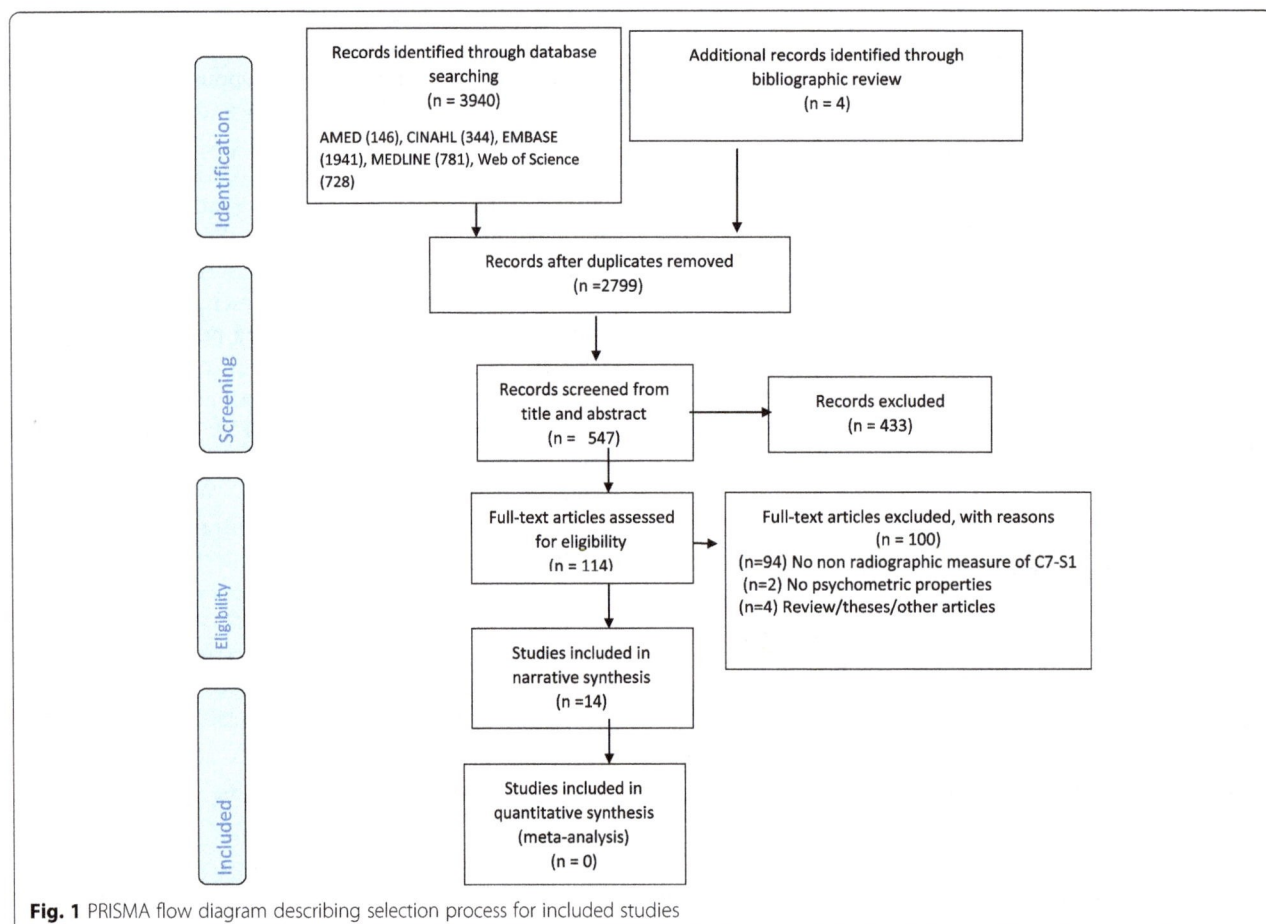

Fig. 1 PRISMA flow diagram describing selection process for included studies

Table 1 Detailed description of non-radiographic measurement methods, equipment and technique used in the included studies

Method	Description of evaluation	Equipment required	Technique	References
Biophotogrammetry	Biophotogrammetric analysis involves measuring, off-lateral posture photographs, the distance from a plumbline to the lordotic and cervical apex [25] or C7, S1 prominences [30].	Digital camera with vertical plumbline reference posterior to the subject within field of view and a known (presized) object within field of view to establish distance scaling. Computer with graphic editing software	Adhesive stickers that can be seen from the lateral margin of the body are placed on the C7 and S1 landmarks. After calibration, the distance from the plumbline to the landmark points are measured using graphic editing software.	[25, 30]
Infra-red motion analysis	Motion analysis computer-interfaced stereovideographic acquisition of infra-red-activated anatomical markers at C7 [21, 26], T1 [28] and S1.	Minimum of three motion analysis cameras linked to a computer via an image processor. Infra-red light reflected on the adhesive markers	Adhesive infra-red markers are affixed to C7/T1 and S1. The markers are activated by infra-red light and the dedicated computer system triangulates the spine data measuring the sagittal arrows.	[21, 26, 28]
Plumbline	A ruler and plumbline to measure the distance to the C7 and L3 [29, 31], or C7 and S1 [21] anatomical points on the body	Ruler and plumbline	The plumbline is held against or very near to the posterior surface of the skin. The distance from the plumbline to C7 and L3 or S1 is measured.	[21, 29, 31]
Spinal mouse	Spinal mouse assessment uses a wireless computer-interfaced rollerball input device to determine the inclination of the spine from C7 to S1 and the vertical.	Spinal Mouse (Idiag, Voletswil, Switzerland) and computer	The spinal mouse is rolled along the contour of the spine from C7 to S1 measuring distance of travel and angulation.	[23, 24]
Surface topography	Surface topography based on Moire stereovideography measures the distortion of a predicted light grid to create a 3D model of the back providing angular or distance offset data from the vertebral prominens (C7 or T1) to the midpoint between the PSIS.	Surface topography machine (Biomod, AXS Ingenierie, Bordeaux, France) [13] formetric (Diers International, Schlangenbad, Germany) [19, 20, 22, 27] and computer interface	Depending on system, optional, infra-red adhesive markers are placed on C7, PSISs and inter-gluteal cleft. Scanning is performed according to the specifications of the manufacturer.	[13, 19, 20, 22, 27]
Freepoint ultrasound	Freepoint ultrasound system emits an ultrasonic signal from the probe to receivers which triangulate the position of T1 and C7 in space.	Freepoint ultrasound system (GTCO Calcomp, Scottsdale, USA) and interfaced computer	The freepoint probe is used to identify the T1 and S1 landmarks, which are triangulated and digitised allowing for computerised 3D reconstruction.	[28]

[13, 21, 25, 29]. These plumbline reference line-to-body surface landmark points are commonly termed "sagittal arrows" in the literature [21]. The horizontal offset between superior and inferior landmarks was measured in seven studies, but there was inconsistency with landmark identification. Three studies used the vertebra prominens and the midpoint of the lumbar dimples [19, 20, 27], one study C7 and the midpoint of the lumbar dimples [21], two studies used C7-S1 [26, 30], and one study used T1-S1 [28].

Quality assessment

The average quality of the 14 studies was 56% (range 44–77%) (Table 2). One validity and reliability study [22], two validity studies [19, 21] and three reliability studies [23, 25, 27] were of high quality, scoring > 60% on the critical appraisal tool. The main items with low scores were a suitable description of the raters (71% of studies unreported), within-rater blinding (77% of studies unreported), variation of testing order between raters (92% of studies unreported) and a suitable explanation of withdrawals from the study (92% of studies unreported).

Participants

Healthy adult participants were evaluated in five studies [20, 24, 27, 28, 30] and healthy children in one study [23]. Four studies evaluated participants with spine deformity or pain; three included adolescents [22, 26, 31] and one involved adults [13]. One study evaluated children, adolescents and adults with spine deformity [19], one study evaluated adults who demonstrated clinical

manifestation of mouth breathing during childhood [25] and another study, adults with camptocormia [21].

Sample sizes for the validity studies ranged from 95 [19] to 326 [13] participants for the two surface topography studies and 49 participants for the plumbline and IR motion study [21]. Reliability study sample sizes ranged from two participants examined once by five raters (inter-rater) and 15 times by one rater (intra-rater) [13] to 180 participants examined by two raters (inter-rater) and then repeated after 5 min by one rater (intra-rater) [29]. Only four studies included participants with a mean age greater than 30 years [13, 21, 24, 30].

Validity and reliability

Validity

Correlations between non-radiographic and radiographic methods of measuring global sagittal balance ranged from low to high (Table 3). Liljenquist et al. [19] compared surface topography sagittal trunk offset distance to radiographic SVA and reported a root mean square deviation (RMSD) of 1.07 cm. Legaye [13] compared surface topography trunk inclination to radiographically determined C7-S1 global sagittal axis and reported a moderate and significant correlation of $r = 0.68$ ($p < 0.001$). Knott et al. [22] compared surface topography sagittal trunk inclination to radiographically determined SVA inclination and reported a low Pearson correlation of 0.49. de Seze et al. [21] compared radiographic SVA to plumbline and IR motion analysis and reported high ICCs of 0.81 and 0.83 respectively.

Table 2 Methodological quality of included studies evaluated using the Brink and Louw critical appraisal tool

Study	Key information	1	2	3	4	5	6	7	8	9	10	11	12	13	High-quality > 60%
1	de Seze [21]	✓	✗	✓	n/a	n/a	n/a	✓	n/a	✓	✗	✓	✗	✓	6/9 = 66%
2	Grosso 2002 [31]	✓	✓	n/a	✗	✗	✗	n/a	✓	n/a	✗	n/a	✗	✓	4/9 = 44%
3	Kellis 2008 [23]	✓	✓	n/a	✓	✓	✗	n/a	✓	n/a	✓	n/a	✗	✓	7/9 = 77%
4	Knott 2016 [22]	✓	✗	✓	✗	✗	✗	✓	✓	✓	✓	✓	✗	✓	8/13 = 62%
5	Legaye 2012 [13]	✓	✗	✓	✗	✗	✗	✗	✗	✓	✓	✓	✗	✓	6/13 = 46%
6	Liljenqvist 1998 [19]	✓	✗	✓	n/a	n/a	n/a	✗	✗	✓	✓	✓	✗	✓	6/9 = 66%
7	Mannion 2004 [24]	✓	✗	n/a	✓	✗	✗	n/a	✗	n/a	✓	n/a	✗	✓	4/9 = 44%
8	Mohokum 2010 [20]	✓	✓	n/a	✗	✗	✗	n/a	✓	n/a	✓	n/a	✗	✓	5/9 = 55%
9	Milanesi 2011 [25]	✓	✗	n/a	✓	✓	✗	n/a	✓	n/a	✓	n/a	✗	✓	6/9 = 66%
10	Negrini 2001 [26]	✓	✗	n/a	✗	✗	✗	n/a	✓	n/a	✓	n/a	✓	✓	5/9 = 55%
11	Schroeder [27]	✓	✓	n/a	✗	✓	✗	n/a	✓	n/a	✓	n/a	✗	✓	6/9 = 66%
12	Zabjek 1999 [28]	✓	✗	n/a	✗	✗	✓	n/a	✓	n/a	✓	n/a	✗	✓	5/9 = 55%
13	Zaina 2012 [29]	✗	✗	n/a	✗	✗	✗	n/a	✓	n/a	✓	n/a	✗	✓	4/9 = 44%
14	Zheng 2010 [30]	✓	✗	n/a	✗	✗	✗	n/a	✓	n/a	✓	n/a	✗	✓	4/9 = 44%

1 description of study population, *2* description of raters, *3* explanation of reference standards (validity only), *4* between rater blinding (reliability only), *5* within rater blinding (reliability), *6* variation of testing order (reliability), *7* time period between index test and reference standard (validity), *8* time period between repeated measures (reliability), *9* independency of reference standard from index test (validity), *10* description of index test procedure, *11* description of reference test procedure (validity), *12* explanation of any withdrawals, *13* appropriate statistics methods. ✓ Reported, ✗ Not reported

Table 3 Study characteristics, reliability, validity and SEM data of included studies

Non-radiographic method	Study	Index test variable	Sample	Age	Methodology description	Validity test variable	Reliability test variable	Statistical measure	Resultant statistical value	SEM
Biophotogrammetric analysis	Milanesi 2011 [25]	Cervical and lumbar lordosis apex arrows	24 adults with clinical manifestation of mouth breathing during childhood	18–30 years	3 raters on 1 occasion		Inter-rater	ICC	>0.75	0.23–0.37 cm (range)
	Zheng 2010 [30]	C7-S1 offset	30 asymptomatic adult participants	35.5 ± 9.4 years	Examined 12 times in neutral standing and hands on clavicles		Intra-rater	Repeatability (mean of the SD ± SD)		6 ± 1.9 mm neutral standing
								As above		7.3 ± 3 mm hands on clavicles
Freepoint (FP) ultrasound system	Zabjeck 1999 [28]	T1-S1 offset	15 adult control participants	25 ± 6 years	Examined 5 times by each system 1 week apart		FP intra-session	Mean ± SD	19.1 ± 7.9 mm	2.03 mm (mean)
							FP inter-session difference	Mean ± SD	–3.2 ± 11.6 mm	2.99 mm (mean)
							MA vs. freepoint	ICC	0.93	
Infra-red motion analysis	de Seze 2015 [21] Elite IR optoelectronic system	C7-S1 offset	43 adults with camptocormia	69 ± 10 years		Validity. Radiographic sagittal vertical axis (SVA)		ICC	0.83	
	Negrini 2001. [26] Auscan optoelectronic 3D IR imaging system with manual landmark identification	C7-S1 offset	97 patients with adolescent idiopathic scoliosis	15.15 ± 2.25 years	Examined twice with 3 time intervals between measurements		Intra-session 6 s interval	Bland and Altman repeatability coefficient		12.52 mm (mean difference)
							Intra-session 24 s interval	As above		14.64 mm (as above)
							Intra-session 167 s interval	As above		22.94 mm (as above)
	Zabjeck 1999 [28] IR motion analysis (MA) system and freepoint (FP) ultrasound system	T1-S1 offset	15 adult control participants	25 ± 6 years	Examined 5 times by each system 1 week apart		MA intra-session difference	Mean ± SD	10.9 ± 7 mm	1.8 mm (mean)

Table 3 Study characteristics, reliability, validity and SEM data of included studies *(Continued)*

	Study	Measurement	Sample	Age	Procedure	Validity	MA inter-session difference	Mean ± SD			
Plumbline testing	de Seze 2015 [21]	C7-S1 Sagittal arrows	43 adults with camptocormia	69 ± 10 years		Validity. Radiographic sagittal vertical axis (SVA)		ICC	2.9 ± 6.9 mm	0.81	1.78 mm (mean)
	Grosso 2002 [31]	C7-L3 sagittal arrows	116 AIS, hyperkyphotic and hyperlordotic adolescents	13.6 ± 2.4 years	2 raters on 2 occasions		Inter-rater	ICC cervical		0.86	
								ICC lumbar		0.76	
	Zaina 2012 [29]	C7 and L3 Sagittal arrows	180 AIS and hyperkyphotic adolescents	Aged 11-16	Examined by 2 raters and then repeated after 5 min by one rater		Intra-rater	Bland and Altman repeatability coefficient			0.9 mm C7 / 1.2 mm L3 (mean difference)
							Inter-rater	As above			1.7 mm C7 / 2.2 mm L3
Spinal mouse	Kellis 2008 [23]	C7-S1 Angular trunk inclination	81 healthy children	10.6 ± 1.7 years	Examined by 3 raters on 2 separate occasions		Intra-rater	ICC		0.67–0.87	1.19°–1.97° (range)
							Inter-rater	ICC		0.77–0.82	0.96°–1.2°
	Mannion 2004 [24]	C7-S1 Angular trunk inclination	29 healthy adult participants	45.4 ± 7.7 years	Examined by 2 raters on 2 separate occasions		Intra-rater	ICC		0.83–0.84	1° (0.8°–1.5°) (mean)(95% CI)
							Inter-rater	ICC		0.71–0.77	1.5° (1.2–2.2 95% CI) (as above)
Surface topography	Knott 2016 [22] Diers formetric surface topography system compared with upright full spine radiographs	VP-DM sagittal trunk inclination. Compared with C7-S1 trunk inclination	193 AIS and hyperkyphotic adolescents	8-18 years	Multicentre trial with same day testing.	Validity. Radiographic sagittal vertical inclination	Three scans repeated within 5 min	Pearson's Correlation		0.49	± 3.7° (SD)
								ICC		0.91	± 1.1° (SD)
	Legaye 2012 [13]. Biomod surface topographical system with manual landmark identification	C7 and superior border of gluteal cleft angular trunk inclination	1 symptomatic male, 1 asymptomatic scoliotic female participant	Both 53-year olds	Examined once by 5 raters (inter-observer) and 15 times by one rater (intra-observer).		Intra-rater	Confidence interval		1°	
							Inter-rater	Confidence interval		1°	
		C7 and superior border of -gluteal cleft (pelvic) sagittal arrows	As above				Intra-rater	Confidence interval		3 mm cervical	
										5 mm pelvic	
							Inter-rater	Confidence interval		4 mm cervical	
										4 mm pelvic	

Table 3 Study characteristics, reliability, validity and SEM data of included studies *(Continued)*

Study	Parameter	Population	Age	Correlation	Validity	Rater/Occasion	Measure	Value	SEM
Liljenqvist 1998 [19] Diers formetric surface topography system compared with upright full spine radiographs	C7 and superior border of -gluteal cleft Angular trunk inclination	326 adults with pain or deformity (kyphosis, fractures, scoliosis)	Range from 7 to 86 years	Correlation between radiographs and surface topography	Validity. Radiographic C7S1 angular axis		Pearson's correlation	R = 0.68 p < 0.001	
	VP-DM sagittal offset distance	95 children, adolescents and adult patients with scoliosis or hyperkyphosis	Mean age 16.5 range 7–30 years	Correlation between radiographs and surface topography examined by 2 raters	Validity. Radiographic sagittal vertical axis (SVA)		Root mean square deviation	1.07 cm	
Mohokum [20] 2010 Diers formetric surface topography system with automatic landmark identification	VP-DM sagittal offset distance[a]	51 healthy adults with normal and high BMI	24.6 ± 5.8 years	Examined 3 times by 3 raters on one occasion		Intra-rater	Cronbach α	0.950–0.985	3.49 mm (mean)
						Inter-rater	Cronbach α	0.97	
Schroeder [27] 2015 Diers formetric surface topography system with automatic landmark identification	VP-DM sagittal offset distance	20 adult participants without back pain	25.4 ± 5.5 years	Within 5 min on 1 day, the following day and the following week		Intra-day	ICC	0.858–0.978	3 mm (mean)
						Inter-day	ICC	0.843–0.977	
						Inter-week	ICC	0.855–0.977	

[a]Erroneously reported as degrees

VP vertebra prominens, *DM* midpoint between *PSIS* dimples, *SEM* standard error of measurement

Reliability

The overall reliability results of all non-radiographic measurements ranged from moderate (ICC 0.67) to very high (Cronbach α 0.98). Spinal mouse methodology rated moderate (ICC 0.67) to high (ICC 0.87) [23, 24], biophotogrammetric (ICC > 0.75) [25] and plumbline measurement (ICC 0.76–0.86) [31] rated high, and surface topography inter- and intra-rater reliability rated high (ICC 0.84) [27] to very high (Cronbach α 0.95) [20]. The repeatability coefficient of the three methods reporting reliability by Bland and Altman statistics ranged from 0.9 mm [29] to 22.9 mm [32]. The results of the descriptive statistics depicting the reliability of the remaining three methods ranged from 3 mm [13] to 19.1 mm [28]. The test-retest order of precision from most to least precise was plumbline (0.9–1.2 mm) [29], surface topography (3–5 mm) [13], bio-photogrammetry (6–7.3 mm) [30], motion analysis (2.9–10.9 mm) [28], freepoint ultrasound (3.2–19.1 mm) [28] and Auscan motion analysis (10.9–22.9 mm) [26]. Study characteristics are shown in Table 3.

Selection of the superior landmark reference point varied within our included studies, with eight studies adopting C7 [13, 21, 23, 24, 26, 29–31], four studies the vertebral prominens [19, 20, 22, 27], and one study adopting T1 [28]. Similar variation was observed in the inferior reference point with two studies adopting L3 [29, 31], five studies S1 [23, 24, 26, 28, 30], five studies the midpoint between the posterior superior iliac spine (PSIS) dimples [19–22, 27], and one study adopting the superior margin of the gluteal cleft [13].

Discussion

The aim of this systematic review was to identify, synthesise and summarise the reliability and validity of the non-radiographic global sagittal balance measurement methods. Several methods that vary widely in cost and technological complexity were identified, including plumbline testing, surface topography and IR motion analysis, which all had the most supporting evidence. Surface topography had low to moderate validity, very high reliability and high, but less than plumbline testing, accuracy. IR motion analysis had high validity and reliability with moderate accuracy. The overall quality rating of the studies was below the 60% threshold for a high rating, and they displayed a lack of homogeneity with regard to participants, reporting variables, and methods of measuring agreement.

The present systematic review noting that the plumbline method, which is the least technologically advanced and least expensive method, has high validity [21] and high reliability [29, 31]. This suggests that the plumbline method, which is easily accessible to clinicians and requires little training, can provide quantifiable data and

offer higher intra-rater reliability precision than the other methods. However, a note of caution is due here as de Seze et al.'s [21] validity results were obtained from a sample of Parkinson's disease patients exhibiting camptocormia (SVA 110 ± 11 mm), limiting generalisability to a different population.

Surface topography, unlike the other methods of measurement and with very little operator involvement, is able to provide, in one scan, the widest variety of sagittal balance measurements, including trunk inclination, distance offset measurements and sagittal arrows distance measurements. The reliability scores for inter-rater, intra-rater, inter-day and intra-day testing, including one from a high-quality study [27] ranged from high to very high reliability (ICC 0.86–0.98). However, the validity scores ranged from moderate (Pearson's r of 0.68) in a low-quality study [13] to low (Pearson r of 0.49) in a high-quality study [22]. There was little consistency with regard to reporting limits of agreement of surface topography to SVA with Liljenqvist et al. [19] reporting a distance offset RMSD of 1.07 cm and Knott [22] an angular average difference of $\pm 3.7°$. This suggests a level of inaccuracy and further work to establish clinical limits of agreement is needed, given that radiographic SVA threshold ranges defining anterior sagittal balance are 3–5 cm [6–9, 13].

Not only are our results confounded by the inconsistent selection of superior and inferior landmarks between our studies, and not all sagittal balance parameters can be measured with the same accuracy and reliability. Furthermore, the surrogate outcomes provided by non-radiographic measurement raises a question whether manually palpated surface landmarks accurately correlate with radiographic landmarks. Robinson et al. reported moderate inter-rater palpation agreement (67% within 10 mm) and moderate agreement with radiographically determined L5 (kappa 0.48) but poor agreement with radiographically determined C7 (kappa 0.18). [33]. Kilby et al. reported wide variability for manual palpation of ultrasonically identified lumbopelvic landmarks (Bland Altman limits of agreement −27 to 26 mm) concluding that manual palpation of lumbopelvic points has limited validity [34]. These validity results suggest that further research needs to be conducted to evaluate if radiographic methods of measuring global sagittal balance can be replaced with non-radiographic methods. This should be conducted with simultaneous non-radiographic evaluation of lumbar lordosis which appears to be, in conjunction with pelvic tilt, the main contributor to global sagittal balance [2, 8, 13].

The reliability of the lower cost and simpler, spinal mouse and biophotogrammetric methods, [16, 32] has been investigated to a lesser extent than plumbline, IR and surface topography. The spinal mouse system, which involves a wirelessly connected trackball, measures global sagittal balance by trunk inclination. Although validity studies are available for spinal mouse determined sagittal and coronal spine parameters, with high to very high correlation with radiographically measured coronal frontal plane Cobb angle (ICC 0.87–0.96) [35], lordosis ($r = 0.73$) and kyphosis ($r = 0.76$) angles [36], none have evaluated the validity of trunk inclination. As the spinal mouse reliability studies included in the current review involved healthy adolescent and young populations, further studies, which involve older populations need to be undertaken. In a systematic review of non-radiographic measurement of thoracic kyphosis, Barrett et al. [16] also identified strong reliability for spinal mouse measurements. Barrett et al. concluded that the flexicurve was the most feasible non-radiographic method of measuring kyphosis, with high levels of reliability and validity; however, the flexicurve cannot be used for measurement of sagittal balance.

There remains considerable debate regarding the most appropriate method of measuring agreement within reliability and validity studies [37]. Only 30% of our studies reported Bland-Altman plots, and this is less than the 85% reported in Zaki et al.'s [37] systematic review of agreement within medical instrumentation testing methods. Zaki et al. cautioned researchers about utilising inappropriate methodologies to measure agreement because they are likely to result in incorrect conclusions and possible detrimental patient care. They recommended reporting results using multiple methods of measuring agreement. The limits of agreement should also be extrapolated into clinically meaningful limits which were not detailed in any of our included studies.

Strengths and limitations
Despite following the PRISMA guidelines, including all stages conducted by two independent reviewers, all languages and participants of any age, as with all such reviews, the possibility exists that not all the available articles were identified by the searches. We recognise that article quality may have been scored higher if the authors had adhered to the critical appraisal tool items but not reported on relevant items. We stress the importance of publication date, especially for the technology-based methods, since progressive technological evolution limits comparison of results and accuracy between and within advancing methods. There are also some limitations to be considered when interpreting our review. Due to significant variability in study methodologies, populations, reporting parameters and statistics, a quantitative meta-analysis could not be conducted.

Conclusion
Sagittal alignment, which is associated with increased pain and reduced quality of life, is an important concept emerging within the field of spine pain and deformity care. Non-radiographic methods of measuring global sagittal balance have low to very high reliability and, limited to plumbline testing, surface topography and IR motion, low to high validity. Thus, although it is currently unclear if these three methods can be used to evaluate sagittal balance pathology, they can be used with relative confidence for the monitoring of global sagittal balance. Further research needs be undertaken to establish the value of non-radiographic methods of measuring global sagittal balance. These future studies should ideally include the ageing population, adhere to best practice research methodology and psychometric agreement statistics reporting.

Abbreviations
AMED: The Allied and Complementary Medicine Database; CINAHL: The Cumulative Index of Nursing and Allied Health Literature database; DM: Midpoint between surface location of PSISs; EMBASE: The Excerpta Medica journal citation database; FP ultrasound: Freepoint ultrasound; ICC: Intra-class correlation coefficient; IR: Infra-red; ISO: International Organization for Standardization; MA: Motion analysis; MEDLINE: The National Library of Medicine journal citation database; PRISMA: The Preferred Reporting Items for Systematic Reviews and Meta-Analyses guidelines; PROSPERO: International prospective register of systematic reviews; PSIS: Posterior superior iliac spine; QUADAS: An assessment tool for the quality of diagnostic accuracy studies; QUAREL: An assessment tool for the quality of diagnostic reliability studies; R: Correlation coefficient; RMSD: Root mean square deviation is a measure of the difference between predicted and observed values; SEM: The standard error of measurement is the standard deviation of errors of measurement; SRS-23: Health-related quality of life questionnaire developed by the Scoliosis Research Society; SVA: Sagittal vertical axis; a measure of the horizontal offset of the midpoint of the C7 vertebrae from the posterior border of S1; T1-Spi: The angle between the midpoint of the fist thoracic vertebrae and a vertical line at the hip axis; VP: Vertabrae prominens: prominent surface location around C7, T1

Acknowledgements
No acknowledgments to declare.

Funding
No funding was received for the preparation and submission of this research report.

Authors' contributions
LC, SK, MS, SD, KR, EP were involved in the conception of the study, design of the study and helped to draft the manuscript. LC, SK, EP were involved with the database searches, record screening and article review process. All authors read and approved the final manuscript.

Competing interests

The authors declare that they have no competing interests.

References

1. Glassman SD, Bridwell K, Dimar JR, Horton W, Berven S, Schwab F. The impact of positive sagittal balance in adult spinal deformity. Spine. 2005;30(18):2024–9.
2. Smith JS, Klineberg E, Schwab F, Shaffrey CI, Moal B, Ames CP, Hostin R, Fu KM, Burton D, Akbarnia B, Gupta M, Hart R, Bess S, Lafage V, International Spine Study G. Change in classification grade by the SRS-Schwab Adult Spinal Deformity Classification predicts impact on health-related quality of life measures: prospective analysis of operative and nonoperative treatment. Spine. 2013;38(19):1663–71.
3. Barreto MVA, Pratali RR, Barsotti CEG, Santos FPE, Oliveira CEAS, Nogueira MP. Incidence of spinal deformity in adults and its distribution according SRS-Schwab classification. Coluna/Columna. 2015;14:93–6.
4. Akbar M, Terran J, Ames CP, Lafage V, Schwab F. Use of Surgimap spine in sagittal plane analysis, osteotomy planning, and correction calculation. Neurosurg Clin N Am. 2013;24(2):163–72.
5. Lafage R, Ferrero E, Henry JK, Challier V, Diebo B, Liabaud B, Lafage V, Schwab F. Validation of a new computer-assisted tool to measure spino-pelvic parameters. Spine J. 2015;15(12):2493–502.
6. Le Huec JC, Charosky S, Barrey C, Rigal J, Aunoble S. Sagittal imbalance cascade for simple degenerative spine and consequences: algorithm of decision for appropriate treatment. Eur Spine J. 2011;20(Suppl 5):699–703.
7. Bess S, Schwab F, Lafage V, Shaffrey CI, Ames CP. Classifications for adult spinal deformity and use of the Scoliosis Research Society-Schwab Adult Spinal Deformity Classification. Neurosurg Clin N Am. 2013;24(2):185–93.
8. Schwab F, Ungar B, Blondel B, Buchowski J, Coe J, Deinlein D, DeWald C, Mehdian H, Shaffrey C, Tribus C, Lafage V. Scoliosis Research Society-Schwab adult spinal deformity classification: a validation study. Spine. 2012;37(12):1077–82.
9. Lee JS, Lee HS, Shin JK, Goh TS, Son SM. Prediction of sagittal balance in patients with osteoporosis using spinopelvic parameters. Eur Spine J. 2013;22(5):1053–8.
10. Mac-Thiong JM, Transfeldt EE, Mehbod AA, Perra JH, Denis F, Garvey TA, Lonstein JE, Wu C, Dorman CW, Winter RB. Can c7 plumbline and gravity line predict health related quality of life in adult scoliosis? Spine. 2009;34(15):E519–27.
11. Lafage V, Schwab F, Patel A, Hawkinson N, Farcy JP. Pelvic tilt and truncal inclination: two key radiographic parameters in the setting of adults with spinal deformity. Spine. 2009;34(17):E599–606.
12. Berjano P, Bassani R, Casero G, Sinigaglia A, Cecchinato R, Lamartina C. Failures and revisions in surgery for sagittal imbalance: analysis of factors influencing failure. Eur Spine J. 2013;22(Suppl 6):S853–8.
13. Legaye J. Follow-up of the sagittal spine by optical technique. Ann Phys Rehabil Med. 2012;55(2):76–92.
14. Damet J, Fournier P, Monnin P, Sans-Merce M, Ceroni D, Zand T, Verdun FR, Baechler S. Occupational and patient exposure as well as image quality for full spine examinations with the EOS imaging system. Med Phys. 2014;41(6):063901.
15. Brink Y, Louw QA. Clinical instruments: reliability and validity critical appraisal. J Eval Clin Pract. 2011;18(6):1126–32.
16. Barrett E, McCreesh K, Lewis J. Reliability and validity of non-radiographic methods of thoracic kyphosis measurement: a systematic review. Man Ther. 2014;19(1):10–7.
17. Munro BH, Visintainer MA. Statistical methods for health care research. Philadephia: Lipincott Williams & Wilkins; 2005.
18. Portney L, Watkins MP. Foundations of clinical research. New Jersey: Pearson Education Inc.; 2009.
19. Liljenqvist U, Halm H, Hierholzer E, Drerup B, Weiland M. 3-Dimensional surface measurement of spinal deformities with video rasterstereography. Z Orthop Ihre Grenzgeb. 1998;136(1):57–64.
20. Mohokum M, Mendoza S, Udo W, Sitter H, Paletta JR, Skwara A. Reproducibility of rasterstereography for kyphotic and lordotic angles, trunk length, and trunk inclination: a reliability study. [Erratum appears in spine (Phila Pa 1976). 2010 Aug 15;35(18):1738 note: Melvin, Mohokum [corrected to Mohokum, Melvin]; Sylvia, Mendoza [corrected to Mendoza, Sylvia]]. Spine. 2010;35(14):1353–8.
21. de Seze MP, Guillaud E, Slugacz L, Cazalets JR. An examination of camptocormia assessment by dynamic quantification of sagittal posture. J Rehabil Med. 2015;47(1):72–9.
22. Knott P, Sturm P, Lonner B, Cahill P, Betsch M, McCarthy R, Kelly M, Lenke L, Betz R. Multicenter comparison of 3D spinal measurements using surface topography with those from conventional radiography. Spine Deformity. 2016;4(2):98–103.
23. Kellis E, Adamou G, Tzilios G, Emmanouilidou M. Reliability of spinal range of motion in healthy boys using a skin-surface device. J Manip Physiol Ther. 2008;31(8):570–6.
24. Mannion A, Knecht K, Balaban G, Dvorak J, Grob D. A new skin-surface device for measuring the curvature and global and segmental ranges of motion of the spine: reliability of measurements and comparison with data reviewed from the literature. Eur Spine J. 2004;13(2):122–36.
25. Milanesi JM, Borin G, Correa EC, da Silva AM, Bortoluzzi DC, Souza JA. Impact of the mouth breathing occurred during childhood in the adult age: biophotogrammetric postural analysis. Int J Pediatr Otorhinolaryngol. 2011;75(8):999–1004.
26. Negrini S, Negrini A, Atanasio S, Carabalona R, Grosso C, Santambrogio GC, Sibilla P. Postural variability of clinical parameters evaluated in orthostatic position in idiopathic scoliosis. Eura Medicophys. 2001;37(3):135–42.
27. Schroeder J, Reer R, Braumann KM. Video raster stereography back shape reconstruction: a reliability study for sagittal, frontal, and transversal plane parameters. Eur Spine J. 2015;24(2):262–9.
28. Zabjek KF, Simard G, Leroux MA, Coillard C, Rivard CH. Comparison of the reliability of two 3D acquisition systems used for the study of anthropometric and postural parameters. Ann Chir. 1999;53(8):751–60.
29. Zaina F, Donzelli S, Lusini M, Negrini S. How to measure kyphosis in everyday clinical practice: a reliability study on different methods. Res Spinal Deformities. 2012;8(176):264–7.
30. Zheng X, Chaudhari R, Wu C, Mehbod AA, Transfeldt EE, Winter RB. Repeatability test of C7 plumb line and gravity line on asymptomatic volunteers using an optical measurement technique. Spine. 2010;35(18):E889–94.
31. Grosso C, Negrini S, Boniolo A, Negrini AA. The validity of clinical examination in adolescent spinal deformities. Stud Health Technol Inform. 2002;91:123–5.
32. Fortin C, Feldman DE, Cheriet F, Labelle H. Clinical methods for quantifying body segment posture: a literature review. Disabil Rehabil. 2011;33(5):367–83.
33. Robinson R, Robinson HS, Bjørke G, Kvale A. Reliability and validity of a palpation technique for identifying the spinous processes of C7 and L5. Man Ther. 2009;14(4):409–14.
34. Kilby J, Heneghan NR, Maybury M. Manual palpation of lumbo-pelvic landmarks: a validity study. Man Ther. 2012;17(3):259–62.
35. Livanelioglu A, Kaya F, Nabiyev V, Demirkiran G, Firat T. The validity and reliability of "Spinal Mouse" assessment of spinal curvatures in the frontal plane in pediatric adolescent idiopathic thoraco-lumbar curves. Eur Spine J. 2016;25(2):476–82.
36. Yousefi MIS, Mehrshad N, Afzalpour M, Naghibi SE. Comparing the validity of non-invasive methods in measuring thoracic kyphosis and lumbar lordosis. Zahedan J Res Med Sc. 2012;14(4):37–42.
37. Zaki R, Bulgiba A, Ismail R, Ismail NA. Statistical methods used to test for agreement of medical instruments measuring continuous variables in method comparison studies: a systematic review. PLoS One. 2012;7(5):e37908.

14

Onset and remodeling of coronal imbalance after selective posterior thoracic fusion for Lenke 1C and 2C adolescent idiopathic scoliosis

Masayuki Ishikawa[1,6], Kai Cao[2], Long Pang[2], Nobuyuki Fujita[2,6], Mitsuru Yagi[3,6], Naobumi Hosogane[4,6], Takashi Tsuji[5,6], Masafumi Machida[3], Shinichi Ishihara[1,6], Makoto Nishiyama[1], Yasuyuki Fukui[1,6], Masaya Nakamura[2,6], Morio Matsumoto[2,6] and Kota Watanabe[2,6,*] [iD]

Abstract

Background: Postoperative coronal imbalance is a significant problem after selective thoracic fusion for primary thoracic and compensatory lumbar curves in adolescent idiopathic scoliosis (AIS). However, longitudinal studies on postoperative behavior of coronal balance are lacking. This multicenter retrospective study was conducted to analyze factors related to onset and remodeling of postoperative coronal imbalance after posterior thoracic fusion for Lenke 1C and 2C AIS.

Methods: Twenty-one Lenke 1C or 2C AIS patients, who underwent posterior thoracic fusion ending at L3 or above, were included with a minimum 2-year follow-up. The mean patients' age was 15.1 years at the time of surgery. Radiographic measurements were performed on Cobb angles of the main thoracic (MT) and thoracolumbar/lumbar (TLL) curves and coronal balance. Factors related to the onset of immediately postoperative coronal decompensation (IPCD) and postoperative coronal balance remodeling (PCBR), defined as an improvement of coronal balance during postoperative follow-up, were investigated using comparative and correlation analyses.

Results: Mean Cobb angles for the MT and TLL curves were 57.3° and 42.3° preoperatively and were corrected to 22.8° and 22.5° at final follow-up, respectively. Mean preoperative coronal balance of −3.8 mm got worse to −21.2 mm postoperatively, and regained to −12.0 mm at final follow-up. Coronal decompensation was observed in two patients preoperatively, in ten patients immediately postoperatively, and in three patients at final follow-up. The preoperative coronal balance and lowest instrumented vertebra (LIV) selection relative to stable vertebra (SV) were significantly different between patients with IPCD and those without. PCBR had significantly negative correlation with immediately postoperative coronal balance.

Conclusions: IPCD after posterior thoracic fusion for Lenke 1C and 2C AIS was frequent and associated with preoperative coronal balance and LIV selection. However, most patients with IPCD regained coronal balance through PCBR, which was significantly associated with immediately postoperative coronal balance. A fixation more distal to SV shifted the coronal balance further to the left postoperatively.

Keywords: Adolescent idiopathic scoliosis, Lenke 1C, Selective thoracic fusion, Posterior spinal fusion, Coronal balance, Coronal imbalance, Coronal decompensation, Remodeling, Surgical outcome, SRS-22

---

* Correspondence: kw197251@keio.jp
[2]Department of Orthopedic Surgery, School of Medicine, Keio University, 35 Shinanomachi, Shinjuku-ku, Tokyo 160-8582, Japan
[6]Keio Spine Research Group, 35 Shinanomachi, Shinjuku-ku, Tokyo 160-8582, Japan
Full list of author information is available at the end of the article

Background

Selective thoracic fusion (STF) has been the gold standard for treating primary thoracic and compensatory lumbar curves in adolescent idiopathic scoliosis (AIS), in which both the thoracic and lumbar curves cross midline, and the lumbar curve is smaller and more flexible than the thoracic curve, since Moe had advocated its concept [1, 2]. For this curve pattern, STF induces spontaneous lumbar curve correction and preserves more mobile lumbar segments than does fusing both the thoracic and lumbar curves [3–8]. However, postoperative coronal imbalance is a significant problem after STF [7, 9–11], which may result in poor surgical outcomes with re-operation. Moreover, reported surgical outcomes have shown that patients with resultant coronal imbalance after surgery tend to have inferior Scoliosis Research Society (SRS) questionnaire score on patients' satisfaction with treatments, compared to balanced patients [12]. Thus, the postoperative behavior of coronal balance is a major concern in the surgical outcomes for primary thoracic and compensatory lumbar curves in AIS. Causative factors reported for postoperative coronal decompensation include excessive correction of the thoracic curve, improper selection of the lowest instrumented vertebra (LIV), pre-existing coronal decompensation, and inappropriate curve identification [7–11, 13]; however, many of previous studies on postoperative behavior of coronal balance after STF are based on various surgical approaches including anterior approach and/or posterior approach with pedicle screw (PS), hook or hybrid constructs [3, 4, 6, 10, 13], and those with PS construct are scant. Apparently, surgical procedures and corrective maneuvers would influence the postoperative course of unfused lumbar curve and coronal balance.

On the other hand, we also experience some improvement of postoperative coronal imbalance during postoperative period after STF; however, some patients persist coronal imbalance. Compared to causative factors for the onset of postoperative coronal decompensation, the factors associated with the improvement of postoperative coronal imbalance during postoperative period have not been well investigated.

Thus, the purposes of this study were (1) to evaluate the postoperative behavior of coronal balance after posterior thoracic fusion with PS construct for Lenke 1C and 2C AIS (Lenke 1C/2C-AIS), in which the thoracolumbar/lumbar (TLL) curve bends less than 25° on side-bending without 20° or more kyphosis between T10 and L2, and the apical vertebra of TLL curve does not touch the center sacral vertical line (CSVL) and (2) to identify factors related to the onset of immediately postoperative coronal decompensation (IPCD) and changes of coronal balance during the follow-up period. In this study, postoperative change of coronal balance (PCCB) was defined as the change of coronal balance between preoperative and immediately postoperative evaluations, whereas postoperative coronal balance remodeling (PCBR) was defined as the improvement of postoperative coronal balance between immediately postoperative and final follow-up evaluations.

We hypothesized that preoperative radiographic measurements, LIV selection, and amount of main thoracic (MT) curve correction would have an impact on IPCD, PCCB, and PCBR.

Methods

This study was designed as a multicenter retrospective study reviewing radiographs and clinical charts. After institutional review board approval by the ethics committee at the International University of Health and Welfare (No. 5-15-19), radiographic measurements and clinical charts review were conducted. Twenty-one patients (twenty females, one male), who underwent posterior thoracic fusion for Lenke 1C or 2C AIS at three institutes, were enrolled in this study. Inclusion criteria were as follows: (1) primary surgery by posterior thoracic fusion with PS construct of LIV ending at L3 or above for Lenke 1C/2C-AIS and (2) patients with minimum 2 years follow-up.

The mean age and Risser grade at the time of surgery were 15.1 ± 2.7 (11–22) years old and 3.4 ± 1.4 (1–5), respectively. The mean follow-up period was 3.1 (2–7.3) years. Investigated clinical data were Lenke classification, number of fused vertebrae, and level of LIV. Radiographic coronal measurements included the Cobb angles of the proximal thoracic (PT), MT, and TLL curves; apical vertebral translations (AVT) of the MT (AVT-MT) and TLL (AVT-TLL) curves; LIV tilt; coronal balance; and trunk shift on preoperative, postoperative (between 1 and 4 weeks after surgery), and final follow-up standing posteroanterior (PA) radiographs. Preoperative curve flexibilities were evaluated on right and left side-bending films. Radiographic sagittal measurements included the proximal thoracic kyphosis between T2 and T5, thoracic kyphosis between T5 and T12, thoracolumbar kyphosis between T10 and L2, lumbar lordosis between T12 and S1, and sagittal balance on preoperative, postoperative, and final follow-up standing lateral radiographs.

Measurements for coronal curvature were performed by the Cobb method. AVT-MT and AVT-TLL were measured with reference to the C7 plumb line or the CSVL, respectively. Coronal balance was measured as the horizontal distance between the C7 plumb line and the CSVL, and trunk shift was measured as the horizontal distance between the center of apex for MT curve and the CSVL. Coronal balance and trunk shift were defined as a negative value when the C7 plumb line or the center of apex for MT curve locates at the left side to the CSVL. Sagittal balance was measured as the horizontal distance between the C7 plumb line and superior-posterior corner of S1 vertebra and was defined as a positive value when the C7 plumb line locates anteriorly to superior-posterior corner of S1 vertebra, and vice versa. Coronal decompensation was defined as the absolute value of coronal balance greater than 2 cm. The ratios of values of MT curve to those of TLL curve in preoperative Cobb angle and AVT were also calculated. Reference vertebrae including the lower end vertebra (EV) and the lower neutral vertebra (NV) of MT curve, the stable vertebra (SV) at thoracolumbar lesion, and the apex of TLL curve (ApexTLL) were recorded, and the gap differences between the LIV and the reference vertebrae were counted (LIV-EV, LIV-NV, LIV-SV, ApexTLL-LIV).

Preoperative radiographic measurements, including the Cobb angles, and flexibilities of the PT, MT, and TLL curves, the AVT of the MT and TLL curves, the ratios of the MT curve to TLL curve in the Cobb angle and AVT, coronal balance, trunk shift and sagittal values, LIV selection, and postoperative correction of MT curve were evaluated whether correlating or not, to PCCB and PCBR.

Additionally, patient-reported clinical outcomes with Scoliosis Research Society-22 (SRS-22) questionnaire scores at the final follow-up were reported.

Surgical procedure

All patients were operated on posteriorly. After exposure of the posterior elements of the spine, removal of inferior facet joints to be fused in all cases was performed. Pedicle screws were inserted bilaterally by free-hand technique, with additional attachment of some hooks in seven cases. For most patients, the LIV was selected at the SV on a PA radiograph; for others, the LIV was selected at a more distal level to partially correct the TLL curve. Corrective maneuver includes rod rotation on the concave side, followed by in-situ rod contouring, placement of a rod on the convex side, and segmental compression and distraction via PS. Intra-operative spinal cord monitoring with motor-evoked potential was routinely performed. Bone grafting was carried out using local bone materials from facetectomies and osteotomies in all cases.

Statistical analyses

Statistical analyses were performed using the software package IBM SPSS Statistics 22 (IBM Japan, Tokyo, JAPAN). Radiographic measurement values at different time points were evaluated by analysis of variance. Unpaired t test was used to compare continuous variables. Correlation analyses were performed using Pearson's correlation coefficients. A P value less than 0.05 was set to be statistically significant.

Results

The Lenke classification was 1C– in three, 1CN in ten, 1C+ in one, 2C– in two, and 2CN in five. The mean

number of fused vertebrae was 9.6 ± 2.4(6–14), and the LIV was T11 in six, T12 in six, L1 in five, L2 in three, and L3 in one (Table 1). Details of each patient are shown at Table 2. The mean Cobb angles for the PT, MT, and TLL curves were 29.4 ± 9.4° (flexibility, 24.7 ± 19.3%), 57.3 ± 12.1° (flexibility, 29.6 ± 16.3%), and 42.3 ± 5.7° (flexibility, 75.0 ± 14.6%) preoperatively and were corrected to 16.1 ± 7.6°, 17.8 ± 7.7°, and 19.3 ± 7.4° immediately postoperatively and 16.9 ± 7.8° (42.8 ± 18.8% correction), 22.8 ± 8.9° (60.4 ± 12.2% correction), and 22.5 ± 7.8° (46.6 ± 17.6% correction) at the final follow-up, respectively (Table 3). The preoperative Cobb angle ratio of the MT curve to the TLL curve was 1.4 ± 0.2. The postoperative changes in the Cobb angles of the PT, MT, and TLL curves were statistically significant (Table 3). The mean AVT-MT and AVT-TLL were 45.2 ± 15.5 mm and 22.0 ± 5.7 mm preoperatively and were corrected to 2.0 ± 11.7 mm and 25.0 ± 7.0 mm immediately postoperatively and 10.0 ± 13.0 mm and 16.8 ± 8.4 mm at the final follow-up (Table 3). The preoperative AVT ratio of the MT curve to the TLL curve was 2.4 ± 1.2. The mean coronal balance and trunk shift were –3.8 ± 10.8 mm and 41.3 ± 20.5 mm preoperatively and were corrected to –21.2 ± 13.6 mm and –19.3 ± 16.7 mm immediately postoperatively and –12.0 ± 11.1 mm and -2.5 ± 17.4 mm at the final follow-up, respectively (Table 3) (Fig. 1). Coronal decompensation was observed in two patients preoperatively, in ten immediately postoperatively, and in three at the final follow-up. No patients required revision surgery. The mean LIV tilt was 24.4 ± 12.3° preoperatively and was corrected to 8.1 ± 6.7° immediately postoperatively and 10.2 ± 5.8° at the final follow-up. The postoperative changes in AVT-MT, AVT-TLL, LIV tilt, coronal balance, and trunk shift at the final follow-up were statistically significant (Table 3).

Preoperative sagittal measurements did not change significantly at the final follow-up (Table 4).

The mean gap differences in LIV-EV, LIV-NV, LIV-SV, and ApexTLL-LIV were 1.0 ± 1.4, 1.1 ± 1.5, 0.6 ± 1.4, and 1.9 ± 1.2, respectively.

Factors associated with IPCD, PCCB, and PCBR

In 20 of 21 patients, coronal balance shifted to the left immediately after surgery. Comparative study showed that among preoperative radiographic measurements, LIV selection and the amount of MT curve correction, the preoperative coronal balance and trunk shift and LIV-SV were significantly different between patients with IPCD and those without (–11.0 ± 7.8 mm vs 2.7 ± 9.0 mm, $p < 0.01$; 30.1 ± 15.1 mm vs 51.5 ± 19.9 mm, $p < 0.05$; 1.3 ± 1.5 vs –0.1 ± 0.9, $p < 0.05$, respectively) (Table 5). PCCB had significant correlation to the LIV selection (LIV-EV $r = -0.58$, $p < 0.01$; LIV-NV $r = -0.47$, $p < 0.05$; LIV-SV $r = -0.48$, $p < 0.05$; ApexTLL-LIV $r =$

Table 1 Patients' demographics

Characteristics	N or mean (SD/range)
Gender	Female 20, male 1
Age (years old)	15.1 ± 2.7
Risser grade	3.4 ± 1.4
Follow-up period (years)	3.1 (2–7.3)
Lenke classification	1C– (3)
	1CN (10)
	1C+ (1)
	2C– (2)
	2CN (5)
Mean fused vertebrae	9.6 ± 2.4
Lowest instrumented vertebra	T11 (6)
	T12 (6)
	L1 (5)
	L2 (3)
	L3 (1)

0.61, $p < 0.01$), whereas PCCB had no significant correlation to the preoperative radiographic measurements or the amount of MT curve correction (Table 6).

On the contrary, PCBR had no significant correlation to the preoperative radiographic measurements, LIV selection, or the amount of MT curve correction, whereas PCBR had significant correlation to the immediately postoperative coronal balance ($r = -0.61$, $p < 0.01$) and trunk shift ($r = -0.57$, $p < 0.01$) (Table 6) (Fig. 2).

SRS-22 questionnaire scores

Domain scores of SRS-22 questionnaire were 4.4 ± 0.2 in Pain, 4.4 ± 0.5 in Function, 3.4 ± 0.9 in Self-Image, 3.9 ± 1.0 in Mental Health, 3.9 ± 0.7 in Satisfaction, and 4.0 ± 0.4 in Total at the final follow-up.

Discussion

The surgical outcomes for a primary thoracic curve with a compensatory lumbar curve remain one of the most controversial issues in surgical AIS treatment. Advantages of STF for this curve pattern are saving more mobile lumbar segments and inducing spontaneous lumbar curve correction; however, the risks of postoperative coronal decompensation and resultant marked lumbar curve

Table 2 Details of each patient

Case no.	Age (y/o)	Gender	Follow-up period (years)	Lenke Classification	Fusion level	MT curve (°) Level	Preop.	Postop.	Final	TLL curve (°) Level	Preop.	Postop.	Final	Coronal balance (mm) Preop.	Postop.	Final
1	12	F	4.0	1CN	T4–T12	T6–T11	52	10	13	T11–L3	47	33	19	−9	−22	−16
2	11	F	5.5	2CN	T3–L1	T5–T11	76	32	39	T11–L4	45	17	20	0	−5	−10
3	15	F	7.3	1CN	T2–L2	T6–T12	60	22	24	T12–L4	42	22	25	10	−5	0
4	14	F	5.0	1C–	T2–L2	T6–T11	55	20	18	T11–L3	32	14	15	−10	−53	−26
5	14	F	4.5	1CN	T2–L1	T5–T11	52	15	12	T11–L4	38	20	26	−12	−22	−2
6	14	F	3.0	1CN	T2–L3	T5–T11	51	15	18	T11–L4	44	25	37	−2	−37	−18
7	17	F	2.0	1CN	T3–L2	T5–T10	47	14	14	T10–L4	44	13	13	−2	−41	−40
8	13	F	5.0	2CN	T5–T12	T6–T12	51	28	28	T12–L4	43	31	32	−22	−30	−33
9	20	F	2.0	2CN	T2–L1	T5–T11	92	33	36	T11–L4	51	13	26	−10	−27	−2
10	12	F	2.3	2CN	T2–T12	T5–T12	76	18	38	T12–L4	55	18	29	14	−8	0
11	14	F	2.3	2C–	T4–T11	T5–T11	50	8	13	T11–L4	42	9	6	−13	−6	−17
12	13	F	2.6	2C–	T5–T11	T5–T11	49	7	17	T11–L3	38	8	17	−25	−26	−17
13	17	M	2.3	2CN	T5–L1	T5–T12	52	14	25	T12–L4	32	25	17	11	−12	−10
14	18	F	2.0	1CN	T5–T12	T5–T11	61	22	21	T11–L4	41	26	26	0	−18	−11
15	15	F	2.0	1CN	T6–T11	T5–T12	39	14	24	T12–L4	40	14	27	−4	−24	−9
16	17	F	2.0	1CN	T5–T12	T5–T11	48	13	16	T11–L4	34	24	22	−14	−44	−11
17	22	F	2.8	1C–	T5–L1	T4–T12	65	20	21	T12–L4	43	13	12	0	−14	−6
18	17	F	3.1	1C–	T3–T11	T3–T11	54	30	32	T11–L4	44	32	31	0	−15	−16
19	15	F	2.3	1CN	T5–T12	T5–T12	58	9	13	T12–L4	48	15	16	−8	−15	−12
20	13	F	2.1	1C+	T5–T11	T4–T12	64	18	35	T12–L4	46	14	32	0	−8	4
21	15	F	2.0	1CN	T5–T11	T4–T11	50	13	23	T11–L4	40	19	26	15	−13	0

MT main thoracic, *TLL* thoracolumbar/lumbar

Table 3 Radiographic coronal measurements

Coronal measurements	Preop.	Postop.	Final follow-up
PT curve (°)	29.4 ± 9.4	16.1 ± 7.6[a]	16.9 ± 7.8[a]
Flexibility (%)	24.7 ± 19.3		
Correction rate (%)			42.8 ± 18.8
MT curve (°)	57.3 ± 12.1	17.8 ± 7.7[a]	22.8 ± 8.9[a]
Flexibility (%)	29.6 ± 16.3		
Correction rate (%)			60.4 ± 12.2
TLL curve (°)	42.3 ± 5.7	19.3 ± 7.4[a]	22.5 ± 7.8[a]
Flexibility (%)	75.0 ± 14.6		
Correction rate (%)			46.6 ± 17.6
AVT-MT (mm)	45.2 ± 15.5	2.0 ± 11.7[a]	10.0 ± 13.0[a]
AVT-TLL (mm)	22.0 ± 5.7	25.0 ± 7.0	16.8 ± 8.4[a]
LIV tilt (°)	24.4 ± 12.3	8.1 ± 6.7[a]	10.2 ± 5.8[a]
Coronal balance (mm)	−3.8 ± 10.8	−21.2 ± 13.6[a]	−12.0 ± 11.1[a]
Trunk shift (mm)	41.3 ± 20.5	−19.3 ± 16.7[a]	−2.5 ± 17.4[a]

Values indicate mean ± standard deviation
PT proximal thoracic, *MT* main thoracic, *TLL* thoracolumbar/lumbar, *AVT* apical vertebral translation, *LIV* lowest instrumented vertebra
[a]Statistical significance

Table 4 Radiographic sagittal measurements

Sagittal measurements	Preop.	Postop.	Final follow-up
T2–T5 (°)	8.8 ± 4.7	11.6 ± 5.1	11.3 ± 5.9
T5–T12 (°)	17.5 ± 10.8	15.8 ± 8.1	18.2 ± 8.1
T10–L2 (°)	−4.9 ± 12.4	−2.8 ± 10.1	−4.0 ± 9.5
T12–S1 (°)	−53.1 ± 12.0	−44.6 ± 12.5	−48.1 ± 10.6
Sagittal balance (mm)	−9.7 ± 23.3	3.2 ± 22.0[a]	−17.1 ± 13.5

Values indicate mean ± standard deviation
[a]Statistical significance

and TLL curves cross midline. In these curve patterns, coronal balance are usually prone to shift to the left preoperatively, and previous studies have shown that coronal balance tends to shift further to the left after STF, which may result in coronal decompensation in some patients [7]. Whereas, it is also known that patients with immediately postoperative coronal imbalance usually regain coronal balance to some degrees during the follow-up period; however, some patients persist coronal imbalance after surgery.

Several causative factors have been reported for postoperative coronal decompensation; however, many of these causative factors were based on not only various surgical approaches but also the evaluation with the change of coronal balance between preoperative and final follow-up evaluations. Detailed analyses to seek the factors associated with the changes of coronal balance between preoperative and immediately postoperative follow-ups and between immediately postoperative

magnitude compared to correction and fusion of both the thoracic and lumbar curves are considered to be shortcomings in STF. The primary thoracic and compensatory lumbar curves are generally classified as King type II or Lenke 1C/2C curves, in which the MT curve is larger and more rigid than the TLL curve and both the MT

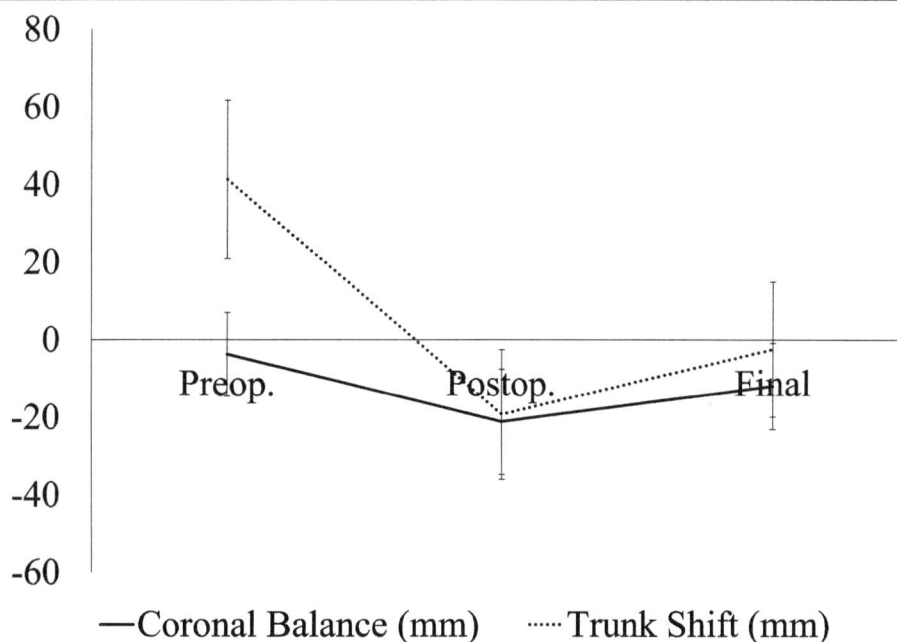

Fig. 1 Postoperative behavior of coronal balance and trunk shift. Preoperative coronal balance and trunk shift were significantly shifted to the left immediately postoperatively; however, both of them regained balance at final follow-up

Table 5 Comparative analyses between patients with IPCD and those without

Parameters		IPCD ($N = 10$)	Non-IPCD ($N = 11$)	P value
PT Cobb (°)	Preop.	27.8 ± 7.2	30.7 ± 11.2	0.50
	Flexibility (%)	15.7 ± 12.8	31.7 ± 21.3	0.10
	Postop.	16.8 ± 8.3	15.5 ± 7.4	0.72
	Final	16.5 ± 6.3	17.3 ± 9.2	0.81
	Correction rate (%)	41.3 ± 17.3	44.3 ± 20.8	0.72
MT Cobb (°)	Preop.	53.6 ± 14.2	60.5 ± 9.2	0.20
	Flexibility (%)	29.2 ± 18.9	29.9 ± 14.7	0.93
	Postop.	16.9 ± 7.9	18.7 ± 7.7	0.59
	Final	19.6 ± 7.8	25.8 ± 9.1	0.11
	Correction rate (%)	63.2 ± 12.4	57.9 ± 12.1	0.33
TLL Cobb (°)	Preop.	41.1 ± 5.8	43.5 ± 5.6	0.36
	Flexibility (%)	76.2 ± 16.2	74.2 ± 14.4	0.81
	Postop.	19.5 ± 8.5	19.1 ± 6.7	0.90
	Final	23.3 ± 7.6	21.7 ± 8.2	0.65
	Correction rate (%)	43.0 ± 17.2	49.8 ± 18.2	0.39
AVT-MT (mm)	Preop.	41.1 ± 16.2	48.8 ± 14.7	0.27
	Postop.	3.9 ± 13.3	0.0 ± 10.2	0.47
	Final	9.3 ± 12.1	10.6 ± 14.3	0.84
AVT-TLL (mm)	Preop.	24.1 ± 6.7	20.1 ± 4.2	0.13
	Postop.	27.2 ± 7.7	23.1 ± 6.1	0.21
	Final	18.5 ± 9.7	15.3 ± 7.4	0.43
LIV tilt (°)	Preop.	18.6 ± 11.2	29.2 ± 11.4	0.05
	Postop.	7.8 ± 7.2	8.4 ± 6.5	0.87
	Final	9.8 ± 6.1	10.5 ± 5.7	0.78
Coronal balance (mm)	Preop.	**−11.0 ± 7.8**	**2.7 ± 9.0**	**<0.01**
	Postop.	**−32.5 ± 10.7**	**−10.8 ± 4.6**	**<0.01**
	Final	**−17.4 ± 12.5**	**−7.1 ± 7.1**	**<0.05**
Trunk shift (mm)	Preop.	**30.1 ± 15.1**	**51.5 ± 19.9**	**<0.05**
	Postop.	**−28.6 ± 17.4**	**−10.8 ± 11.0**	**<0.05**
	Final	−9.0 ± 15.9	3.5 ± 17.2	0.10
LIV-EV		1.6 ± 1.7	0.5 ± 0.9	0.09
LIV-NV		1.5 ± 1.8	0.7 ± 1.1	0.24
LIV-SV		**1.3 ± 1.5**	**−0.1 ± 0.9**	**<0.05**
ApexTLL-LIV		1.4 ± 1.3	2.3 ± 1.0	0.10

Values indicate mean ± standard deviation. Bold values indicate a statistical significance
IPCD immediately postoperative coronal decompensation, *PT* proximal thoracic, *MT* main thoracic, *TLL* thoracolumbar/lumbar, *AVT* apical vertebral translation, *LIV* lowest instrumented vertebra, *EV* end vertebra, *NV* neutral vertebra, *SV* stable vertebra

and final follow-ups are still lacking. PCBR, defined as the improvement of coronal balance between immediately postoperative and final follow-ups, is another aspect of the postoperative behavior of coronal balance, compared to the onset of postoperative coronal decompensation.

Thus, we attempted to define the correlative factors to IPCD, PCCB, and PCBR after posterior thoracic fusion with PS construct in Lenke 1C/2C-AIS.

As demonstrated in the results, coronal balance tends to shift to the left preoperatively, and it shifts further to the left immediately postoperatively in 20 of 21 patients. To detect the causative factors for the onset of IPCD, we performed comparative and correlation analyses. From the comparative study, preoperative coronal balance and trunk shift, and LIV-SV were found to be significantly different between compensated and decompensated patients immediately postoperatively, whereas correlation

Table 6 Correlation analyses on PCCB and PCBR

Parameters		PCCB		PCBR	
		r	P value	r	P value
PT Cobb	Preop.	0.27	0.23	−0.20	0.39
	Flexibility	0.02	0.93	−0.13	0.63
	Postop.	−0.04	0.87	−0.05	0.84
	Final	0.16	0.48	−0.14	0.54
	Correction rate	0.16	0.50	−0.09	0.71
MT Cobb	Preop.	0.16	0.49	0.05	0.84
	Flexibility	0.13	0.59	0.02	0.92
	Postop.	−0.01	0.95	−0.04	0.86
	Final	0.10	0.66	−0.11	0.65
	Correction rate	0.00	0.99	0.15	0.53
TLL Cobb	Preop.	0.27	0.24	−0.28	0.22
	Flexibility	0.02	0.95	0.02	0.96
	Postop.	−0.14	0.54	−0.09	0.72
	Final	−0.16	0.48	0.28	0.23
	Correction rate	0.28	0.22	−0.41	0.07
AVT-MT	Preop.	0.12	0.62	0.16	0.49
	Postop.	−0.03	0.90	−0.12	0.62
	Final	0.16	0.50	−0.24	0.30
AVT-TLL	Preop.	−0.14	0.57	0.31	0.20
	Postop.	0.25	0.30	0.07	0.77
	Final	0.16	0.50	−0.02	0.93
LIV tilt	Preop.	0.18	0.44	−0.27	0.25
	Postop.	−0.46	0.05	0.03	0.89
	Final	−0.38	0.10	0.12	0.62
Coronal balance	Preop.	−0.33	0.14	−0.12	0.60
	Postop.	**0.66**	**<0.01**	**−0.61**	**<0.01**
	Final	0.26	0.26	0.25	0.28
Trunk shift	Preop.	−0.09	0.71	0.06	0.81
	Postop.	**0.51**	**<0.05**	**−0.57**	**<0.01**
	Final	0.32	0.15	0.01	0.98
LIV-EV		**−0.58**	**<0.01**	0.24	0.29
LIV-NV		**−0.47**	**<0.05**	0.18	0.44
LIV-SV		**−0.48**	**<0.05**	0.17	0.47
ApexTLL-LIV		**0.61**	**<0.01**	−0.31	0.17

A r indicates Pearson's correlation coefficient. Bold values indicate a statistical significance

PCCB postoperative change of coronal balance, *PCBR* postoperative coronal balance remodeling, *PT* proximal thoracic, *MT* main thoracic, *TLL* thoracolumbar/lumbar, *AVT* apical vertebral translation, *LIV* lowest instrumented vertebra, *EV* end vertebra, *NV* neutral vertebra, *SV* stable vertebra

analysis found that PCCB was significantly correlated to the LIV selection relative to the EV, NV, SV, and ApexTLL. Regarding LIV selection, only the LIV-SV was found to be significantly associated with both the onset of IPCD and PCCB. These results indicate that the immediately postoperative change of coronal balance depends only on LIV selection, and not on preoperative radiographic measurements or the amount of MT curve correction, and that a fixation more distal to the SV shifts the coronal balance even further to the left immediately postoperatively. Moreover, a patient with a pre-existing coronal imbalance to the left tends to be decompensated to the left immediately postoperatively if the LIV is selected at a level more distal to the SV. It is important to note that coronal balance shifted further to the left immediately postoperatively in majority of patients even when the LIV was selected at the SV, indicating that STF may itself produce an immediately postoperative leftward shift of the coronal balance [11]. Accordingly, patients with preoperative coronal imbalance further to the left and inappropriate selection of LIV, such as fixation distal to the SV would be at a high risk of IPCD. These findings suggest that selecting the LIV at the SV would minimize the risk of IPCD for patients with Lenke 1C/2C-AIS.

Regarding PCBR, this study demonstrated that PCBR occurred in majority of patients more than 5 mm during postoperative periods and the deterioration of immediately postoperative coronal balance occurred in only limited cases (four cases) at the final follow-up and also found that PCBR had significantly negative correlation to the immediately postoperative coronal balance and trunk shift. These results indicate that patients with coronal balance shifted further to the left immediately postoperatively tend to compensate more balance during the follow-up period, which may be attributed to a postural reflex, potentially existing in the relatively flexible lumbar curves (Lenke 1C/2C-AIS), although three patients persisted coronal decompensation at the final follow-up. That is, PCBR is dependent on the immediately postoperative condition in coronal balance and trunk shift. Coronal decompensation at the final follow-up was observed in three patients, so comparative analysis to detect the causative factors for coronal decompensation at the final follow-up was not performed because of the limited number of patients, although the LIV-SV tended to be larger in patients with coronal decompensation at the final follow-up, compared to those without (2.3 vs 0.3). Patients with coronal decompensation at the final follow-up were all decompensated immediately postoperatively, and none of the compensated patients immediately postoperatively were decompensated at the final follow-up. Accordingly, optimal curve identification and surgical strategy to minimize the risk of IPCD may be more beneficial to prevent coronal decompensation at the final follow-up. The current study suggests that selecting the LIV at the SV minimizes the risk of postoperative coronal decompensation after posterior thoracic fusion using PS construct for Lenke 1C/2C-AIS and results in acceptable patients-reported outcomes.

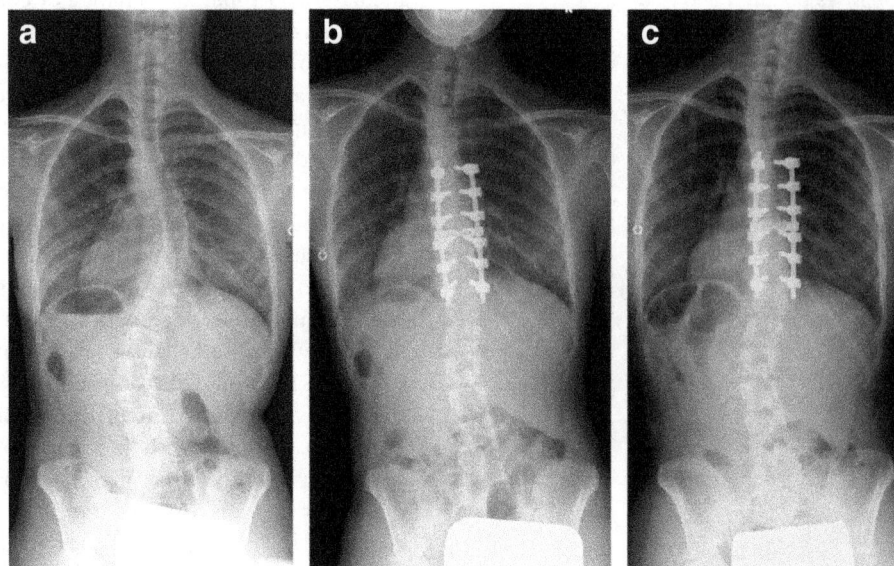

Fig. 2 A representative case (Case No. 15). A 15-year-old female with Lenke 1CN adolescent idiopathic scoliosis underwent selective posterior thoracic fusion from T6 to T11. The preoperative coronal balance of −4 mm (**a**) worsened to −24 mm immediately after surgery (**b**), but recovered to −9 mm with remodeling, as seen 2 years after surgery (**c**)

Further studies to determine the optimal candidate for STF based on the preoperative characteristics of the TLL curve and coronal balance are needed to prevent postoperative coronal decompensation in the primary thoracic and compensatory lumbar curves.

This retrospective study has several limitations, including the small sample size and relatively short follow-up period. As for the follow-up period, observation with longer postoperative period is critical in the evaluation of clinical and radiographic outcomes, especially in treating young patients. However, the postoperative spontaneous unfused lumbar curve correction and remodeling of trunk shift after STF are reported to occur usually within 2 years after surgery [14], so a minimum 2-year follow-up observation may minimize these concerns.

Conclusions

The onset of IPCD was associated with the preoperative coronal balance and trunk shift, and the LIV selection relative to the SV, whereas PCBR was associated with the immediately postoperative coronal balance and trunk shift in patients treated by posterior thoracic fusion using PS construct for Lenke 1C/2C-AIS. Selecting the LIV at the SV would be optimal in treating Lenke 1C/2C-AIS in terms of avoiding postoperative coronal decompensation.

Abbreviations
AIS: Adolescent idiopathic scoliosis; AVT: Apical vertebral translation; CSVL: Center sacral vertical line; EV: End vertebra; IPCD: Immediately postoperative coronal decompensation; LIV: Lowest instrumented vertebra; MT: Main thoracic; NV: Neutral vertebra; PA: Posteroanterior; PCBR: Postoperative coronal balance remodeling; PCCB: Postoperative change of coronal balance; PS: Pedicle screw;

PT: Proximal thoracic; SRS: Scoliosis Research Society; STF: Selective thoracic fusion; SV: Stable vertebra; TLL: Thoracolumbar/lumbar

Acknowledgements
There was no acknowledgment for this study.

Funding
There was no funding for this study.

Authors' contributions
MI made the study design and wrote the initial protocol. MI, KC, LP, NF, MY, and KW collected the data for all the patients. MI evaluated the results, and the final statistical analyses were performed by MI. MI drafted the manuscript. MM (the thirteenth author) revised the manuscript critically and gave final approval of the version to be published. All authors contributed and approved the final manuscript.

Competing interests
The authors declare that they have no competing interests.

Author details
[1]Spine and Spinal Cord Center, Mita Hospital, International University of Health and Welfare, 1-4-3 Mita, Minato-ku, Tokyo 108-8329, Japan. [2]Department of Orthopedic Surgery, School of Medicine, Keio University, 35 Shinanomachi, Shinjuku-ku, Tokyo 160-8582, Japan. [3]Department of Orthopedic Surgery, Murayama Medical Center, 2-37-1 Gakuen, Musashimurayama-shi, Tokyo 208-0011, Japan. [4]Department of Orthopedic Surgery, National Defense Medical College, 3-2 Namiki, Tokorozawa-shi, Saitama 359-8513, Japan. [5]Department of Orthopedic Surgery, Kitasato University, Kitasato Institute Hospital, 5-9-1 Shirokane, Minato-ku, Tokyo 108-8642, Japan. [6]Keio Spine Research Group, 35 Shinanomachi, Shinjuku-ku, Tokyo 160-8582, Japan.

References

1. Moe JH. A critical analysis of methods of fusion for scoliosis. An evaluation in two hundred and sixty-six patients. J Bone Joint Surg Am. 1958;40:529–54.
2. King HA, Moe JH, Bradford DS, Winter RB. The selection of fusion levels in thoracic idiopathic scoliosis. J Bone Joint Surg Am. 1983;65:1302–13.
3. Lenke LG, Betz RR, Bridwell KH, Harms J, Clements DH, Lowe TG. Spontaneous lumbar curve coronal correction after selective anterior or posterior thoracic fusion in adolescent idiopathic scoliosis. Spine (Phila Pa 1976). 1999;24:1663–72.
4. Dobbs MB, Lenke LG, Walton T, Peelle M, Rocca GD, Steger-May K, Bridwell KH. Can we predict the ultimate lumbar curve in adolescent idiopathic scoliosis patients undergoing a selective fusion with undercorrection of the thoracic curve? Spine (Phila Pa 1976). 2004;9:277–85.
5. Chang KW, Chang KI, Wu CM. Enhanced capacity for spontaneous correction of lumbar curve in the treatment of major thoracic-compensatory C modifier lumbar curve pattern in idiopathic scoliosis. Spine (Phila Pa 1976). 2007;32:3020–9.
6. Takahashi J, Newton PO, Ugrinow VL, Bastrom TP. Selective thoracic fusion in adolescent idiopathic scoliosis. Factors influencing the selection of the optimal lowest instrumented vertebra. Spine (Phila Pa 1976). 2011;36:1131–41.
7. Lenke LG, Bridwell KH, Baldus C, Blanke K. Preventing decompensation in King type II curves treated with Cotrel-Dubousset instrumentation. Strict guidelines for selective thoracic fusion. Spine (Phila Pa 1976). 1992;17:S274–81.
8. Ishikawa M, Cao K, Pang L, Watanabe K, Yagi M, Hosogane N, Machida M, Shiono Y, Nishiyama M, Fukui Y, Matsumoto M. Postoperative behavior of thoracolumbar/lumbar curve and coronal balance after posterior thoracic fusion for Lenke 1C and 2C adolescent idiopathic scoliosis. J Orthop Sci. 2015;20:31–7.
9. Thompson JP, Transfeldt EE, Bradford DS, Ogilvie JW, Boachie-Adjei O. Decompensation after Cotrel-Dubousset instrumentation of idiopathic scoliosis. Spine (Phila Pa 1976). 1990;15:927–31.
10. McCance SE, Denis F, Lonstein JE, Winter RB. Coronal and sagittal balance in surgically treated adolescent idiopathic scoliosis with the King II curve pattern. A review of 67 consecutive cases having selective thoracic arthrodesis. Spine (Phila Pa 1976). 1998;23:2063–73.
11. Wang Y, Bünger CE, Wu C, Zhang Y, Hansen ES. Postoperative trunk shift in Lenke 1C scoliosis. What causes it? How can it be prevented? Spine (Phila Pa 1976). 2012;37:1676–82.
12. Schulz J, Asghar J, Bastrom T, Shufflebarger H, Newton PO, Sturm P, Betz RR, Samdani AF, Yaszay B, Harms Study Group. Optimal radiographical criteria after selective thoracic fusion for patients with adolescent idiopathic scoliosis with a C lumbar modifier. Does adherence to current guidelines predict success? Spine (Phila Pa 1976). 2014;39:E1368–73.
13. Demura S, Yaszay B, Bastrom TP, Carreau J, Newton PO, Harms Study Group. Is decompensation preoperatively a risk in Lenke 1C curves? Spine (Phila Pa 1976). 2013;38:E649–55.
14. Wang Y, Bünger CE, Zhang Y, Wu C, Hansen ES. Postoperative spinal alignment remodeling in Lenke 1C scoliosis treated with selective thoracic fusion. Spine J. 2012;12:73–80.

15

Current knowledge of scoliosis in physiotherapy students trained in the United Kingdom

D.A. Jason Black[1*], Christine Pilcher[1], Shawn Drake[2], Erika Maude[1] and David Glynn[3]

Abstract

Background: It has been highlighted in both Poland and the United States of America (USA) that knowledge of idiopathic scoliosis (IS) among physiotherapy students is limited with respect to the 2011 International Society on Scoliosis Orthopaedic and Rehabilitation Treatment (SOSORT) guidelines. Early detection of scoliosis and correct initial management is essential in effective care, and thus physiotherapists should be aware of the basic criteria for diagnosis and indications for treatment. The aim of this study was to evaluate the basic knowledge of IS in physiotherapy students trained in the United Kingdom (UK).

Methods: A previously designed and tested 10-question survey, including knowledge of the 2011 SOSORT guidelines, was transcribed onto an online-survey platform. Questions were designed to analyse knowledge of definition, cause, development, prevalence, diagnosis, treatment and bracing of scoliosis.

All UK universities offering physiotherapy degrees were invited to participate, with the programme lead of each institution asked to distribute the questionnaire to all penultimate and final year physiotherapy students (bachelor's and master's degrees). The final number of students who received the study invitation is unknown. The survey link closed after 8 weeks of data collection.

Results : Two hundred and six students, split over 12 institutions, successfully completed the questionnaire. Analysis showed that 79% of students recognised when IS is likely to develop, yet only 52% recognised that IS's aetiology is unknown. Eighty-eight percent of students incorrectly defined IS as a 2-dimensional deformity, with only 24% successfully recognising the prevalence of IS within the scoliosis population. Just 12% knew the criteria for diagnosis; however, 93% were unable to recognise the appropriate treatment approach through therapeutic exercise. Finally, 54% of students managed to identify correctly when bracing is recommended for IS.

In comparison to previous studies within the USA, students in the UK performed worse in relation to all questions except treatment (7% answered correctly vs 3% in the American study).

Conclusion: With only 7% of students able to answer > 50% of the survey questions correctly, there is a clear lack of knowledge of appropriate IS diagnosis and care which could directly impact the information these patients are given within the first contact primary care in the UK.

Keywords: Scoliosis, Physiotherapy, University, Knowledge, Education, Treatment, Bracing, Causes, Screening, Diagnosis

* Correspondence: jasonblack@scoliosissos.com
D.A. Jason Black is the lead author
[1]Scoliosis SOS Clinic, 63 Mansell Street, London E1 8AN, UK
Full list of author information is available at the end of the article

Background

Scoliosis refers to a 3-dimensional deformity of the spine [1] and is a condition which is generally accepted as affecting 2–3% of children aged 12–16 years old [2]. The current knowledge of scoliosis, including its diagnosis and management among physiotherapy students' in UK, is not known. A few previous studies completed outside the UK have investigated this, largely reporting a poor result.

Drake et al. designed a 10-question multiple choice survey to establish the knowledge of scoliosis diagnosis and treatment in 178 physiotherapy students in the USA. Results were poor, showing a mean overall correct score of 43%, with only 15 students answering over 70% correctly [3].

A study completed in Poland by Ciazynski et al. also tested the knowledge of physiotherapy students in this field using a similar questionnaire format to the study by Drake et al. [4]. Apart from the much smaller subject numbers in this study (37), the students had already covered conservative treatment methods for scoliosis in their syllabus. These students generally performed more favourably in comparison to those in the study by Drake et al. [3], noting scoliosis as a 3-dimensional deformity (81.3 versus 29%) and how to confirm diagnosis (62.2 versus 20%). Most participants (90.5%) in the study by Drake et al. [3] were not familiar with any conservative treatment methods, whereas most students (94.6%) were aware of at least one conservative treatment method in the study by Ciazynski et al. [4], who recommends that education for scoliosis among physiotherapy students should be comprehensive and cover the current SOSORT guidelines.

With an increase in self-referral to physiotherapy in the UK [5], the likelihood of a physiotherapist being the first point of contact for a patient with scoliosis is increased. For this reason, it could be considered particularly important that physiotherapists have the knowledge and understanding to be able to screen and recognise the symptoms of a patient with scoliosis effectively. Furthermore, it is crucial for physiotherapists to know when it is appropriate to refer on and what treatment options are available.

Few text books from the recommended reading lists for physiotherapy degree courses in the UK mention scoliosis and most universities do not cover scoliosis as part of their syllabus or recommend specific reading on this topic. Therefore, it is unlikely many physiotherapy students in the UK will have adequate knowledge to be able to recognise and effectively manage patients with scoliosis. No study has verified the knowledge of IS diagnosis and management in physiotherapy students in the UK; therefore, this study has chosen to establish this in students in their penultimate and final years of physiotherapy degrees across different universities in the UK.

Objectives

The aim of this study is to analyse the current knowledge of physiotherapy students at a university within the UK on their understanding of IS referring to the 2011 SOSORT guidelines. Thereby, investigating their proficiency as physiotherapists to provide screening, advice and exercise prescription to self-referring patients with IS.

Methods

Questionnaire development

Development of a questionnaire was completed by Drake et al. [3] using a theoretical framework from a previously completed student survey by Cziazynski et al. [4] and utilising the information provided within the 2011 SOSORT guidelines [1]. The survey was split into two distinct sections: seven questions based on analysing knowledge of scoliosis (definition, cause, development, prevalence, diagnosis, treatment and bracing) and three multiple choice questions looking at the students' opinions on what exercises they thought might be beneficial or detrimental to a patient's scoliosis, as well as their familiarity with accepted physiotherapy treatment methods for scoliosis.

The initial survey drafts were reviewed by colleagues at the Department of Physical Therapy at Arkansas State University. Following this, the second draft was reviewed by a panel of content experts, consisting of physical therapists specialising in treatment of scoliosis.

Following validation of the initial survey, a pilot study was completed with 27 physical therapy students at Arkansas State University.

Questionnaire distribution

Taking this validated and tested questionnaire, the 10-question survey [Additional file 1] was transcribed onto an online-survey platform. All UK universities offering physiotherapy degrees were invited to participate in the study through an introductory email to the programme lead of each institution. Supportive programme leads were asked to distribute the questionnaire to all students who met the inclusion criteria. The online questionnaire was accessible for a period of 8 weeks in the period of Autumn 2015, at which point the survey link was closed and all data were accumulated for analysis.

Inclusion and exclusion

The inclusion criteria consisted of UK students who were in their penultimate or final year for either a bachelor's or master's physiotherapy degree. Excluded from the study were any students who had recently graduated or were unable to complete the entire questionnaire.

All students were initially asked for their consent to participate in the study and then requested to complete the survey in one independent sitting without the use of external resources. The information collected from the student was their initials, current degree and stage of degree completion, university attended and if they had any previous experience with scoliosis.

Ethical approval

The need for ethical approval was waived by the Council for Allied Health Professions Research. Permission to distribute the survey was obtained from the the the Subject/Clinical Lead at each institution that participated.

Results

Following completion of the study period, 206 students had attempted the questionnaire and met the required inclusion criteria, with 165 completing the questionnaire fully and thus being included in all further analysis. The students were spread across 12 different universities in the UK, encompassing Scotland, England, Wales and Northern Ireland.

To remain in-line with the methods used by Drake et al. [3], and to enable a direct comparison between the results of these two studies, the 31 students that responded 'I Do Not Know' were removed from the analysis of that question. Therefore in order to allow comparison to previous research, the '% of Correct Responses' when discussed within each item section below was the percentage of students who selected the commonly accepted answer to each question, posed against those who provided an attempted response and removing 'I Do Not Know' as an option (Column F). The table below for reference also has an analysis of those subjects who answered as 'I Do Not Know' as a demonstration of ignorance to the topic and a more true representation of correct responses for future research (Column E) (Table 1).

Question 1 (definition): what is idiopathic scoliosis?

Within this question, students were asked to recognise that scoliosis is a 3-dimensional deformity [6]. One

hundred and forty-five of the 164 students (88%) who attempted an answer to this question selected scoliosis to either be a 2-dimensional or a lateral curvature of the spine (Fig. 1).

Question 2 (cause): what causes idiopathic scoliosis?

When considering the potential aetiology specifically to 'idiopathic scoliosis', 52% of respondents highlighted that the accepted cause of IS is unknown [7] (Fig. 2).

Question 3 (development): when does idiopathic scoliosis commonly develop?

One area well recognised by the students within the study was the period within which IS most commonly develops and is diagnosed. When given the options of either a period in adulthood, childhood/adolescence, in utero or as compensation to another disease, the students did correctly recognise that IS most commonly develops between a period in childhood and adolescence. Thus, they were able to identify correctly the patient group at most risk of diagnosis [8] (Fig. 3).

Question 4 (prevalence): how prevalent is idiopathic scoliosis among patients with scoliosis?

Nearly a quarter (24%) of participants correctly identified the prevalence of IS within the scoliosis population as 80%. This figure is significant as it shows that when a patient is diagnosed with scoliosis, only in 20% of cases will the therapist/practitioner be able to identify a definite cause towards the development of the condition [9] (Fig. 4).

Question 5 (diagnosis): how is the diagnosis of idiopathic scoliosis commonly confirmed?

In order to diagnose IS formally, a patient must present with a minimum of 10° of lateral curvature on radiography, alongside an evident and measurable amount of axial rotation [10]. The use of the Cobb angle is widely accepted as the diagnostic tool taken from radiographs, but for a conclusive diagnosis, the Cobb angle should be

Table 1 Results of survey per question

Column A Question	Column B Number of answer attempted (%)	Column C Number of responses removing 'I Do Not Know'	Column D Number of correct responses	Column E Percent of correct responses (excluding unanswered)	Column F Percent of correct responses (excluding unanswered and 'I Do Not Know')
1—Definition	190 (92%)	164	19	10	12
2—Cause	183 (89%)	137	71	39	52
3—Development	173 (84%)	134	106	61	79
4—Prevalence	170 (83%)	95	23	14	24
5—Diagnosis	167 (81%)	93	11	7	12
6—Treatment	166 (81%)	116	8	5	7
7—Bracing	165 (80%)	70	38	23	54

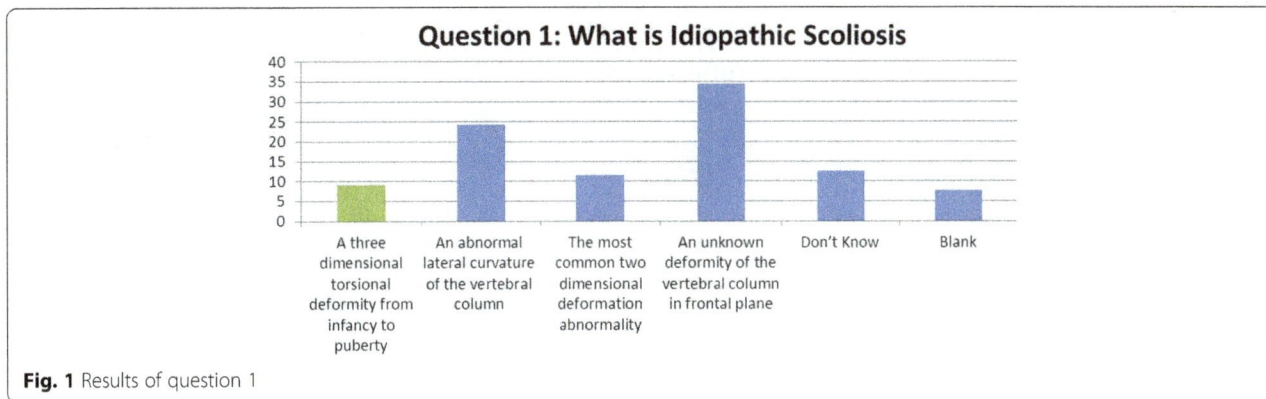

Fig. 1 Results of question 1

considered alongside a physical assessment and analysis of the structural rotation of the patient's spine [1]. This strict procedure will limit any false-positive diagnostics and also provide the therapist and practitioner with more accurate information regarding the development and severity of the patient's condition. Only 12% of respondents were able to recognise these diagnostic criteria (Fig. 5).

Question 6 (treatment): what should the treatment of idiopathic scoliosis using therapeutic exercise include?
There are currently, and have been historically, many different approaches to conservative management of scoliosis internationally. The wide variation in approaches and lack of availability of treatment facilities has resulted in a dilution of correct information and loss of clear management and treatment pathways in scoliosis care (Fig. 6).

With this wide gulf in different approaches, it is still largely accepted that all therapeutic exercise should be based on the recognised methods with addition of new

ideas, but all based upon correction in 3-dimensions with the aim of preventing or limiting progression [11].

There is yet to be any universal approach and any self-limiting therapy such as stretching of concavities or core stabilisation exercises should always be developed with consideration to the 3-dimensional aspect of scoliosis [1].

Just 7% of respondents recognised this specific accepted view that all exercises should be based around 3-dimensional correction and aim at limiting/preventing progression.

Question 7 (bracing): when is bracing recommended for patients with idiopathic scoliosis?
Following a multi-centred, partially randomised study in 2014 [12], bracing has become an integral and decisive part of conservative management of scoliosis and its correct application is key to the benefit achieved. It is widely accepted that patients should be recommended for bracing treatment if their Cobb angle is greater than 20° and their condition is highlighted as having an

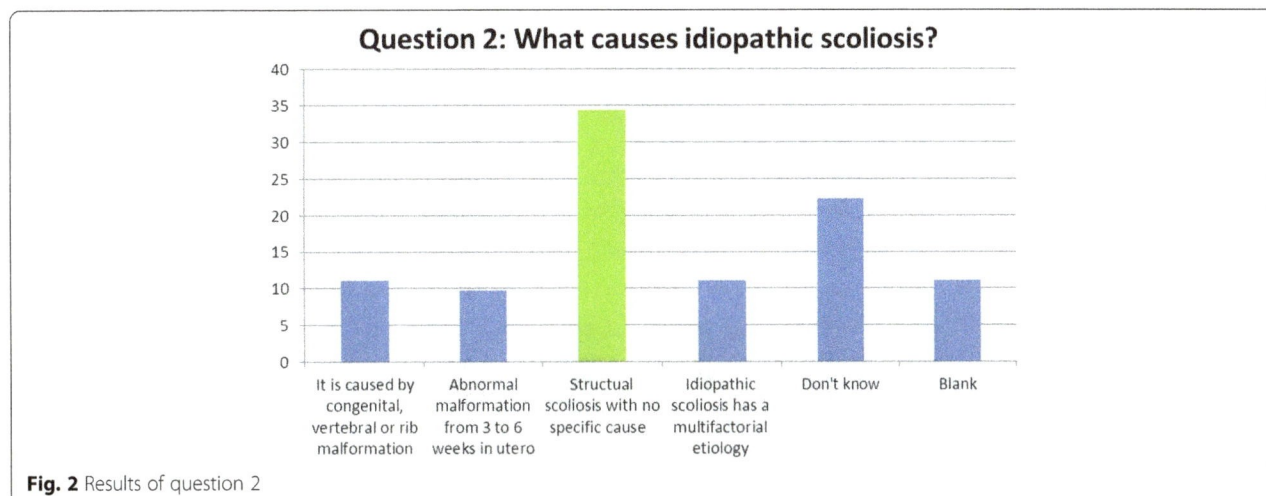

Fig. 2 Results of question 2

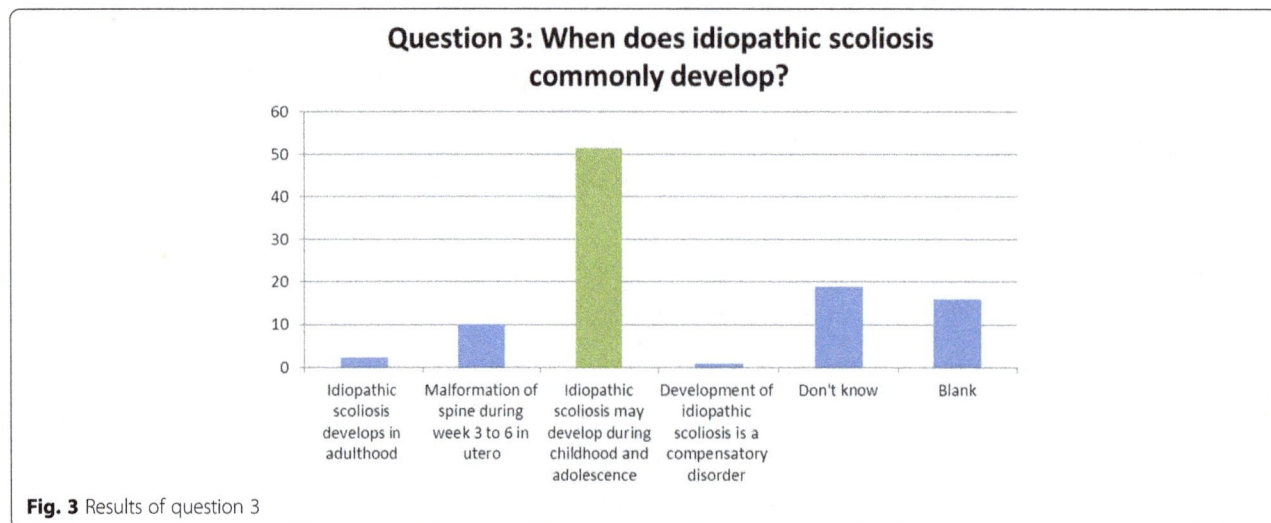

Fig. 3 Results of question 3

elevated risk of progression, whether this be through their age, maturity level, degree of angle or physical characteristics [13] (Fig. 7).

Fifty-four percent of respondents recognised the potential use of bracing in patients with a moderate and potentially progressive curvature when offered with alternatives such as a leg length discrepancy, severe curvature (> 45°) and mild curvatures (5–10°). As bracing therapy use alongside physiotherapy has been neglected in the past, it is essential that therapists and practitioners recognise when this approach is recommended [14].

Point of interest

As an opinion-based end point for the survey, the students within the study were asked three questions to highlight which physical activity they felt was most beneficial, and conversely least beneficial, for patients with scoliosis. It was also used to evaluate the

participant's knowledge of the treatment modalities highlighted as being recommended by the 2011 SOSORT guidelines. The results are highlighted in Figs. 8, 9 and 10. Subjects believed Pilates and swimming to be the most beneficial and gymnastics and martial arts to be the most detrimental and this study also demonstrates that students' knowledge of the SOSORT recommended modalities for conservative management was very minimal. SOSORT has developed a review looking at seven different, widely accepted scoliosis schools, but 84% of students were unable to recognise any of the four most popular methods [15].

Discussion

Our results showed a disappointing 7% of the students were able to answer more than 50% of the survey questions correctly in relation to the widely accepted guidelines on IS management. The results of the survey were

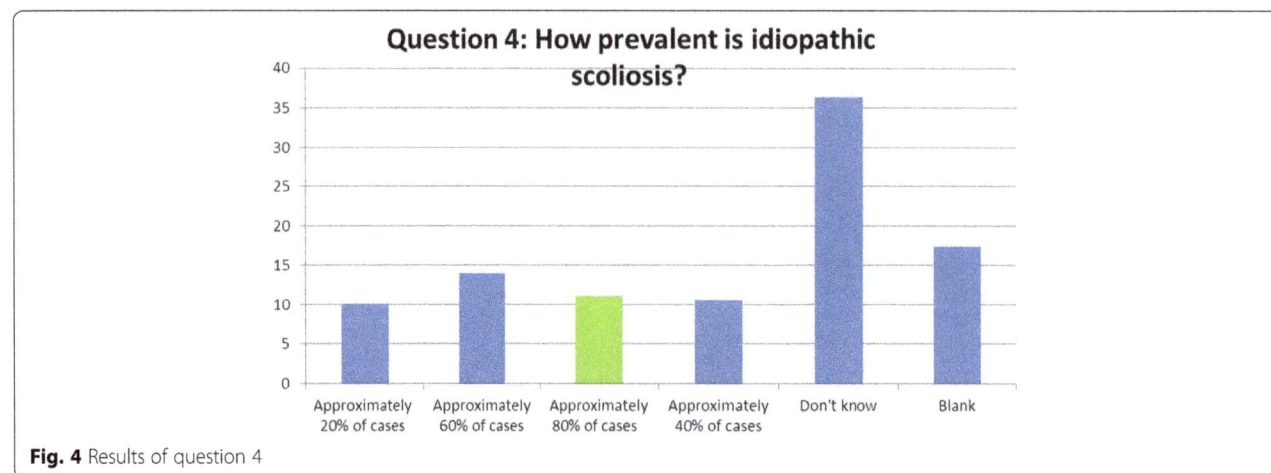

Fig. 4 Results of question 4

Question 5: How is diagnosis confirmed?

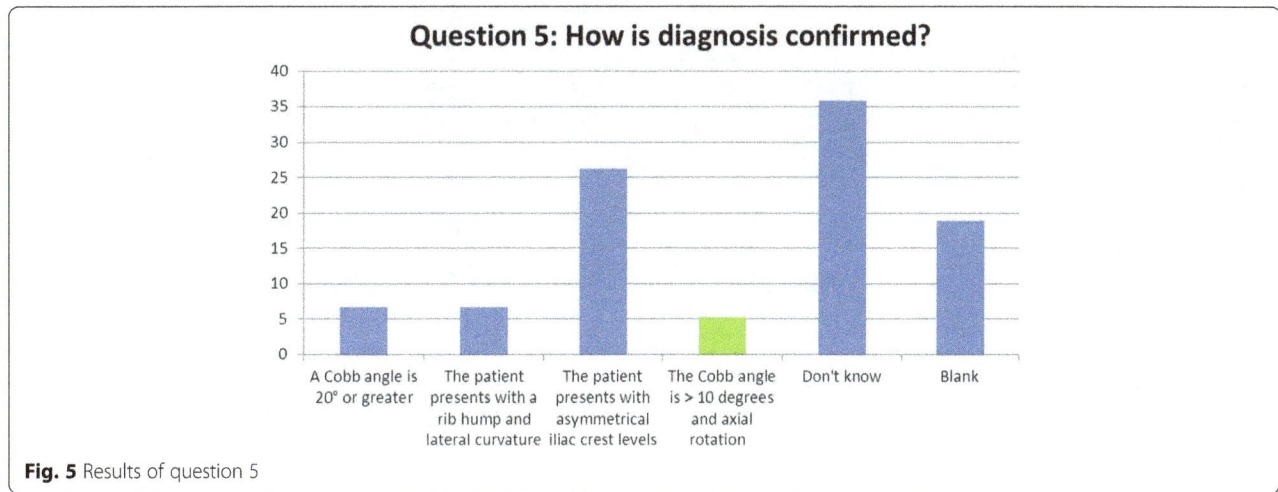

Fig. 5 Results of question 5

particularly poor in relation to recognition of scoliosis as a 3-dimensional condition, and the application of this knowledge into their rehabilitation planning. The participants were capable of recognising the patient group and age range of patients that were likely to present with structural or developing scoliosis; however, their ability to take this a step further into diagnosis, further referral, provision of advice and prescription of exercises suitable for their patients' scoliosis was very limited.

When comparing our results directly to previous studies on this topic, the subjects of this study performed worse in relation to their USA counterparts in all aspects except when asked, 'What should treatment of Idiopathic Scoliosis using therapeutic exercise include?' 6% answered correctly compared to 3% in the American study [3]. This indicates that our trainee physiotherapists in the UK are being poorly equipped to provide a satisfactory level of care to patients with scoliosis in day-to-day clinical practice. Research has shown, in Poland, physiotherapists are taught in line with the 2011 SOSORT guidelines and thus are much more familiar with the aetiology of scoliosis along with the treatment approaches available to this patient group [4].

Re-introduction of school screening has been raised in recent times, with a report in 2011 stating the reasoning behind its cessation to be very complex, involving many factors, such as the lack of accurate and reliable screening procedures, the frequency of false positives, the lack of knowledge into the natural history of scoliosis, especially in milder curves, and the evidence to support provision of efficient and effective rehabilitation protocols, again for milder curves predominantly. It reports a minimal amount of research comparing bracing or exercise therapies in relation to surgery and a lack of standardised care provision [16].

Question 6: The treatment of idiopathic scoliosis should include?

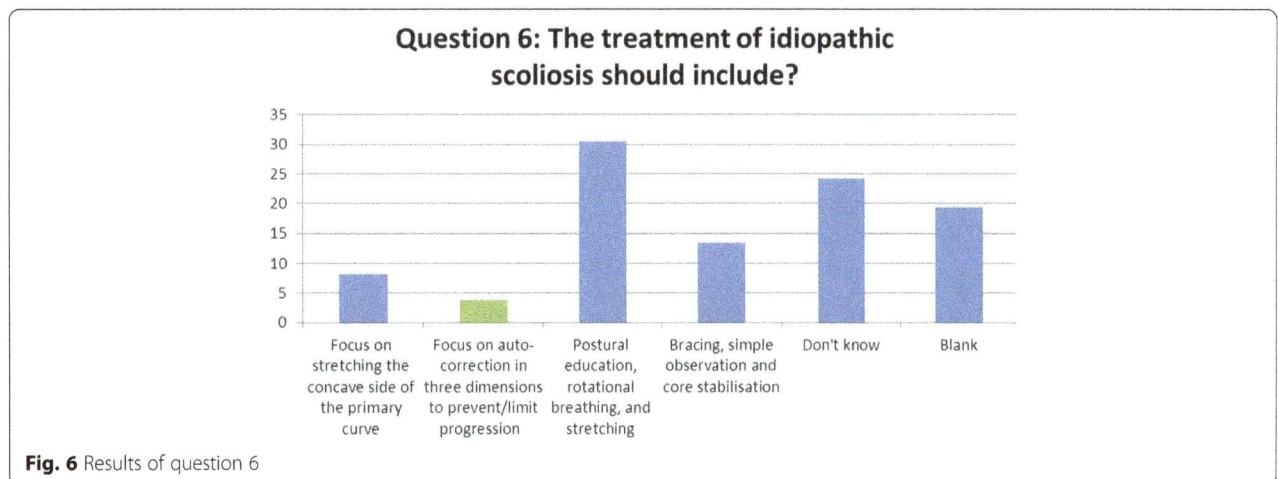

Fig. 6 Results of question 6

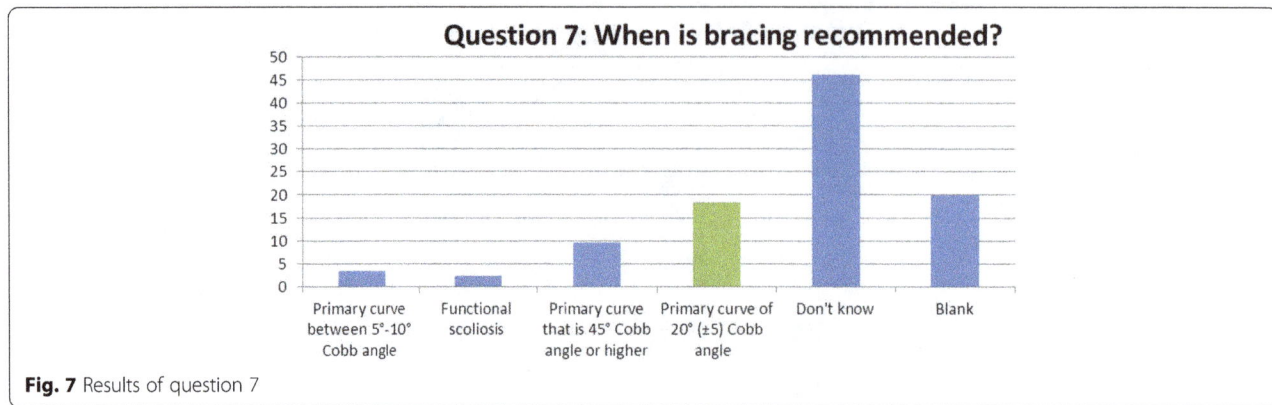

Fig. 7 Results of question 7

This lack of evidence, traditional non-provision of services and sparse background research into the topic has led to a severe absence in the development of education surrounding scoliosis in physiotherapists trained in the UK. This takes on even greater importance when placed in the context of the current drive towards self-referral to physiotherapy for musculoskeletal disorders. One in three clinical commissioning groups in England are now allowing for direct access to physiotherapy through self-referral [5]. This means that more and more frequently, physiotherapists will become the first point-of-contact for patients presenting with the first signs of scoliosis. Based on our results, it appears that physiotherapists in the UK are ill-equipped to provide this first point of care in relation to scoliosis and they are unlikely to be able to provide the standard of care, advice, onward referral and exercise prescription that is required to manage such a progressive and time sensitive condition.

The primary limitation to this study was the inability of the author to control the distribution of the questionnaire towards the target population. Distribution relied upon the programme lead from each individual institution to issue the questionnaire. Three leads actually refused to distribute the survey because they reported that scoliosis was not covered on their syllabus and thus their students would likely provide an unfavourable response. Without knowing the full demographic of students completing the survey and size of the population to which the questionnaire was distributed, there can be no definitive conclusion drawn on the entire UK-based student population and no comparisons can be drawn between universities.

Within the 'Point of Interest' questions, the respondants were asked to provide an opinion based view on physical activity with scoliosis; however, as yet there is no noted evidence to suggest whether any physical activity is beneficial for scoliosis.

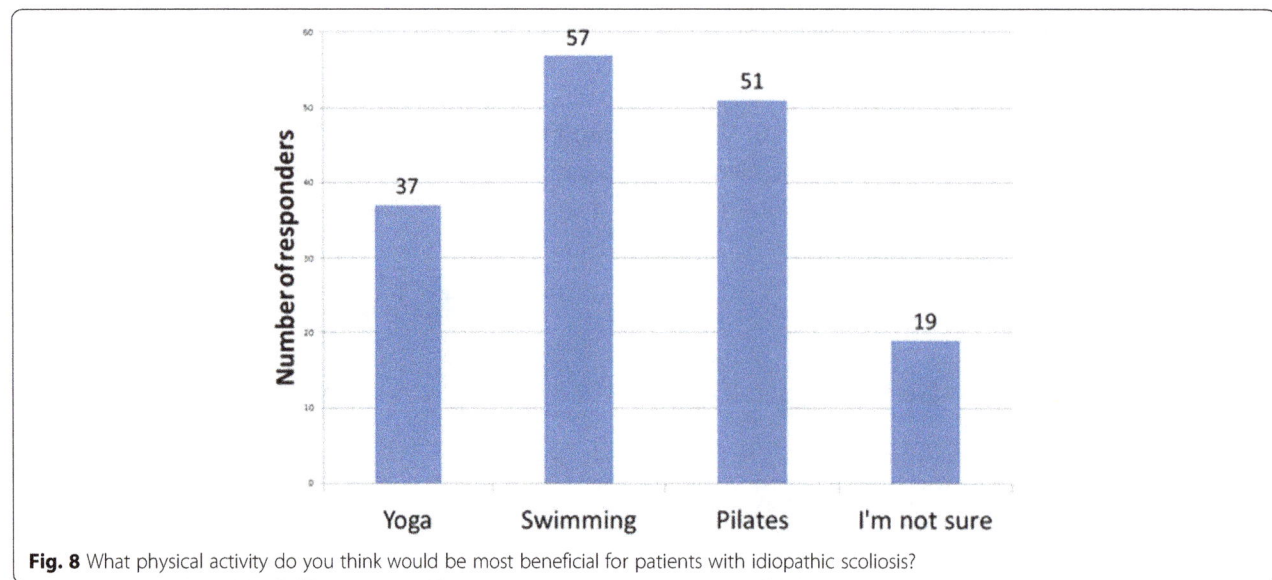

Fig. 8 What physical activity do you think would be most beneficial for patients with idiopathic scoliosis?

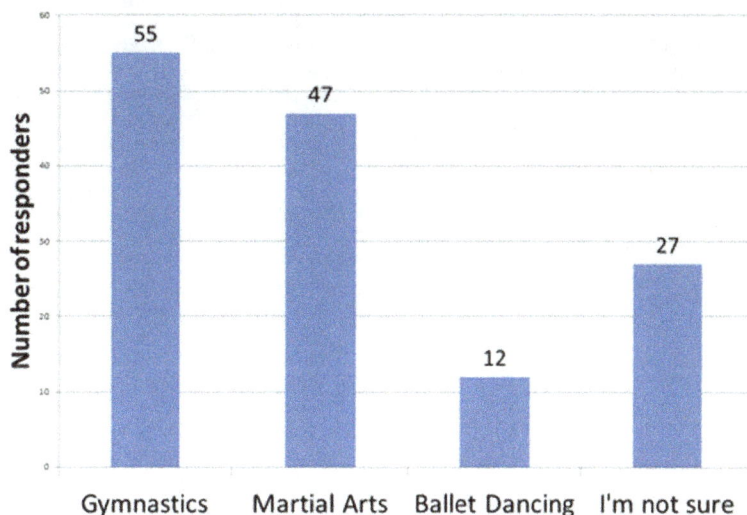

Fig. 9 What physical activity do you think would be most harmful for patients with idiopathic scoliosis?

Going forward, this study could be expanded to include post-graduate physiotherapists, especially focussing on the physiotherapists who are currently working within a self-referral system. This would enable analysis to be undertaken to rate the ability of these physiotherapists to identify effectively and manage scoliosis patients on a day-to-day basis within the NHS.

Conclusion
Physiotherapy students in the UK are being let down by poor training and poor provision of information in a condition that affects 3–4% of the population. Scoliosis is a musculoskeletal condition that progresses dramatically during the adolescent years of a patient's development, and thus should be managed with experience, knowledge and, essentially, with speed. Currently physiotherapy students are leaving university without even the most basic appreciation of scoliosis as a 3-dimensional condition and therefore are unprepared to provide accurate information in practice to patients and their families. This could potentially lead to a large number of patients being left undiagnosed or diagnosed much later, and so becoming more at risk of surgical intervention or from physical and emotional dysfunctions.

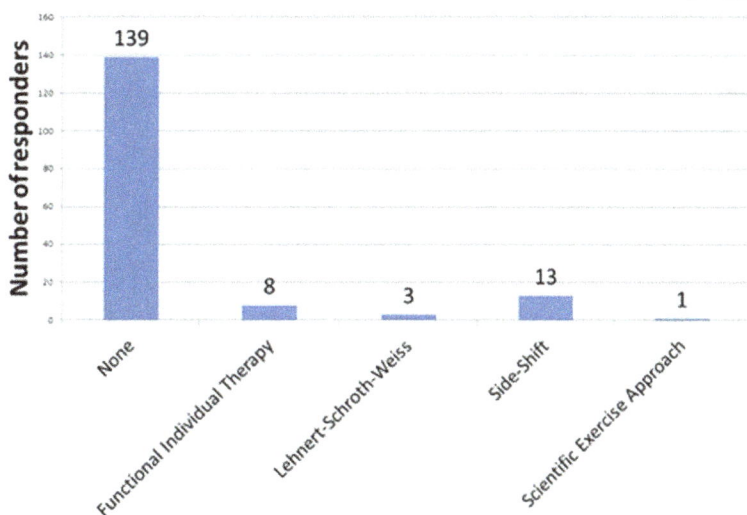

Fig. 10 What method of conservative treatment for idiopathic scoliosis are you most familiar with?

Abbreviations

AIS: Adolescent idiopathic scoliosis; GP: General practitioner; IS: Idiopathic scoliosis; NHS: National Health Service; SOSORT: International Society on Scoliosis Orthopaedic and Rehabilitation Treatment; UK: United Kingdom; USA: United States of America

Acknowledgements

We would like to acknowledge the hard work done by Shawn Drake, Arkansas State University, in the development of the survey questionnaire and her agreement to distribute this questionnaire among our target population. Thanks also to all programme leads of the universities who helped in the distribution of the questionnaire within their institutions.

Funding

Not applicable. Publication fee provided by Scoliosis SOS Limited.

Authors' contributions

DAJB and CP contributed to completion of the study and drafting of the manuscript. EM was involved with proof reading and guidance. SD provided development of survey questionnaire and DG completed all statistical analysis and amalgamation of results. All authors read and approved the final manuscript.

Competing interests

DAJB and CP are employees of Scoliosis SOS (Physiotherapy Clinic) and are members of SOSORT.
EM is a Clinic Principal and Founder of Scoliosis SOS (Physiotherapy Clinic) and is a member of SOSORT.
DG and SD declare that they have no competing interests.

Author details

[1]Scoliosis SOS Clinic, 63 Mansell Street, London E1 8AN, UK. [2]Arkansas State University, PO Box 910, Jonesboro, AR 72467, USA. [3]Independent, York, UK.

References

1. Negrini S, Aulisa AG, Aulisa L, Circo AB, de Mauroy JC, Durmala J, Grivas TB, Knott P, Kotwicki T, Maruyama T, Minozzi S, O'Brien JP, Papadopoulos D, Rigo M, Rivard CH, Romano M, Wynne JH, Villagrasa M, Weiss HR, Zaina F. 2011 SOSORT guidelines: orthopaedic and rehabilitation treatment of idiopathic scoliosis during growth. Scoliosis. 2012;7:3.
2. Reamy BV, Slakey JB. Adolescent idiopathic scoliosis: review and current concepts. Am Fam Physician. 2001;64:111–6.
3. Drake S, Glidewell MA, Thomas J. Current knowledge of scoliosis in physical therapy students trained in the United States. Scoliosis. 2014;9(Suppl 1):O64.
4. Ciazynski D, Czernicki K, Durmala J. Knowledge about idiopathic scoliosis among students of physiotherapy. Stud Health Technol Inform. 2008;140:281–5.
5. Self-referral: key to improving access to physiotherapy [http://www.csp.org. uk/professional-union/practice/self-referral] Accessed 2 Dec 2016.
6. Grivas TB, Vasiliadis ES, Rodopoulos G. Aetiology of idiopathic scoliosis. What have we learned from school screening? Stud Health Technol Inform. 2008;140:240–4.
7. Rogala EJ, Drummond DS, Gurr J. Scoliosis: incidence and natural history. A prospective epidemiological study. J Bone Joint Surg Am. 1978;60(2):173–6.
8. Negrini S, Aulisa L, Ferraro C, Fraschini P, Masiero S, Simonazzi P, Tedeschi C, Venturin A. Italian guidelines on rehabilitation treatment of adolescents with scoliosis or other spinal deformities. Eura Medicophys. 2005;41(2):183–201.
9. Asher MA, Burton DC. Adolescent idiopathic scoliosis: natural history and long term treatment effects. Scoliosis. 2006;1:2.
10. Janicki JA, Alman B. Scoliosis: review of diagnosis and treatment. Paediatr Child Health. 2007;12(9):771–6.
11. Weiss H, Negrini S, Hawes M, Rigo M, Kotwicki T, Grivas T, members of the SOSORT. Physical exercises in the treatment of idiopathic scoliosis at risk of brace treatment—SOSORT consensus paper 2005. Scoliosis. 1:6.
12. Weinstein SL, Dolan LA, Wright JG, Dobbs MB. Effects of bracing in adolescents with idiopathic scoliosis. N Engl J Med. 2013;369:1512–21.
13. Negrini S, Grivas TB, Kotwicki T, Rigo M, Zaina F. Guidelines on "Standards of management of idiopathic scoliosis with corrective braces in everyday clinics and in clinical research": SOSORT Consensus 2008. Scoliosis. 2009;4(1):2.
14. Negrini S. Approach to scoliosis changed due to causes other than evidence: patients call for conservative (rehabilitation) experts to join in team orthopaedic surgeons. Disabil Rehabil. 2008;30(10):731–41.
15. Berdishevsky H, Lebel VA, Bettaby-Saltikov J, Rigo M, Lebel A, Hennes A, Romano M, Bialek M, M'hango A, Betts T, de Mauroy JC, Durmala J. Physiotherapy scoliosis-specific exercises—a comprehensive review of seven major schools. Scoliosis and Spinal Disorders. 2016;11:20.
16. UK National Screening Committee: Screening for adolescent idiopathic scoliosis. External review against programme appraisal criteria for the UK National Screening Committee (UK NSC): Bazian Ltd ;2011: 1-46. 3 [http://www.britscoliosissoc.org.uk/data/documents/1466-13.pdf] Accessed 28 Nov 2016.

16

3D correction of AIS in braces designed using CAD/CAM and FEM

Nikita Cobetto, Carl-Éric Aubin[*], Stefan Parent, Soraya Barchi, Isabelle Turgeon and Hubert Labelle

Abstract

Background: Recent studies showed that finite element model (FEM) combined to CAD/CAM improves the design of braces for the conservative treatment of adolescent idiopathic scoliosis (AIS), using 2D measurements from in-brace radiographs. We aim to assess the immediate effectiveness on curve correction in all three planes of braces designed using CAD/CAM and numerical simulation compared to braces designed with CAD/CAM only.

Methods: SRS standardized criteria for bracing were followed to recruit 48 AIS patients who were randomized into two groups. For both groups, 3D reconstructions of the spine and patient's torso, respectively built from bi-planar radiographs and surface topography, were obtained and braces were designed using the CAD/CAM approach. For the test group, 3D reconstructions of the spine and patient's torso were additionally used to generate a personalized FEM to simulate and iteratively improve the brace design with the objective of curve correction maximization in three planes and brace material minimization.

Results: For the control group (CtrlBraces), average Cobb angle prior to bracing was 29° (thoracic, T) and 25° (lumbar, L) with the planes of maximal curvature (PMC) respectively oriented at 63° and 57° on average with respect to the sagittal plane. Average apical axial rotation prior to bracing was 7° (T) and 9° (L). For the test group (FEMBraces), initial Cobb angles were 33° (T) and 28° (L) with the PMC at 68° (T) and 56° (L) and average apical axial rotation prior to bracing at 9° (T and L). On average, FEMBraces were 50% thinner and had 20% less covering surface than CtrlBraces while reducing T and L curves by 47 and 48%, respectively, compared to 25 and 26% for CtrlBraces. FEMBraces corrected apical axial rotation by 46% compared to 30% for CtrlBraces.

Conclusion: The combination of numerical simulation and CAD/CAM approach allowed designing more efficient braces in all three planes, with the advantages of being lighter than standard CAD/CAM braces. Bracing in AIS may be improved in 3D by the use of this simulation platform. This study is ongoing to recruit more cases and to analyze the long-term effect of bracing.

Keywords: Computer-aided design/computer-aided manufacturing, Scoliosis, Thoraco-lumbo-sacral orthosis, Finite element model (FEM), RCT

* Correspondence: carl-eric.aubin@polymtl.ca
Department of Mechanical Engineering, Polytechnique Montreal, P.O. Box 6079, Downtown Station, Montreal, Quebec H3C 3A7, Canada

Background

Orthopedic bracing is the conservative treatment generally prescribed to control curve progression in adolescent idiopathic scoliosis (AIS) showing curves between 20° and 40° of Cobb angle [1]. AIS is a three-dimensional (3D) deformity of the spine which includes a deviation in the coronal plane, changes in the sagittal curves, and an axial rotation of the vertebrae [2, 3]. Bracing was demonstrated as an effective treatment to prevent curve progression, as assessed using 2D coronal X-ray measurements, and immediate in-brace correction was found to be correlated to long-term effectiveness [4–7]. The treatment outcomes rely on multiple factors such as timing with adolescent growth spurt, spine flexibility, and patient compliance to treatment [8–11].

However, bracing is not always successful and there is a lack of knowledge regarding the correction in the sagittal and transverse planes [12]. Studies reported that brace wear tends to create a hypokyphotic effect and provide a non-significant correction of vertebral axial rotation [13, 14], as well as having no effect on the orientation of the planes of maximum curvature (PMC), which are defined by the planes passing through the apex and the end vertebrae of a given curve [2, 13, 15].

Traditional vs. CAD/CAM brace fabrication

Computer-aided design/computer-aided manufacturing (CAD/CAM) systems are now frequently used for brace design and have proven to be as effective compared to the traditional plaster-cast methods, using 2D metrics [16]. Traditional brace fabrication of rigid thoraco-lumbo-sacral orthosis (TLSO) is based on craftsmanship and involves plaster molding, which requires time and material consumption and presents a low accuracy [17]. However, the CAD/CAM design technique does not have an impact on brace effectiveness' improvement. For this purpose, finite element models (FEM) have been developed to analyze brace biomechanics [18–23]. More recently, a simulation platform was created by combining CAD/CAM system and FEM [24, 25]. It allows the simulation of brace installation on the patient before its fabrication and the iterative improvement of its design and biomechanical efficiency [24, 25]. A randomized controlled trial (RCT) using this simulation platform was previously realized to evaluate the effectiveness of braces designed using this platform compared to standard braces designed with the plaster-cast technique and the CAD/CAM technology only [26]. Braces designed with the simulation platform were found to be more effective than the standard braces for correcting the major thoracic curve. Yet, measurements of brace effectiveness were done in 2D using the postero-anterior and lateral radiographs, and it remained to be demonstrated that

the 3D correction of the curve could also be improved by the use of this simulation platform.

The objective of this study was to revisit the data from the previous RCT study to assess the 3D immediate effectiveness of braces designed using CAD/CAM and FEM compared to CAD/CAM only.

Methods

Study design

Inclusion criteria for this study were based on the SRS standardized criteria for bracing, and patients were consecutively recruited at our scoliosis clinic [27]. Inclusion criteria were AIS diagnosis (Cobb angle between 20° and 40°), a Risser sign of 0–2, and a full-time TLSO prescription. The study was approved by our institutional ethical committee, and each participant and their parents gave a written consent.

A simple randomization sequence was prepared by a biostatistician not involved in the recruitment and follow-up of the patients and was generated by a randomization table (simple block randomization list with a block size of 4). Patients were assigned to their group using the randomization sequence. The caregivers were blinded but not the orthotist. All patients had their brace designed by one of the two participating orthotists having more than 10 years of experience with TLSO and 2 years of experience with CAD/CAM technology. The patients from the control group received a TLSO designed and fabricated using the CAD/CAM approach only (CtrlBrace) while the patients from the test group received a TLSO designed and fabricated using the CAD/CAM approach but additionally simulated using a patient-specific FEM (FEMBrace).

Brace design and fabrication

For all patients, simultaneous calibrated bi-planar postero-anterior (PA) and lateral (LAT) radiographs were taken during the patient's first visit and after the brace installation using a low-dose digital radiography system (EOS™, EOS imaging, Paris, France). The 3D reconstruction was done with a custom-developed software using a semi-automated method based on 19 anatomical control points on the vertebral bodies, pedicles, and posterior arches [28]. The following indices were computed using the initial and in-brace 3D reconstructions using a custom measurement software: main thoracic (T) and lumbar (L) Cobb angles, kyphosis (T4–T12) and lordosis (L1–S1) angles, apical rotation at the apex of both T and L curves, and orientation of the PMC for T and L curves [29]. The precision using this software has been shown to be less than 1.5 mm for mean point-to-surface error and inferior to 5° for angular measurements compared to computed tomographic scan reconstructions [30].

For all patients, the external torso geometry was acquired using a surface topography system (3-dimensional Capturor, Creaform Inc., Levis, Canada) [31, 32]. Modification of the external torso geometry was done by the orthotists using a CAD/CAM software (Rodin4D, Bordeaux, France) to design the shape of the brace by virtually adding or removing material to introduce pressure and relief areas and corrective translations. Braces were then fabricated using a numerically controlled carver (Model C, Rodin 4D, Bordeaux, France) linked to the CAD/CAM software. A polyurethane foam bloc was carved according to the CAD model, and brace shell thermoforming was done using a heated copolymer sheet. The fabricated brace was trimmed and adjusted by the orthotist, and brace effectiveness was assessed using the 3D reconstruction of the spine obtained from calibrated PA and LAT in-brace radiographs [28]. The brace covering surface area was computed by importing the STL file of the brace design in a CAD/CAM software (CATIA V5R21, Dassault Sytemes, Vélizy-Villacoublay, France). Brace shell thickness and corrective pad thickness were measured by the orthotist following brace adjustment using a caliper tool [26].

Additional steps for the test group (FEMBrace)

Radiopaque markers visible on X-rays and trunk surface were a priori positioned on anatomical points of the patient's torso (vertebrae T1 and L5, sternum jugular notch and xiphoid process, right and left anterior iliac spines) and were used to register the 3D reconstruction and the external torso geometry using a point-to-point least square algorithm. Using a previously validated method, the registered geometry was used to create a personalized FEM using Ansys 14.5 software package (Ansys Inc., Canonsburg, PA, USA) [7, 33]. The FEM includes the vertebrae T1 to L5, intervertebral discs, ribs, sternum, costal cartilages, ligaments, abdominal cavity, and soft external tissues (Fig. 1). Mechanical properties of the anatomical structures were taken from published data obtained on typical human cadaveric spine segments [20, 21, 33–37].

For FEMBraces, during the brace design process, the 3D reconstruction of the initial patient's spinal geometry (previously obtained for the FEM generation) was available and imported as an STL file in the CAD/CAM software to help position the corrective translation and pressure areas on the torso geometry. A brace FEM using polyethylene mechanical properties was then created. The orthotist selected nodes on the brace FEM to define the strap localization and virtually positioned the brace on the patient's FEM. The brace installation was then simulated using a point-to-surface contact interface between the brace and the trunk models to represent friction and force transfer from the brace shell to the patient's trunk surface [33, 38]. During the brace installation simulation, the brace was opened by applying displacement on nodes of the brace posterior opening. The brace was then placed on the trunk model, and sets of co-linear forces were applied at the strap fixation sites as previously determined by the orthotist [33]. During all simulation steps, the pelvis was fixed in space and the first thoracic vertebra (T1) was allowed to rotate and translate longitudinally. For a given simulation, the correction was assessed using post-processed Cobb angles, lordosis and kyphosis, vertebral axial rotation, and the orientation of the PMC, as well as the distance between patient's skin and brace shell (brace fitting) (Fig. 2). Following the brace simulation, it was possible to modify the brace design to improve brace correction. To improve 3D correction, the brace design was iteratively modified by the orthotist in the CAD/CAM software by varying mainly the corrective pressure area localization and depth, as well as the trim lines, relief zones, side of trochanteric pressure area, and openings on the brace, and was simulated. The brace effectiveness was computationally assessed by the orthotist to maximize the correction using post-processed 3D indices. The strategy

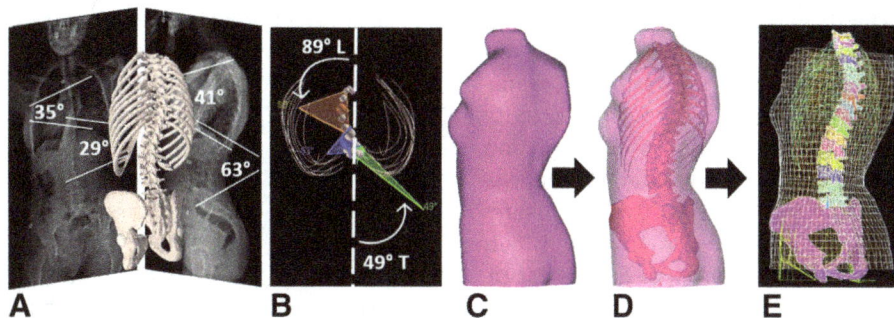

Fig. 1 a Acquisition of the calibrated bi-planar radiographs and view of the corresponding 3D reconstruction of the spine, rib cage, and pelvis. **b** Top view of the planes of maximal curvature. **c** Torso 3D geometry following surface topography acquisition. **d** 3D geometric registration of the spine and torso geometry. **e** Finite element model of the trunk: vertebrae, intervertebral discs, ribs, sternum, costal cartilages, ligaments, and soft external tissues

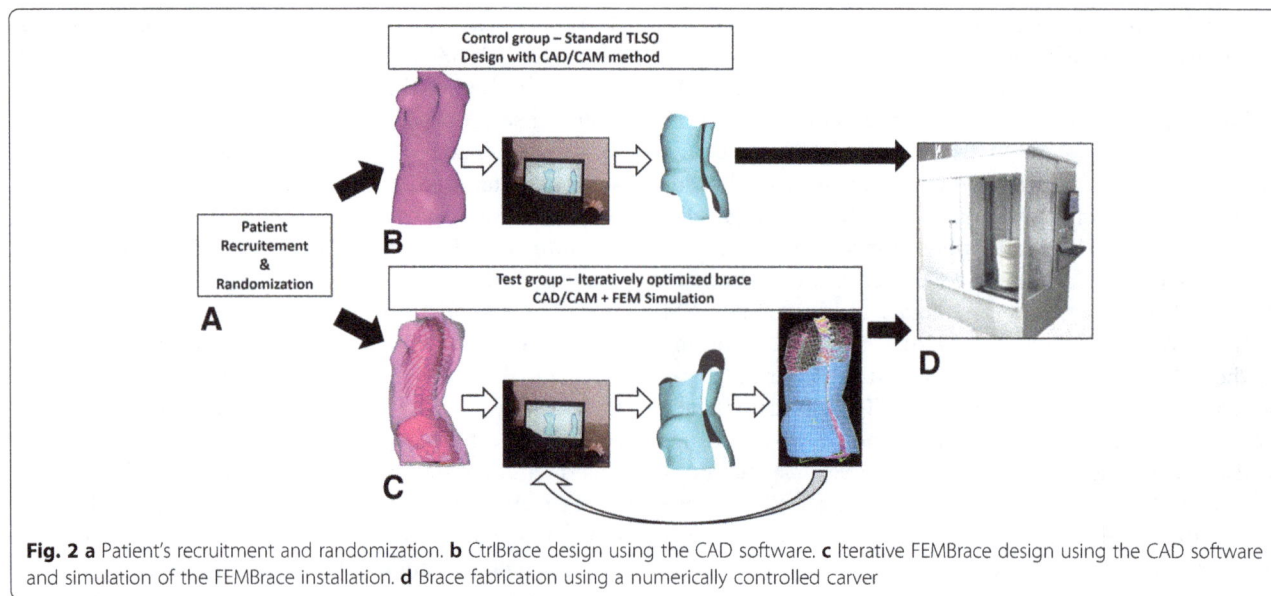

Fig. 2 a Patient's recruitment and randomization. **b** CtrlBrace design using the CAD software. **c** Iterative FEMBrace design using the CAD software and simulation of the FEMBrace installation. **d** Brace fabrication using a numerically controlled carver

for correction maximization was to incrementally accentuate pad depth by 5 mm until simulated spinal correction remained stable even with the corrective area depth increasing (2° Cobb angle) [25]. The numerical process required an average of 3 iterations per patient (minimum 2, maximum 6). The strategy for minimizing the brace surface contact was to create openings in the brace shell at locations where the simulated distance between brace material and patient's skin was more than 6 mm.

The optimal FEMBrace was then fabricated using the same numerical controlled carver and thermoforming process as for the control group (CtrlBrace). The FEMBrace was trimmed by the orthotist, and brace effectiveness was assessed using the 3D reconstruction of the spine computed from simultaneous PA and LAT radiographs. Brace covering surface and brace thickness were measured using the same methods as for CtrlBrace.

Statistical analysis

Statistical analysis was performed using STATISTICA 10.0 software package (Statistica, StatSoft Inc., Tulsa, Oklahoma, USA). To verify that both groups were statistically comparable, a paired Student t test (95% significance level) was applied to compare the curve severity, T4–T12 kyphosis, L1–S1 lordosis, apical axial rotation, and the orientation of the PMC between both groups. A statistical analysis was also realized using a paired Student t test (95% significance level) to analyze if there was a significant difference between both groups for in-brace indices.

Results

Twenty-five patients and 23 patients were respectively recruited in the control group and the test group.

Following statistical analysis, both groups were found comparable and had non-statistically different age, sex, weight, height, skeletal maturity, curve type, curve severity, and initial 3D parameters (Table 1). For the control group, average Cobb angle prior to bracing was 29° (T) and 25° (L) and the apical axial rotation was of 7° for the T curve and 9° for the L curve with respective PMC oriented at 63° and 57° with respect to the sagittal plane. For the test group, average Cobb angle prior to bracing was 33° (T) and 28° (L) and the average apical axial rotation was of 9° for both T and L curves, with respective PMC of 68° and 56°. For both groups, average initial T4–T12 kyphosis was 25° and average L1–S1 lordosis was 66°.

The coronal plane correction was statistically significantly greater in the test group vs. the control group ($p < 0.05$): FEMBraces reduced T Cobb angle by 47% while it reduced the L Cobb angle by 48% vs. 25 and 26% respectively for the CtrlBraces (Table 2). The actual FEMBrace Cobb angle correction was predicted with an average difference inferior to 5° by the simulation.

In the transverse plane, the correction also was statistically significantly greater in the test group vs. the control group ($p < 0.05$): apical axial rotation was corrected by 46% for FEMBraces vs. 30% for CtrlBraces for both T and L curves (Table 2). A statistically significant corrective effect was found between the in-brace-corrected PMC and the out of brace initial PMC for the L curve (p value = 0.01) for both groups. However, the orientation of the PMC of the T curve was not really modified in both groups, but with larger variability in the control group.

In the sagittal plane, the kyphosis was significantly less reduced in the test vs. control group ($p < 0.05$)

Table 1 Patient data at initial visit (measurements in the three planes computed using the 3D reconstruction of the spine)

		Test group $N = 25$			Difference between groups	CtrlBrace $N = 23$		
		Mean	SD	N	Paired t test[a]	Mean	SD	N
Coronal plane	T Cobb angle	33°	8°	23	$p = 0.06$	29°	8°	20
	L Cobb angle	28°	9°	21	$p = 0.14$	25°	10°	17
Transverse plane	T apical axial rotation	9°	3°	23	$p = 0.41$	7°	6°	20
	L apical axial rotation	9°	5°	21	$p = 0.60$	9°	6°	17
	T plane of maximum curvature (angle with respect to the sagittal plane)	68°	17°	23	$p = 0.28$	63°	23°	20
	L plane of maximum curvature (angle with respect to the sagittal plane)	56°	19°	21	$p = 0.66$	57°	26°	17
Sagittal plane	T4–T12 kyphosis	25°	15°	25	$p = 0.91$	25°	12°	23
	L1–S1 lordosis	66°	9°	25	$p = 0.91$	66°	11°	23

[a]Statistically significantly different for $p < 0.05$

(2 vs. 16%), but there was no significant difference for the change of lordosis (21 vs. 16%) (Table 2). Detailed statistical results including the p values are described in Table 2.

FEMBraces had an average of 20% less covering surface than the CtrlBraces. The brace shell thickness was the same for both groups (4 mm), but 13-mm-thick pads were added to the CtrlBraces (no foam pad (liner) was necessary for the FEMBraces). As CtrlBrace foam pads were covering on average 34% of the brace area, we estimated globally FEMBraces to be 50% thinner than CrtlBraces (Fig. 3).

The time needed for the orthotists to complete the iterative brace design process was of 5 min to start the simulation (manipulations to prepare and position the brace model on the trunk model, selection of the strap fixation sites) and 10–15 min per iteration to perform the modifications on the brace design in the CAD/CAM software for the next simulation. However, the time needed for the brace fitting was reduced by approximately 30 min as compared to the CtrlBraces.

Discussion

This study demonstrated a clinically and statistically significant greater 3D immediate in-brace effectiveness for braces designed using a new design platform combining CAD/CAM and FEM compared to CAD/CAM only. The main strength of this study is the 3D analysis and the RCT design, which confirms and supports previous feasibility studies with CAD/CAM and FEM simulations for brace design in AIS. It distinguishes from previous studies for which brace effectiveness was only evaluated in 2D using only the PA and LAT radiographs.

Using this simulation platform, it is possible to simulate/test different brace designs and better define the treatment plan to include the sagittal and transverse plane correction parameters. We believe that having access to spinal 3D reconstructions and FEM combined with CAD/CAM techniques allows orthotists to better visualize and address the sagittal, transverse, and coronal profiles of the spine. This could improve brace design with better 3D fitting to correct efficiently the spinal deformity in the frontal plane, as well as in the transverse

Table 2 In-brace results for T and L Cobb angles, apical axial rotation for T and L apex, and orientation of the planes of maximal curvature and kyphosis and lordosis angles

		FEMBrace (test group)		Difference between groups	CtrlBrace (control group)	
		Mean	SD	Student's t test[a]	Mean	SD
Coronal plane	T Cobb angle reduction (%)	47	20	$p = 0.01$	25	18
	L Cobb angle reduction (%)	48	24	$p = 0.04$	26	27
Transverse plane	T curve apical axial rotation correction (%)	46	24	$p = 0.004$	30	17
	L curve apical axial rotation correction (%)	46	22	$p = 0.003$	30	23
	T plane of maximum curvature reduction (degrees)	0	18	$p = 0.28$	3	30
	L plane of maximal curvature reduction (degrees)	11	40	$p = 0.66$	11	46
Sagittal plane	T4–T12 kyphosis reduction (degrees)	−2	6	$p = 0.02$	−16	28
	L1–S1 lordosis reduction (degrees)	12	25	$p = 0.44$	11	24

[a]Significant difference between both groups for $p < 0.05$

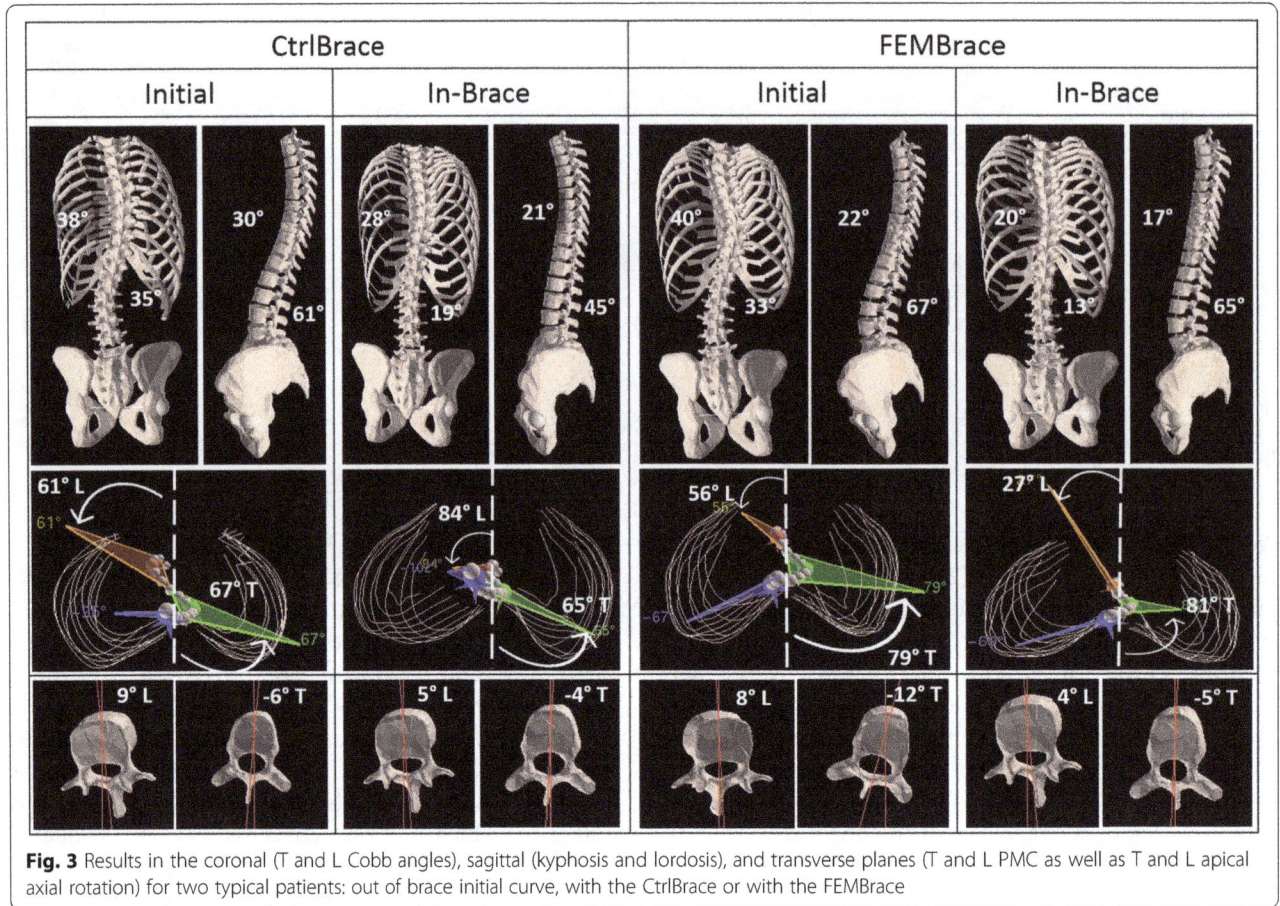

Fig. 3 Results in the coronal (T and L Cobb angles), sagittal (kyphosis and lordosis), and transverse planes (T and L PMC as well as T and L apical axial rotation) for two typical patients: out of brace initial curve, with the CtrlBrace or with the FEMBrace

plane, while preserving the kyphosis and lordosis curvatures in the sagittal plane.

Furthermore, by performing the measurements using the 3D reconstruction instead of radiographs, it was possible to assess additional 3D parameters, which were not evaluated in previous studies [24–26] such as the axial rotation at the apex of the curves and the orientation of the PMC for both T and L curves. Vertebral axial rotation is possibly associated with curve progression [39], and correcting or controlling this parameter could improve brace effectiveness for the long-term results.

The limited action of the CtrlBraces on the orientation of the PMC was also reported in previous studies [13, 37]. The PMC combines the regional description of the spine curvature in both the sagittal and the coronal planes; therefore, it is not an independent index as compared to the vertebral axial rotation, which is a measurement of the mechanical torsion in the spine. The components of brace design that could address the residual regional deformity of the PMC remain to be dealt with. The use of the patient-specific FEM could be useful to further improve the 3D effectiveness of braces.

However, there are limitations to this trial. The detailed muscles and muscular activation were not modeled in the

FEM but were indirectly represented through a global evaluation of forces required to maintain the balance at T1. In this study, we only addressed the immediate effect of wearing a brace. Since a correlation has been reported between immediate in-brace correction and brace treatment long-term effectiveness [5] and that 3D parameters related to curve progression seem to be better controlled, it suggests that FEMBraces may also improve the long-term treatment efficacy in all three planes. A study of long-term effects in a larger cohort appears warranted to evaluate if the 3D correction of the deformity influence the treatment's outcomes.

The use of the simulation platform allowed orthotists to analyze the contact surface between brace and patient's skin, in order to adjust the openings and relief zones on the brace to obtain less covering surface and thinner braces. The addition of FEM to CAD/CAM techniques was not more time-consuming and did not add complexity to brace fabrication as the brace was optimized.

This simulation platform allowed to test any rigid brace design; therefore, it could also be used to study or improve any other braces like the ones with an anterior opening, orthoses used to treat scoliotic thoraco-lumbar curves or orthoses presenting possible 3D spinal correction in the sagittal and the transverse planes [40].

Conclusions

Combining the CAD/CAM approach with FEM simulation allowed the design of more efficient braces to correct the scoliotic spinal deformities in all three planes at the first immediate in-brace evaluation, with lighter design than standard CAD/CAM braces. These results suggest that long-term 3D effect of bracing in AIS may be improved by the use of this new platform, but this should be further tested as part of an ongoing RCT study. We feel that the ability to assess the biomechanical effects of bracing in 3D is becoming important.

Abbreviations

3D: Three-dimensional; AIS: Adolescent idiopathic scoliosis; CAD/CAM: Computer-aided design/computer-aided manufacturing; FEM: Finite element model; L: Lumbar; LAT: Lateral; PA: Postero-anterior; PMC: Plane of maximum curvature; RCT: Randomized controlled trial; T: Thoracic; TLSO: Thoraco-lumbo-sacral orthosis

Acknowledgements

Special thanks to Marie-Chantal Bolduc and Benoit Bissonnette from Orthèse-Prothèse Rive-Sud who contributed to the design and fabrication of the braces and delivery to the patients.

Funding

This project was funded by the Natural Sciences and Engineering Research Council of Canada (RGPIN 239148-11) and the Canadian Institutes of Health Research (MOP-119455).

Authors' contributions

NC built the finite element models of the test group patients for the orthotists simulations, analyzed and interpreted the radiological patient data and statistical analysis, and was a major contributor in writing the manuscript. CEA interpreted the radiological and statistical analysis and was a major contributor in writing the manuscript. SP and HB were the attending physicians for the study and interpreted the radiological patient data. SB was responsible for the ethical procedures and patient recruitment for the study and was a major contributor in writing the manuscript. IT was responsible for the ethical procedures and patient recruitment for the study. All authors read and approved the final manuscript.

Competing interests

Research and development contract was obtained with Groupe Lagarrigue to develop and transfer a license of the simulation platform. Money was given to the university, and the contract was not directly related to the presented RCT study. The RCT study presented in this paper was funded by a peer-reviewed grant from the Canadian Institutes of Health Research. The participating orthotists from Orthèse-Prothèse Rive-Sud received nothing of value to realize this study.

References

1. Nachemson AL, Peterson LE. Effectiveness of treatment with brace in girls who have adolescent idiopathic scoliosis. A prospective, controlled study based on data from the Brace Study of the Scoliosis Research Society. J Bone Joint Surg. 1995;77:815–22.
2. Trobisch P, Suess O, Schwab F. Idiopathic scoliosis. Dtsch Arztebl Int. 2010;107(49):875–83.
3. Labelle H, Aubin CE, Jackson R, Lenke L, Newton P, Parent S. Seeing the spine in 3D: how will it change what we do? J Pediatr Orthop. 2011;31(1 Suppl):S37–45.
4. Castro F. Adolescent idiopathic scoliosis, bracing, and the Hueter-Volkmann principle. Spine. 2003;3:182–5.
5. Weinstein SL, Dolan LA, Wright JG, Dobbs MB. Effects of bracing in adolescents with idiopathic scoliosis. N Engl J Med. 2013;369(16):1512–21.
6. Landauer F, Wimmer C, Behensky H. Estimating the final outcome of brace treatment for idiopathic thoracic scoliosis at 6-month follow-up. Pediatric rehabilitation. 2003;6:201–7.
7. Clin J, Aubin CE, Sangole A, Labelle H, Parent S. Correlation between immediate in-brace correction and biomechanical effectiveness of brace treatment in adolescent idiopathic scoliosis. Spine. 2010;35(18):1706–13.
8. Nault M, Parent S, Phan P, Roy-Beaudry M, Labelle H, Rivard M. A modified Risser grading system predicts the curve acceleration phase of female adolescent idiopathic scoliosis. J Bone Joint Surg Am. 2010;92:1073–81.
9. Lusini M, Donzelli S, Minnella S, Zaina F, Negrini S. Brace treatment is effective in idiopathic scoliosis over 45°: an observational prospective cohort controlled study. Spine J. 2010;14(9):1951–6.
10. Brox JI, Lange JE, Gunderson RB, Steen H. Good brace compliance reduced curve progression and surgical rates in patients with idiopathic scoliosis. Eur Spine J. 2012;21:1957–63.
11. Aulisa GO, Giordano M, Falciglia F, et al. Correlation between compliance and brace treatment in juvenile and adolescent idiopathic scoliosis: SOSORT 2014 award winner. Scoliosis. 2014;9:6.
12. Courvoisier A, Drevelle X, Vialle R, Dubousset J, Skalli W. 3D analysis of brace treatment in idiopathic scoliosis. Eur Spine J. 2013;22:2449–55.
13. Labelle H, Dansereau J, Bellefleur C, Poitras B. Three-dimensional effect of the Boston brace on the thoracic spine and rib cage. Spine. 1996;21:59–64.
14. Schmitz A, Kandyba J, Koenig R, Jaeger UE, Gieseke J, Schmitt O. A new method of MR total spine imaging for showing the brace effect in scoliosis. J Orthop Sci. 2001;6:316–9.
15. Sangole AP, Aubin CE, Labelle H, Stokes IA, Lenke LG, Jackson R, Newton P. Three-dimensional classification of thoracic scoliotic curves. Spine. 2009;34:91–9.
16. Wong MS. A comparison of treatment effectiveness between the CAD/CAM method and the manual method for managing adolescent idiopathic scoliosis. Prosthet Orthot Int. 2005;29(1):105–11.
17. Wong MS. Computer-aided design and computer-aided manufacture (CAD/CAM) system for construction of spinal orthosis for patients with adolescent idiopathic scoliosis. Physiother Theory Pract. 2011;27(1):74–9.
18. Gignac D, Aubin CE, Dansereau J, Labelle H. Optimization method for 3D bracing correction of scoliosis using a finite element model. Eur Spine J. 2000;9:185–90.
19. Wynarsky GT, Schultz AB. Optimization of skeletal configuration: studies of scoliosis correction biomechanics. J Biomech. 1991;24(8):721–32.
20. Perie D, Aubin CE, Lacroix M, Lafon Y, Labelle H. Biomechanical modelling of orthotic treatment of the scoliotic spine including a detailed representation of the brace-torso interface. Med Biol Eng Comput. 2004;42:339–44.
21. Perie D, Aubin CE, Petit Y, Labelle H, Dansereau J. Personalized biomechanical simulations of orthotic treatment in idiopathic scoliosis. Clin Biomech. 2004;19:190–5.
22. Clin J, Aubin CE, Labelle H. Virtual prototyping of a brace design for the correction of scoliotic deformities. Med Biol Eng Comput. 2007;45:467–73.
23. Clin J, Aubin CE, Parent S, Labelle H. Biomechanical modeling of brace treatment of scoliosis: effects of gravitational loads. Med Biol Eng Comput. 2011;49:743–53.
24. Desbiens-Blais F, Clin J, Parent S, Labelle H, Aubin CE. New brace design combining CAD/CAM and biomechanical simulation for the treatment of adolescent idiopathic scoliosis. Clin Biomech. 2012;27:999–1005.
25. Cobetto N, Aubin CE, Clin J, Le May S, Desbiens-Blais F, Labelle H, Parent S. Braces optimized with computer-assisted design and simulations are lighter, comfortable and more efficient than plaster-casted braces for the treatment of adolescent idiopathic scoliosis. Spine Deformity. 2014;2(4):276–84.

26. Cobetto N, Aubin CE, Parent S, Clin J, Barchi S, Tirgeon I, Labelle H. Effectiveness of braces designed using computer aided design and manufacturing (CAD/CAM) and finite element simulation compared to CAD/CAM only for the conservative treatment of adolescent idiopathic scoliosis: a prospective randomized controlled trial. Eur Spine J. 2016 [Epub ahead of print].

27. Richards BS, Bernstein RM, D'Amato CR, Thompson GH. Standardization of criteria for adolescent idiopathic scoliosis brace studies: SRS Committee on Bracing and Nonoperative Management. Spine. 2005;30(18):2068–75.

28. Humbert L, De Guise JA, Aubert B, Godbout B, Skalli W. 3D reconstruction of the spine from bi-planar x-rays using parametric models based on transversal and longitudinal inferences. Med Eng Phys. 2009;31:681–7.

29. Sangole A, Aubin CE, Labelle H, Stokes AF, Lenke L, Jackson R, Newton P. Three-dimensional classification of thoracic scoliotic curves. Spine. 2008;34:91–9.

30. Pomero V, Mitton D, Laporte S, de Guise JA, Skalli W. Fast accurate stereoradiographic 3D-reconstruction of the spine using a combined geometric and statistic model. Clin Biomech. 2004;19(3):240–7.

31. Pazos V, Cheriet F, Dansereau J, Ronsky J, Zernicke RF, Labelle H. Reliability of trunk shape measurements based on 3-D surface reconstructions. Eur Spine J. 2007;16:1882–91.

32. Raux S, Kohler R, Garin C, Cunin V, Abelin-Genevois K. Tridimensional trunk surface acquisition for brace manufacturing in idiopathic scoliosis. Eur Spine J. 2014;4:S419–23.

33. Clin J, Aubin CE, Parent S, Labelle H. A biomechanical study of the Charleston brace for the treatment of scoliosis. Spine (Phila Pa 1976). 2010;35(19):E940–7.

34. Aubin C, Descrimes JL, Dansereau J, et al. Geometrical modeling of the spine and the thorax for the biomechanical analysis of scoliotic deformities using the finite element method. Ann Chir. 1995;49:749–61.

35. Aubin CE, Dansereau J, de Guise JA, Labelle H. A study of biomechanical coupling between spine and rib cage in the treatment by orthosis of scoliosis. Ann Chir. 1996;50:641–50.

36. Howard A, Wright JG, Hedden D. A comparative study of TLSO, Charleston and Milwaukee braces for idiopathic scoliosis. Spine. 1998;23:2404–11.

37. Aubin CE, Dansereau J, de Guise JA, Labelle H. Rib cage-spine coupling patterns involved in brace treatment of adolescent idiopathic scoliosis. Spine. 1996;22:629–35.

38. Zhang M, Mak A. In vivo friction properties of human skin. Prosthetics Orthot Int. 1999;23:135–41.

39. Nault ML, Mac-Thiong JM, Roy-Beaudy M, Turgeon I, Deguise J, Labelle H, Parent S. Three-dimensional spinal morphology can differentiate between progressive and non-progressive patients with adolescent idiopathic scoliosis at the initial presentation: a prospective study. Spine. 2014;39:E601–6.

40. Al-Aubaidi Z, Shin EJ, Howard A, Zeller R. Three dimensional analysis of brace biomechanical efficacy for patients with AIS. Eur Spine J. 2013;22(11):2445–8.

17

Torsion bottle, a very simple, reliable, and cheap tool for a basic scoliosis screening

Michele Romano* (ID) and Matteo Mastrantonio

Abstract

Background: One of the reasons that make scoliosis a disease that scares so much the parents is its specific characteristic of being difficult to detect on its onset.

The aim of this paper is to check the possible usefulness of a simple tool (the torsion bottle) that has been developed with the aim to offer an instrument for home use by parents but also for screening purposes in the low-income countries.

Methods: Study design: retrospective analysis to evaluate intra-operator reliability of the tools and inter-operator repeatability using the torsion bottle.

For the first and the second part of the study, 35 subjects were measured.

The goal of the first experiment was to evaluate the reliability of the torsion bottle to identify all individuals who experienced a thoracic or lumbar prominence equal or greater than 7°.

The secondary aim was to verify the reliability of blinded inter-operator assessments, performed with the torsion bottle by two physiotherapists on the same patients.

Results: The reliability of the assessments of the torsion bottle has been performed with the Kappa statistic to evaluate the measurement agreement.

The results have shown that the intra-operator reliability of the tool is very high between the measurements collected with the scoliometer® and those collected with the torsion bottle (kappa = 0.9278; standard error = 0.7094).

The data of the second part of the study show that the inter-operator reliability is good (kappa = 0.7988; standard error 0.1368).

Conclusion: The collected data showed that the torsion bottle revealed itself as an efficient tool to execute a basic screening to identify the presence of a prominence in a significant group of adolescents.

Keywords: Prominence, Scoliometer®, Measurement

Background

One of the reasons that make scoliosis a disease that scares so much the parents is its specific characteristic of being difficult to detect on its onset.

Too often, it is possible to recognize the appearance of the spinal curves when the disease is already severe.

The reason is due to the typical, slow, and insidious debut of the symptoms.

Being able to identify early the first signs of misalignment of the spine is one of the most effective treatment keys.

Obviously, a frequent monitoring of the clinical signs of scoliosis is the simplest solution [1–3].

One of the most important clinical signs of this disease is the prominence [4]. The presence of the prominence is internationally recognized as an indisputable element of the pathology [5–7].

For the prominence assessment, a scoliometer® is usually used [8, 9].

The scoliometer® is a professional tool used in the medical field by physicians and physical therapists.

Obviously, in a domestic field, the scoliometer® is not available.

For this reason, a very simple tool called torsion bottle, cheap and easy to create, has been developed.

The aim of this paper is to check the possible usefulness of this simple tool (the torsion bottle) that has been

* Correspondence: michele.romano@isico.it
ISICO (Italian Scientific Spine Institute), Via Bellarmino 13/1, Milan, Italy

developed with the aim to offer an instrument for home use by parents but also for screening purposes in the low-income countries.

Methods

Study design: retrospective analysis to evaluate intra-operator reliability of the tool and inter-operator repeatability.

The study was divided into two parts. The main aim was to compare the measurements collected with the torsion bottle and the same measurements collected with the scoliometer® (gold standard) in a population of patients accessing our clinic for the rehabilitation treatment, measured according to our standard evaluation protocol.

The secondary aim was to verify the reliability of blinded inter-operator assessments, performed with the torsion bottle by two physiotherapists on the same patients. These double-blinded measurements were taken periodically for a short time interval in our clinic to verify measurement accuracy in the everyday clinical activities.

The tool

The torsion bottle is composed of a plastic water bottle of 500 ml.

The perfect accuracy of the amount of water to be used is not an essential element. On the outer surface of the bottle, it will be marked with a series of four landmarks that will be essential for its use. These landmarks will be marked only after the bottle is partially emptied and carefully closed.

These landmarks will be adjusted only to the particular amount of water contained in that bottle. In any case, it is recommended to fill approximately half of the bottle.

The torsion bottle is used in a horizontal position as a scoliometer®.

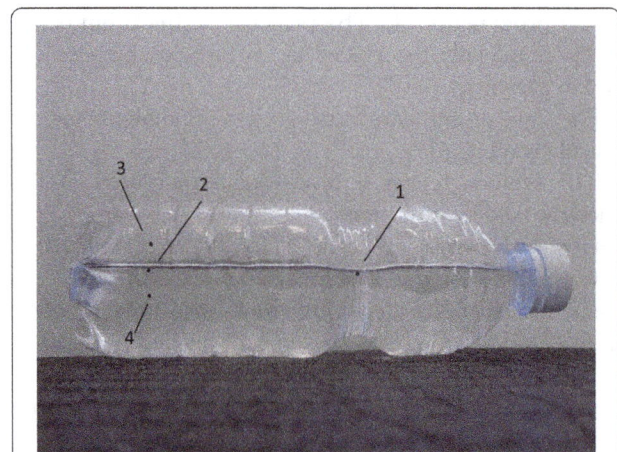

Fig. 2 The distances (in mm) between the landmarks

The rationale of the preparation of the torsion bottle is the variation of the position of the little quantity of water inside the bottle, when the bottle is tilted.

The essential reference signs are:

– Landmarks 1 and 2 which should coincide with the water surface.
– Landmark 3 is the limit of the 7° of the bottle's tilt, and it represents the cutoff to identify the subjects with a prominence less, equal, or greater than this value (Fig. 1).
– Landmark 2 is marked at a distance of 80 mm with respect to landmark 1.
– Landmark 3 is marked 10 mm from the landmark 2 in the orthogonal direction (Fig. 2).

How to use the torsion bottle

How to use the torsion bottle is as follows:

– Forward bending of the patient's trunk to perform an Adam test [10].
– The torsion bottle positioned crosswise on the patient's back with the landmark 1 positioned over

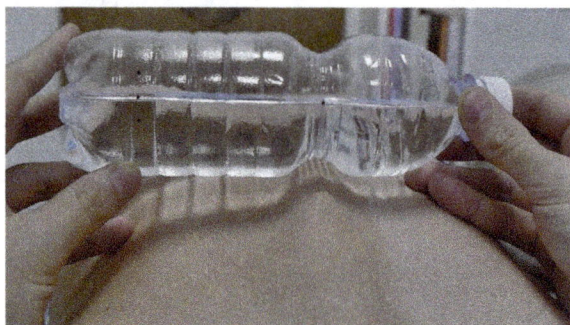

Fig. 1 The four landmarks marked on the torsion bottle

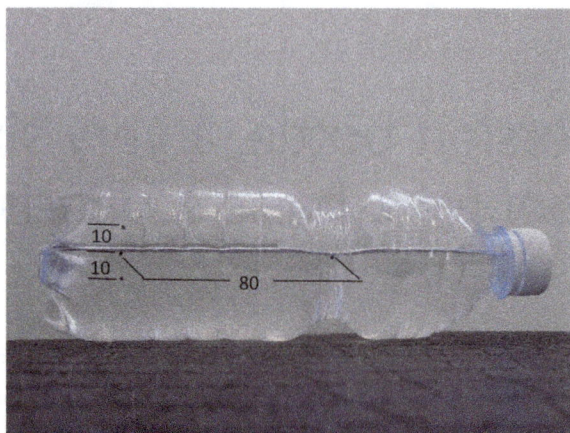

Fig. 3 Use of the torsion bottle. Positioning of the tool

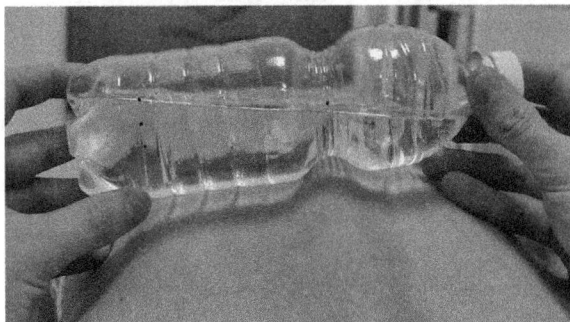

Fig. 4 Tilt of the torsion bottle toward the concavity of the curve

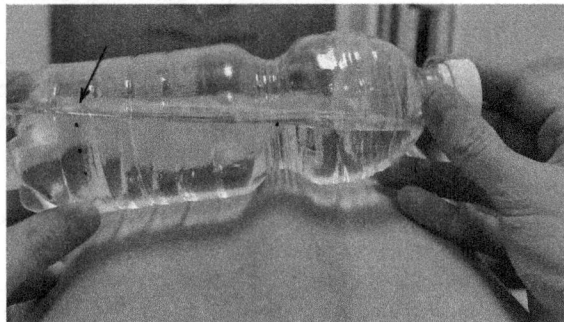

Fig. 6 Check of the position of the water surface respect the landmark number 3

the line of bony prominences and the water surface coinciding with landmarks 1 and 2 (Fig. 3).

- Tilt the bottle until it touches the patient's back (Fig. 4).
- Rotate the bottle until the surface of the water coincides with the position of landmark 1 (Fig. 5).
- Observe the position of the surface of the water with respect to landmarks 3 or 4 (Fig. 6).

Instructions for the preparation and the use of the torsion bottle

https://drive.google.com/file/d/0B2u_ASmUxo0_bj-BiQ0ptTUl5M3M/view?ts=57d16f0e.

The water surface slope, with respect to the reference point, corresponds precisely to 7125°.

The following table shows the variability linked to the potential errors in the mark of the reference points (Table 1).

For the first part of the study, 35 subjects were measured. This group included consecutive adolescents of both genders who attend a specialized clinic for the conservative treatment of scoliosis to perform their medical examinations.

The goal of the experiment was to evaluate the reliability of the torsion bottle to identify all individuals who experienced a prominence equal or greater than 7°.

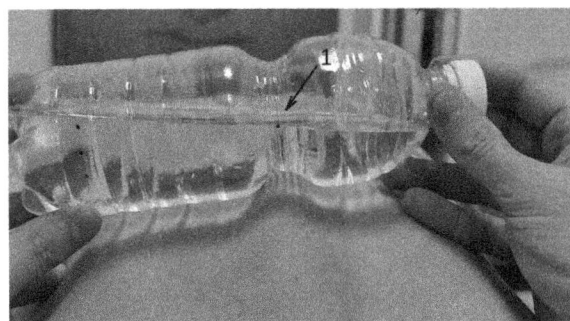

Fig. 5 Rotation of the torsion bottle and realignment of the water surface with the landmark number 1

The presence of a prominence higher than 7° is considered a clinical sign very likely linked to a scoliosis that requires a medical treatment [1].

The assessment was performed by the same evaluator.

The evaluator asked the patient to bend the trunk forwards to perform an Adam test.

As a first action, he performed the measurement with the torsion bottle, and in a second time, the

Table 1 Distances between reference points and relative degrees

Dots 1-2 (cm)	Dots 2-3 (cm)	Degree
8	1	7,125
8	0,7	5,001
8	0,8	5,711
8	0,9	6,419
7,9	0,7	5,064
7,9	0,8	5,782
7,9	0,9	6,499
7,8	0,7	5,128
7,8	0,8	5,856
7,8	0,9	6,582
7,7	0,7	5,194
7,7	0,8	5,932
7,7	0,9	6,667
8,1	0,7	4,939
8,1	0,8	5,641
8,1	0,9	6,340
8,2	0,7	4,879
8,2	0,8	5,572
8,2	0,9	6,263
8,3	0,7	4,821
8,3	0,8	5,505
8,3	0,9	6,189
8	1,2	8,531

measurement with the scoliometer® precisely performed on the same point of the trunk.

For the second part of the study, the assessors measured the prominences of 35 consecutive patients who attended the same clinic for a session of conservative treatment based on Physioterapic Scoliosis Specific Exercises (PSSE).

Measurements were collected blinded by two physiotherapists and processed by a third operator.

The first assessor performed the first evaluation.

The evaluator asked the patient to bend the trunk forwards to perform an Adam test.

The assessor used the torsion bottle to measure the prominence.

The evaluator made a small sign at the back where the measurement had been taken, to enable the second prominence assessment on the same spot (Fig. 7).

The subject was accompanied to another room to carry out a second evaluation performed by the second evaluator.

The data collected in two different files have been handed over to a third operator who performed the comparison and the statistical tests.

Results

The following table shows the detail of the measurements taken for the first part of the study (Table 2):

Column 1: gender of the subject
Column 2: the result of the measurement performed with the torsion bottle and the positive or negative hypothesis of the presence of a prominence equal to or greater than 7°
Column 3: the measurement of the angle trunk rotation performed with the scoliometer®

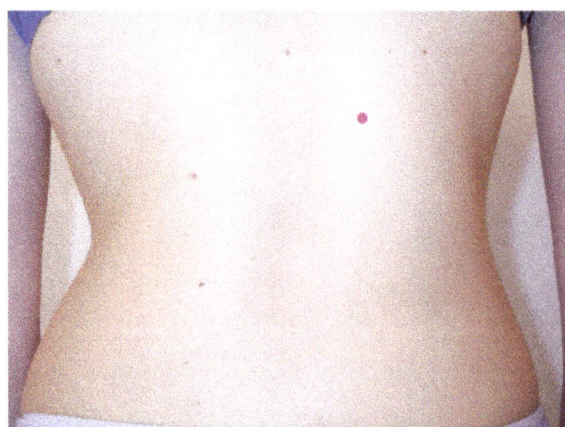

Fig. 7 Landmark on the prominence to made the measure on the same point

Column 4: the agreement of the measurement performed with the torsion bottle and the scoliometer®

Table 3 shows the details of the measurements of the second part of the study:

Column 1: gender of the subject

Table 2 Concordance between Torsion Bottle and Scoliometer assessments

Gender	Torsion Bottle Assessment	Scoliometer Assessment	Concordance
Female	Positive	13	YES
Female	Positive	8	YES
Female	Positive	11	YES
Female	Positive	7	YES
Female	Negative	5	YES
Female	Positive	10	YES
Female	Positive	10	YES
Female	Positive	7	YES
Male	Negative	3	YES
Female	Positive	8	YES
Female	Positive	8	YES
Female	Positive	7	YES
Female	Positive	11	YES
Female	Positive	8	YES
Female	Negative	3	YES
Female	Negative	8	NO
Female	Positive	7	YES
Female	Positive	9	YES
Male	Positive	12	YES
Male	Positive	9	YES
Female	Positive	8	YES
Female	Positive	8	YES
Female	Positive	8	YES
Female	Negative	4	YES
Female	Positive	7	YES
Female	Positive	10	YES
Female	Negative	5	YES
Female	Positive	10	YES
Female	Negative	5	YES
Male	Negative	6	YES
Female	Negative	6	YES
Female	Positive	8	YES
Female	Positive	7	YES
Female	Negative	5	YES
Female	Positive	11	YES

Table 3 Agreement between Torsion Bottle assessment performed by blinded assessors

Gender	Assessor 1	Assessorr 2
Female	Positive	Positive
Female	Positive	Positive
Female	Positive	Positive
Female	Positive	Positive
Female	Positive	Positive
Female	Negative	Negative
Female	Positive	Positive
Male	Positive	Positive
Female	Positive	Positive
Female	Positive	Positive
Female	Positive	Positive
Male	Negative	Negative
Male	Positive	Positive
Male	Positive	Negative
Female	Positive	Positive
Female	Positive	Positive
Female	Positive	Positive
Female	Positive	Positive
Female	Positive	Positive
Female	Negative	Negative
Female	Positive	Positive
Female	Positive	Positive
Female	Positive	Positive
Female	Positive	Positive
Female	Positive	Positive
Female	Positive	Positive
Male	Negative	Negative
Female	Positive	Positive
Female	Positive	Positive
Female	Positive	Positive
Female	Negative	Positive
Female	Positive	Positive
Female	Negative	Negative
Female	Positive	Positive

Column 2: results of the first assessor
Column 3: results of the second assessor

The reliability of the assessments of the torsion bottle has been performed with the Kappa statistic to evaluate the measurement agreement.

The results have shown that the intra-operator reliability of the tool is very high between the measurements collected with the scoliometer® and those collected with the torsion bottle (kappa = 0.9278; standard error = 0.7094).

The data of the second part of the study show that the inter-operator reliability is good (kappa = 0.7988; standard error 0.1368).

Discussion

The collected data showed that the torsion bottle revealed itself as an efficient tool to execute a basic screening to identify the presence of a prominence in a significant group of adolescents.

The basic scoliosis screening is a very simple process but is not performed regularly because, in many countries, the health policy of this disease is based on the concept of "wait and see." Unfortunately, this does not help in prevention but too often leads to surgical intervention, when the severity of the disease is serious.

This torsion bottle has not been conceived for a professional use because the torsion bottle does not quantify the degree of the prominence, unlike the scoliometer®.

It is considered more useful for a domestic use after having trained the parents. This makes it possible to achieve greater awareness and more frequent monitoring in situations of young patients at risk of evolution.

Conclusion

The torsion bottle is useful to perform a pre-investigation of the presence of a prominence, permitting a simplified assessment of its value thus directing to a specialist for a medical assessment.

Another use of the torsion bottle may be provided for screening to be carried out in countries where due to the low-income problems it is difficult to find a scoliometer® or where the presence of health professionals is not so widely distributed.

The water plastic bottles do not have the same shape in all countries. In some countries, it is typical to find this small bottle with a hollow in the upper part (Fig. 1).

This hollow is useful because it avoids a contact with the bony prominences of the spinous processes. When such a tool is not available and it is necessary to use a bottle with a straight profile, it is important to pay attention to the spinous processes to avoid that the contact with the bottle falses the measurement.

Acknowledgements
Not applicable

Funding
No funding was received.

Authors' contributions
MR performed the paper design and wrote and revised the manuscript. He is the author of the pictures. MM revised the manuscript. Both authors read and approved the final manuscript.

Competing interests
Michele Romano is the stockholder of ISICO (Italian Scoliosis Spine Institute). The other author declares that he has no competing interests.

References
1. Negrini S, et al. 2011 SOSORT guidelines: orthopaedic and rehabilitation treatment of idiopathic scoliosis during growth. Scoliosis. 2012;7:3. https://doi.org/10.1186/1748-7161-7-3.
2. Weiss H, et al. Indications for conservative management of scoliosis (guidelines). Scoliosis. 2006;1(1):5.
3. Negrini S, et al. Italian guidelines on rehabilitation treatment of adolescents with scoliosis or other spinal deformities. Eura Medicophys. 2005;41(2):183–201.
4. Zaina F, et al. Clinical evaluation of scoliosis during growth: description and reliability. Stud Health Technol Inform. 2008;135:125–38.
5. Parent EC, et al. Identifying the best surface topography parameters for detecting idiopathic scoliosis curve progression. Stud Health Technol Inform. 2010;158:78–82.
6. Aulisa AG, et al. Correlation between hump dimensions and curve severity in idiopathic scoliosis before and after conservative treatment Spine (Phila Pa 1976). 2018;43(2):114-119.
7. Ferraro C, et al. Hump height in idiopathic scoliosis measured using a humpmeter in growing subjects: relationship between the hump height and the Cobb angle and the effect of age on the hump height. Eur J Phys Rehabil Med. 2017;53(3):377-389.
8. Amendt LE, et al. Validity and reliability testing of the Scoliometer®. Phys Ther. 1990;70(2):108–17.
9. Murrell GA, et al. An assessment of the reliability of the Scoliometer®. Spine (Phila Pa 1976). 1993;18(6):709–12.
10. Côté P, Kreitz B, Cassidy JD, Dzus AK, Martel J. A study of the diagnostic accuracy and reliability of the scoliometer® and Adam's forward bend test. Spine 1998; 1;23(7):796-802.

18

A retrospective analysis of health-related quality of life in adolescent idiopathic scoliosis children treated by anterior instrumentation and fusion

Balaji Zacharia *(ID), Dhiyaneswaran Subramaniyam and Sadiqueali Padinharepeediyekkal

Abstract

Background: Idiopathic scoliosis is the most common type of spinal deformity. Scoliosis is defined as a lateral curvature of the spine greater than 10° accompanied by rotation of the vertebrae. The treatment available for adolescent idiopathic scoliosis is observation, orthosis, and surgery. The surgical options include open anterior release and instrumentation, posterior instrumentation, and thoracoscopic approaches. The Scoliosis Research Society Questionnaire (SRS-30) is a specific instrument to measure health-related quality of life in patients with scoliosis, who had or had not undergone surgery. The purpose was to assess the post-operative functional outcome using SRS-30 in children who underwent anterior release, instrumentation, and fusion using autogenous rib graft for adolescent idiopathic scoliosis (AIS).

Methods: In a retrospective cohort study, 25 patients between the ages of 11 and 17 years, who underwent anterior release, instrumentation, and fusion using autogenous rib graft for adolescent idiopathic scoliosis (AIS) between 2008 and 2014, were included in the study.

Results: The total average score was 4.26 with a SD of 0.014 and had maximum average score 4.5 (for pain) and minimum average score 3.8 (for self-image).

Conclusion: Anterior release, instrumentation, and fusion using autogenous rib graft is having good functional outcome in all domains.

Keywords: Health-related quality of life, Adolescent idiopathic scoliosis, Anterior instrumentation and fusion, SRS-30

Background

Idiopathic scoliosis is the most common type of spinal deformity attended by orthopedic surgeons [1]. Scoliosis is defined as a lateral curvature of the spine greater than 10° accompanied by rotation of vertebrae [2].The prevalence of radiographic curve measuring up to 10° ranges from 1.5 to 3% and that of the curve exceeding 10° is from 0.3 to 0.5%. The prevalence of the curve exceeding 30° is 0.2 to 0.3% [3]. For curves less than 10°, there is an equal prevalence in both sexes, but the higher the degree of curves, the more is the prevalence in females [4, 5]. The etiology of idiopathic scoliosis remains unknown. There are many proposed etiological factors like genetic and neurological disorders, hormonal and metabolic dysfunction, and biomechanical and environmental factors [6].

In structural scoliosis, the vertebral body is rotated towards the convex side of the curve, so the spinous process is rotated towards the concave side of the curve. The asymmetric deformities seen within the vertebral bodies of scoliosis differ significantly from its normal counterpart. The compressive and the distractive force acting on the growing spine produces wedging of the vertebrae. The rotation of the vertebrae produces a hypokyphotic or lordotic curvature of the spine in the sagittal plane. This three-dimensional deformity is better termed as the torsion of the spine and is maximum at

* Correspondence: balaji.zacharia@gmail.com
Department of Orthopedics, Government Medical College, Kozhikode, Kerala 673008, India

the apex of the curve [7–9]. The aorta is usually positioned more laterally and posteriorly in idiopathic adolescent scoliosis [10]. Thoracic cavity is asymmetrical in shape with increased capacity on the concave side and decreased on the convex side. There will be rib prominence on the convex side-rib hump, and breast on the concave side will be more prominent.

There is no definite definition regarding curve progression in the literature but an increase of more than 5–6° over 6 months is considered to be an indicator of progression by most of the studies. Factors such as family history of scoliosis, patient's height to weight ratio, thoracic kyphosis, lumbosacral transition anomaly, spinal balance, and lumbar lordosis are having high predictive value for curve progression in skeletally immature patients [11–13].

Curves less than 40° at maturity may progress to an average of 9° during adulthood and curves more than 40° progress to an average of 20° [14]. Adolescent idiopathic curve does not produce long-term pulmonary functional abnormalities, even though it can produce some restrictive disease. But untreated infantile and juvenile curves and severely lordotic thoracic curves of high degree can result in pulmonary problems [15]. In about 32% of AIS, back pain is reported with increased incidence towards maturity. There is no association between the degree of curvature and back pain [16].

There are different systems to classify scoliosis like Ponseti and Fredman classification, King Classification, and Lenke classification. Lenke is the most recent and commonly used classification system. There are three steps involved in this classification system: identification of the primary curve, assignment of the lumbar modifier, and assignment of the thoracic sagittal modifier [17–19].

The treatment options available for adolescent idiopathic scoliosis are observation, non-surgical intervention, and surgical intervention. In general, no treatment is needed for curves less than 25° regardless of the patient maturity, but follow-up examinations are necessary at regular intervals. Bracing is recommended for skeletally immature patients having curves between 25° and 45° [20, 21]. Numerous authors have challenged the effectiveness of bracing for AIS [22, 23]. The BRAIST study found that bracing significantly reduces the progression of high-risk curve to the threshold for surgery [24].

In skeletally immature patients in whom the curve reaches 40° to 50°, or skeletally mature patients with curves greater than 50°, surgery is a reasonable option [6]. The primary aim of surgical intervention is to reduce the magnitude of the deformity and to obtain solid fusion for prevention of further progression of curve. It results in a well-balanced spine in which head, shoulders, and trunk are centered over the pelvis. Open posterior instrumentation and fusion, open anterior instrumentation and fusion, and thoracoscopic techniques are used for achieving solid arthrodesis and obtaining a balanced three-dimensional correction of the spine. The primary concern of posterior instrumentation in very young patients is the occurrence of crankshaft phenomenon [25]. The risk of crankshaft phenomenon with modern posterior pedicle screw instrumentation has been very minimal in the recent years [26]. Therefore, the anterior surgery for prevention of crankshaft has got limited role in recent years.

The correction and stabilization for scoliosis through anterior approach is introduced by Dwyer in 1964 [27]. Later several modifications of the Dwyer system were done like the Zidelke system (1970), TSRH system (1980), dual-rod dual-screw technique (1990), and L plate system (2006). The advantages of anterior correction include fewer number of fusion levels, excellent correction of deformity, maintaining dorsal kyphosis, implants not prominent under the skin, and preventing crankshaft phenomenon. There is a cosmetic advantage of having smaller scar compared to the posterior approach. However, its limitations are reduction of segmental lumbar lordosis and substantial pseudarthrosis [28]. The indications for anterior fixation are single structural thoracic or thoracolumbar curve (Lenke types I and V), curves less than 70°, and severe thoracic hypokyphosis. It is contraindicated in patients with pulmonary compromise, severe intra-thoracic scarring, small patient size, and severe osteopenia.

Patient-reported health-related quality of life (HRQOL) outcome questionnaires have gained popularity as the method to objectively assess baseline pathology and to measure the effectiveness of an intervention [29]. The Scoliosis Research Society Questionnaire (SRS-30) is a specific instrument to measure health-related quality of life in patients with scoliosis who had undergone surgery or had not [30]. The SRS-30 is well-known as a standard assessment tool to evaluate patients' quality of life across five domains: function/activity, pain, self-image/appearance, mental health, and satisfaction with management [31]. It was Haher [32] who initiated the development of the disease-specific HRQOL instrument SRS-24,consisting of 24 items, to measure many aspects of spinal deformity. Later in 2000, Asher et al. merged similar domains and the new questionnaire SRS-23 was formed [33]. In 2006, Asher et al. again refined the questionnaire to address the diminishing of internal consistency for the function domain in adolescent idiopathic scoliosis [34]. Various versions, scoring instruction, and detailed bibliography of the development of the SRS-HRQOL can be found on the scoliosis research society website www.srs.org [29].

We have conducted a retrospective cohort study to assess the functional outcome of adolescent idiopathic scoliosis (Lenke types I and V) patients treated by anterior release, instrumentation, and fusion using autogenous rib graft.

Methods

After obtaining institutional research committee and ethics committee approval of Government Medical College Kozhikode [Ref no: GMCKKD/RP 2014/IEC/34/03 dtd 17 March 2014], we conducted a retrospective cohort study in a consecutive series of children with adolescent idiopathic scoliosis who underwent anterior release, instrumentation, and fusion using autogenous rib graft in the orthopedic department of our institution. The primary indication for surgery was cosmetic correction of the deformity. There were no cases with back pain. All patients included in the study were concerned about the physical appearance of the back and that was the main indication for surgery. They were included after obtaining the written informed consent from the parents. There were 30 patients who underwent surgical treatment during the period from August 2008 to December 2014. Out of the 30 patients, one patient expired due to unrelated problem and we lost follow-up of four patients. The remaining 25 patients included in the study were having either type I or type V curve after obtaining informed consent from their parents. No children with thoracic insufficiency syndrome was included in our study, and those who underwent posterior procedure were excluded.

All surgery were done under general anesthesia, and preoperative prophylactic antibiotics were given. The patients were positioned laterally with convex side up and thoracotomy/thoracolumbar approach was used. Exposure was completed by removing the rib of one level above the most proximal instrumented vertebrae. After exposing the vertebrae, the anterior release was done by removing disc material and endplate. Correction was done by derotating the apical vertebrae and fixation using pedicle screw and rod instrumentation. Fusion was aided with the help of autogenous rib graft. The whole procedure was done under motor-evoked potential surveillance. Suture removal was done on the 14th day, and patients were discharged with thoracolumbosacral orthosis, which they wore till complete fusion, that was achieved in 9 months.

The age of patients at the time of final evaluation was between 11 and 17 years. SRS-30 was used to measure the patient outcome at the time of the final follow-up. It was divided into five domains according to question type—pain, function /activity, self-image/appearance, mental health, and satisfaction with management. All questions had scores from 1 to 5. The mean score of each domain was used for analysis. The best score is 5 and the worst score is 1.

Results

Our study included 17 girls and 8 boys (Fig. 1). Average duration of follow-up was 4 years and 4 months with SD of 2 years and 3 months [4.3 ± 2.25] (Table 1). There

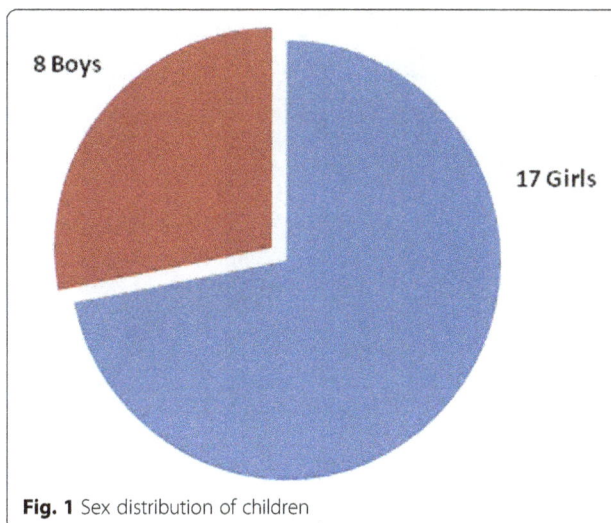

Fig. 1 Sex distribution of children

were 13 children with a pre-operative Cobb angle between 45° and 50°, 9 patients with an angle 50°–60°, 2 patients with an angle between 60° and 65°, and 1 patient with a Cobb angle of above 70° (72°). Post operatively, 21 patients were having a Cobb angle of less than 20° and remaining patients had between 20° and 25°. Out of the five domains of SRS-30, we got maximum average score 4.5 for pain domain and minimum 3.8 for self-image/appearance. For functional activity domain, average score was 4.3. The average scores for mental health and satisfaction with management were 4.4 and 4.3 respectively (Fig. 2). The total average score was 4.26 with a SD of 0.014 (Table 2).

Discussion

In this study, we retrospectively analyzed functional outcome of 25 patients with adolescent idiopathic scoliosis, who underwent anterior release, instrumentation, and fusion using autogenous rib graft. All the surgeries were done by a single surgeon. We got grade 1 fusion in 84% of the cases, grade 2 in 12% of the cases, and grade 3 in 4% of the cases, using Newton et al. grading system for spinal fusion [35]. No case of pseudarthrosis or instrumentation failure was detected in our study. Currently,

Table 1 Case follow-up

Year of surgery	Number of cases	Duration in years at final follow-up after surgery
2008	4	7
2009	3	6
2010	4	5
2011	3	4
2012	4	3
2013	4	2
2014	3	1

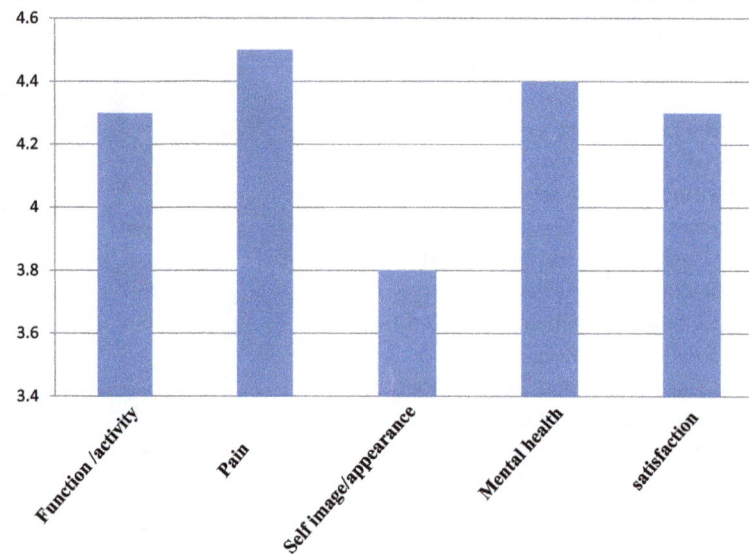

Fig. 2 Average SRS-30 score in each domain

there is an increasing awareness among orthopedic surgeons for evaluating functional over the radiological outcome. There are three types of outcome measures used in orthopedic surgery generic, disease-specific, and anatomy- or joint-specific outcome measures. These outcome measures must have appropriate content for relevant disease or process, reproducibility of results, and responsiveness which is sufficient to detect clinically important change and ease of use for clinicians and patients [36]. In 2013, Sudo et al. conducted a study on the long-term outcome of anterior correction of scoliosis. Their average total SRS score was 4.2 [37]. A study by Sweet et al. in 2001 came to the conclusion that anterior instrumentation and fusion for AIS using a single solid rod has good radiological and clinical outcomes. Poor radiological outcome did not correlate with final Scoliosis Research Society score [38]. Kelly et al. reported an absolute SRS score of 98 of 115 points without much postoperative complication on an average follow-up of 16.97 years [39]. After evaluating the clinical outcome of anterior endoscopic instrumentation for

scoliosis, using SRS-24 showed a significant improvement in pain, self-image, and function in a 2-year follow-up period [40]. In a study by Chan et al., using the results of SRS-22 and SRS-24, to compare the clinical results of various treatment methods, the conclusion was that the values of the scores of these two questionnaires cannot be used interchangeably despite the similarities in the questions and domains [41].

The results of our study cannot be compared with other similar studies conducted to find out HRQL of children with adolescent idiopathic scoliosis treated by using braces and corrective surgeries through anterior or posterior approach because of sociocultural difference among different population. The sociocultural differences will affect the domain of SRS. We have no such similar studies from our population for comparison. This is the first ever attempt to find out HRQL of adolescent idiopathic scoliosis children post-operatively from an Indian subcontinent.

Our study has several limitations. We have conducted this study in a small number of patients. The follow-up of patients varied from 1 to 7 years. We did not have a preoperative patient-based questionnaire, so longitudinal analysis of this measure was not possible.

Table 2 SRS -30 data

Domain	Average score	Standard deviation (SD)	Maximum	Minimum
Function/activity	4.3	0.18	4.6	4.0
Pain	4.5	0.18	4.9	4.3
Self-image/appearance	3.8	0.2	4.2	3.4
Mental health	4.4	0.3	5.0	3.8
Satisfaction with management	4.3	0.3	4.8	3.5
Total	4.26	0.014	4.5	4.0

Conclusion

From our study, using the SRS-30 scoring system in Lenke I and V, we found that anterior release, instrumentation, and fusion using autogenous rib graft is having good functional outcome in all domains: function, pain, self-image, mental health, and satisfaction with management.

Abbreviations
AIS: Adolescent idiopathic scoliosis; HRQOL: Health-related quality of life

Acknowledgements
We are grateful to K I Koshy, Dr. Anu Koshy, and Dr. Ramya Thangavelu for editing this manuscript.

Funding
We have not accepted any financial assistance from within or outside of our institution for collecting data, writing the manuscript, and for its publications.

Authors' contributions
BZ conceived the presented the idea, developed the study design, encouraged SPP to conduct the study by providing him the cases, and also supervised and guided the investigation. DS was assisting and guiding SPP throughout the study. SPP was actively involved in data collection and its analysis and did the statistical work. All the authors equally contributed in the analysis of results and discussion. BZ and DS wrote and revised the manuscript with assistance of SPP. All authors read and approved the final manuscript.

Competing interests
The authors declare that they have no competing interests.

References
1. Lonstein JE. Idiopathic scoliosis. In: Lonstein JE, Bradford DS, Winter RB, Ogilvie J, editors. Moe's textbook of scoliosis and other spinal deformities. 3rd ed. Philadelphia: WB Saunders; 1995. p. 219–56.
2. Brian V. REAMY, LT COL, USAF, MC, Malcolm Grow Medical Center, Andrews Air Force Base, Maryland JOSEPH B. SLAKEY, CDR, MC, USNR, Naval Medical Center, Portsmouth, Virginia Am Fam Physician. Adolescent idiopathic scoliosis: review and current concepts. 2001;64(1):111–7.
3. William C, Warner, Jeffery R, Sawyer, Kelly DM. Scoliosis and kyphosis. Campbell's operative orthopaedics, twelfth edition Chapter 41. 2012. p. 1703–54.
4. Rogala EJ, Drummond DS, Gurr J. Scoliosis: incidence and natural history—a prospective epidemiological study. J Bone Joint Surg Am. 1978;60(2):173–6.
5. Lonstein JE, Bjorklund S, Wanninger MH, et al. Voluntary school screening for scoliosis in Minnesota. J Bone Joint Surg Am. 1982;64(4):481–8.
6. Miyanji F. Adolescent idiopathic scoliosis: current perspectives. Orthopedic Res Rev Dovepress J. 2014;6:17–26.
7. Stephens Richards B, Sucato DJ, Johnston CE. Scoliosis. Tachdjian's paediatric orthopaedics, vol. 1. 5th ed; 2014. p. 206–13. chapter 12
8. Liljenqvist U, Lepsien U, Hackenberg L, et al. Comparative analysis of pedicle screw and hook instrumentation in posterior correction and fusion of idiopathic thoracic scoliosis. Eur Spine J. 2002;11(4):336–43.
9. Liljenqvist UR, Link TM, Halm HF. Morphometric analysis of thoracic and lumbar vertebrae in idiopathic scoliosis. Spine. 2000;25(10):1247–53.
10. Sevastik B, Xiong B, Hedlund R, et al. The position of the aorta in relation to the vertebra in patients with idiopathic thoracic scoliosis. SurgRadiolAnat. 1996;18(1):51–6.
11. Bunnell WP. The natural history of idiopathic scoliosis before skeletal maturity. Spine. 1986;11:773–6. 70
12. Lonstein JE, Carlson JM. The prediction of curve progression in untreated idiopathic scoliosis during growth. J Bone Joint Surg Am. 1984;66:1061–71.
13. Nachemson AL, Peterson LE. Effectiveness of treatment with a brace in girls who have adolescent idiopathic scoliosis. A prospective, controlled study based on data from the brace study of the Scoliosis Research Society. J Bone Joint Surg Am. 1995;77(6):815–22.
14. Ascani E, Bartolozzi P, Logroscino CA, Marchetti PG, Ponte A, Savini R, Travaglini F, Binazzi R, Di Silvestre M. (Phila Pa 1976)Natural history of untreated idiopathic scoliosis after skeletal maturity. Spine. 1986;11(8):784–9.
15. Pehrsson K, Danielsson A, Nachemson A. Pulmonary function in adolescent idiopathic scoliosis: a 25 year follow up after surgery or start of brace treatment. Thorax. 2001;56(5):388–93. https://doi.org/10.1136/thorax.56.5.388.
16. Ramirez N, Johnston CE, Browne RH. The prevalence of back pain in children who have idiopathic scoliosis. J Bone Joint Surg Am. 1997;79(3):364–8.
17. Ponseti IV, Friedman B. Prognosis in idiopathic scoliosis. J Bone Joint Surgery American. 1950;32:381–95.
18. King HA, Moe JH, Bradford DS, Winter RB. The selection of fusion levels in thoracic idiopathic scoliosis. J Bone Joint Surg Am. 1983;65(9):1302–13.
19. Lenke LG, Betz RR, Harms J, et al. Adolescent idiopathic scoliosis: a new classification to determine extent of spinal arthrodesis. J Bone Joint Surg Am. 2001;83(8):1169–81. urg Am. 1997 Mar;79(3):364–8
20. Nachemson AL, Peterson LE. Effectiveness of treatment with a brace in girls who have adolescent idiopathic scoliosis: a prospective, controlled study based on data from the brace study of the Scoliosis Research Society. J Bone Joint Surg Am. 1995;77(6):815–22.
21. Danielsson AJ, Hasserius R, Ohlin A, Nachemson AL. A prospective study of brace treatment versus observation alone in adolescent scoliosis: a follow-up means of 16 years after maturity. Spine (Phila Pa 1976). 2007;32(20):2198–207.
22. Focarile FA, Bonaldi A, Giarolo MA, Ferrari U, Zilioli E, Otta-viani C. Effectiveness of nonsurgical treatment for idiopathic scoliosis: overview of available evidence. Spine (Phila Pa 1976). 1991;16(4):395–401.
23. Goldberg CJ, Moore DP, Fogarty EE, Dowling FE. Adolescent idiopathic scoliosis: the effect of brace treatment on the incidence of surgery. Spine. 2001;26(1):42–7.
24. Weinstein SL, Dolan LA, Wright JG, Dobbs MB. Effects of bracing in adolescents with idiopathic scoliosis. N Engl J Med. 2013;369(16):1512–21.
25. Dubousset J, Herring JA, Shufflebarger H. The crankshaft phenomenon. J PediatrOrthop. 1989;9(5):541–50.
26. Tao F, Zhao Y, Wu Y, et al. The effect of differing spinal fusion instrumentation on the occurrence of postoperative crankshaft 75 phenomenon in adolescent idiopathic scoliosis. J Spinal Disord Tech. 2010; 23(8):e75–80.
27. Dwyer AF. Experience of anterior correction of scoliosis. Clin Orthop. 1973; 93:191–206.
28. Keith H, Bridwell MD. Surgical Treatment of Idiopathic Adolescent Scoliosis; SPINE, vol. 24: Lippincott Williams & Wilkins, Inc; 1999. p. 2607–16. Number 24. https://doi.org/10.1097/00007632-199912150-00008.
29. Baldus C, et al. The Scoliosis Research Society Health-Related Quality Of Life (SRS-30) age–gender normative data an analysis of 1346 adult subjects unaffected by scoliosis. SPINE, vol. 36: Lippincott Williams & Wilkins; 2011. p. 1154–1162©. Number 14. https://doi.org/10.1097/brs.0b013e3181fc8f98.
30. H Yilmaz corresponding author1 and T Kuru2. A comparison of results of SRS-30 questionnaire in scoliosis patients treated surgically or conservatively. Scoliosis. 2012;7(1) https://doi.org/10.1186/1748-7161-7-S1-P15. P15.Published online 2012 Jan27
31. Kin B. et al.HRQoL assessment by SRS-30 for Chinese patients with surgery for Adolescent Idiopathic Scoliosis (AIS). Scoliosis. 2015;10(2) https://doi.org/10.1186/1748-7161-10-S2-S19. S19.Published online 2015 Feb 11
32. Haher T, GorupJ, Shin T, et al. Results of the Scoliosis Research Society instrument for evaluation of surgical outcome in adolescent idiopathic scoliosis. Spine. 1999;24:1435–40.
33. Asher M, Lai S, Burton D. Further development and validation of the Scoliosis Research Society (SRS) outcomes instrument. Spine. 2000;25:2381–6.
34. Asher M, Lai S, Glattes C, et al. Refinement of the SRS-22 health-related quality of life questionnaire function domain. Spine. 2006;31:593–7.
35. Newton PO, White KK, Faro F, Gaynor T. The success of thoracoscopic anterior fusion in a consecutive series of 112 pediatric spinal deformity cases. Spine (Phila Pa 1976). 2005;30(4):392–8.
36. Dodd A1, Osterhoff G1, Guy P1, Lefaivre KA1Assessment of functional outcomes of surgically managed acetabular fractures: a systematic review.Bone Joint J. 2016; 98-B(5):690–695. doi: https://doi.org/10.1302/0301-620X.98B5.36292
37. Sudo H, Ito M, Kaneda K, Shono Y, Abumi K. Long-term outcomes of anterior dual-rod instrumentation for thoracolumbar and lumbar curves in adolescent idiopathic scoliosis a twelve to twenty-three year follow-up study. J Bone Joint Surg Am. 2013;95(8):e49. 1–8

38. Sweet FA, Lenke LG, Bridwell KH, Blanke KM, Whorton J. Prospective radiographic and clinical outcomes and complications of single solid rod instrumented anterior spinal fusion in adolescent idiopathic scoliosis. Spine (Phila Pa 1976). 2001;26(18):1956–65.

39. Kelly DM, McCarthy RE, McCullough FL, Kelly HR. Long-term outcomes of anterior spinal fusion with instrumentation for thoracolumbar and lumbar curves in adolescent idiopathic scoliosis. Spine (Phila Pa 1976). 2010;35(2):194–8.

40. Crawford JR, Izatt MT, Adam CJ, Labrom RD, Askin GN. A prospective assessment of SRS-24 scores after endoscopic anterior instrumentation for scoliosis. Spine (Phila Pa 1976). 2006;31(21):E817–22.

41. Chan CYW, Ortho MS, et al. Comparison of Srs-24 and Srs-22 scores in thirty eight adolescent idiopathic scoliosis patients who had undergone surgical correctional. Malaysian Orthopaedic Journal. 2009;3:56–9. No 1

19

Sagittal plane assessment of spino-pelvic complex in a Central European population with adolescent idiopathic scoliosis

Máté Burkus[1,2]*⦿, Ádám Tibor Schlégl[1], Ian O'Sullivan[1], István Márkus[1], Csaba Vermes[1] and Miklós Tunyogi-Csapó[1]

Abstract

Background: Scoliosis is a complex three-dimensional deformity. While the frontal profile is well understood, increasing attention has turned to balance in the sagittal plane. The present study evaluated changes in sagittal spino-pelvic parameters in a large Hungarian population with adolescent idiopathic scoliosis.

Methods: EOS 2D/3D images of 458 scoliotic and 69 control cases were analyzed. After performing 3D reconstructions, the sagittal parameters were assessed as a whole and by curve type using independent sample t test and linear regression analysis.

Results: Patients with scoliosis had significantly decreased thoracic kyphosis ($p < 0.001$) with values T1–T12, $34.1 \pm 17.1°$ vs. $43.4 \pm 12.7°$ in control; T4–T12, $27.1 \pm 18.8°$ vs. $37.7 \pm 15.1°$ in control; and T5–T12, $24.9 \pm 15.8°$ vs. $32.9 \pm 15.0°$ in control. Changes in thoracic kyphosis correlated with magnitude of the Cobb angle ($p < 0.001$). No significant change was found in lumbar lordosis and the pelvic parameters. After substratification according to the Lenke classification and individually evaluating subgroups, results were similar with a significant decrease in only the thoracic kyphosis. A strong correlation was seen between sacral slope, pelvic incidence, and lumbar lordosis, and between pelvic version and thoracic kyphosis in control and scoliotic groups, whereas pelvic incidence was also seen to be correlated with thoracic kyphosis in scoliosis patients.

Conclusion: Adolescent idiopathic scoliosis patients showed a significant decrease in thoracic kyphosis, and the magnitude of the decrease was directly related to the Cobb angle. Changes in pelvic incidence were minimal but were also significantly correlated with thoracic changes. Changes were similar though not identical to those seen in other Caucasian studies and differed from those in other ethnicities. Scoliotic curves and their effect on pelvic balance must still be regarded as individual to each patient, necessitating individual assessment, although changes perhaps can be predicted by patient ethnicity.

Keywords: EOS 2D/3D, Sagittal alignment, Spino-pelvic parameters, Adolescent idiopathic scoliosis

* Correspondence: burkusmate@gmail.com
[1]Department of Orthopedics, Medical School, University of Pécs, Akác st. 1, Pécs H-7623, Hungary
[2]Department of Traumatology and Hand Surgery, Petz Aladár County Teaching Hospital, Vasvári Pál st. 2-4, Győr H-9023, Hungary

Background

Scoliosis is a rotational deformity of the curvature of the spinal column. Although deformity is most marked in the frontal plane, growing evidence indicates that a detailed sagittal evaluation is necessary in addition to anteroposterior imaging for optimizing treatment planning [1–3].

The sagittal spino-pelvic parameters have been assessed in numerous publications with normal, disease-free populations [4–8] and in spine deformities, including scoliosis [9–11]. While many of these studies found alterations in sagittal alignment in scoliotic patients [9, 10, 12], a notable number reported no significant difference [13].

The dynamic relationship between the sagittal position of the pelvis and the spine is also evident during imaging in spine deformities such as spondylolisthesis and intervertebral disc abnormalities [6, 14, 15]. Changes are seen during growth, too, with all parameters evolving and developing throughout childhood and puberty until their attainment of mature adult values [16–18].

Despite growing agreement on the importance of sagittal alignment in scoliosis treatment, uncertainty exists in the literature about their values in health and in disease. Possible contributing factors are the limitations associated with single-plane image assessment modalities, in addition to inter-individual and even possible inter-ethnic variability [19]. In recent years, studies using the EOS 2D/3D scanner have gained popularity, as the scanner allows improved characterization of complex deformities in three dimensions. The EOS 2D/3D scanner captures standing images with minimal vertical distortion and in combination with its reconstruction software has contributed to our understanding of the biomechanical and anatomical parameters of the spine, pelvis, and lower extremities [18, 20–23].

The current study aims to assess and present data on the sagittal position of the spine and pelvis in a large sample of Central European adolescents and young adults with adolescent idiopathic scoliosis using high accuracy and low radiation EOS imaging and evaluate the relationships within the spino-pelvic complex.

Methods

Our clinic's radiological records were retrospectively examined for the period from 2007 to 2012, and EOS 2D/3D images for 511 AIS patients, defined as Cobb angle > 10°, were found. Patients with any other spinal deformity or those with previous spinal or lower extremity surgical intervention were excluded. Finally, 458 patients (82 male, 376 female) were available, with mean age 16.8 ± 4.7 years, range 12–26 years.

For control, 69 individuals (28 male, 41 female) free from any spinal deformity were randomly collected from our database. EOS 2D/3D scans had been indicated in these individuals due to suspected scoliosis, though this was not found to be present, or for joint pain, which was later found to lack any bone involvement. The mean age was 17.1 ± 4.4 years, range 12–26 years.

All patients or their parents/guardians gave written consent at the time of imaging for future use in clinical research. According to Hungarian regulations for retrospective analysis, further ethical permission was not required.

All images were recorded with the EOS 2D/3D system during routine clinical work, using the standard step-forward position defined by the EOS operating manual (right foot 5–10 cm forward, hands raised to the face with flexed elbows). After scans were collected, 3D reconstruction was performed using the sterEOS software package (v1.3.4.3740, EOS Imaging, Paris, France) (see Fig. 1). During the reconstruction process, an examiner must provide assistance to mark reference points on the images, and so, intra-observer reliability was evaluated to ensure consistency of results. The examiner reviewed 25 randomly selected cases on three separate occasions, and the intraclass correlation coefficient was calculated. Results were assessed as per the Winer criteria in which 0–0.24 is regarded as "weak or absent" reliability, 0.25–0.49 "low," 0.50–0.69 "medium," 0.70–0.89 "high," and 0.90–1.0 "excellent" [24].

The following parameters were evaluated (see Figs. 2 and 3):

- Cobb angle: the angle formed between the superior endplate of the uppermost vertebra of the scoliotic curve and the inferior endplate of the lowest vertebra of the curve;
- T1–T12 kyphosis (kyphosis and lordosis parameters are defined as the angle between the superior endplate of the upper vertebra and inferior endplate surface of the lower vertebra);
- T4–T12, T5–T12 kyphosis;
- L1–L5 and L1–S1 lordosis;
- Pelvic tilt (PT): the angle between a line running from the center of the S1 endplate to the center of the femoral head and the vertical axis (also termed the pelvic version);
- Sacral slope (SS): angle between the S1 endplate and the horizontal axis;
- Pelvic incidence: angle between a perpendicular line through the center of the first sacral vertebral endplate in the sagittal plane and a line passing from the center of the sacral plate to the center of the femoral head.

Patients were also stratified by frontal curve appearance as per the Lenke scoliosis classification [25]. Subgroups and average Cobb angles are shown in Table 1.

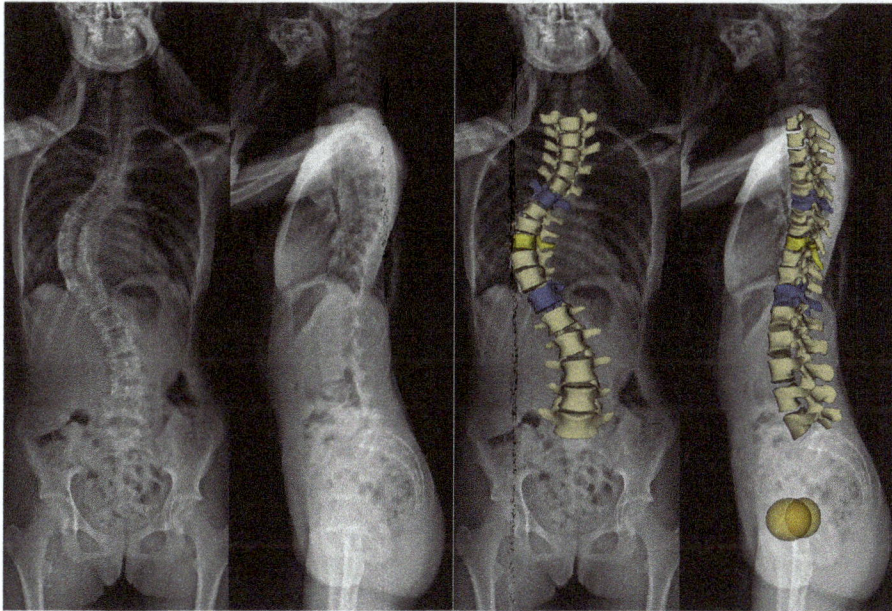

Fig. 1 EOS 3D reconstruction. EOS scan and 3D reconstruction of a 16-year-old female patient with AIS. Cobb angle 67°; Lenke classification, 1AN

For the Lenke subclassification, the central sacral vertical line (CSVL) and sagittal plane curvature of T2–T5 kyphosis, T5–T12 kyphosis, and T10–L2 kyphosis were also evaluated.

The differences between the control and scoliosis groups as a whole, and by each Lenke curve type, were assessed using an independent t test. Linear regression was performed to evaluate the relationship between individual parameters. $p < 0.05$ was considered significant. The normalcy of distribution was assessed by the Kolmogorov–Smirnov test. All statistical analysis of the parameters was done using SPSS v22 (IBM Corp., Armonk, NY, USA) and Microsoft Office Professional Plus v14.0.6112.5000 (Microsoft Corp., Redmond, WA, USA) program packages.

Results

Intra-observer reliabilities for 3D reconstructions were all greater than 0.9, regarded as "excellent." The results of sagittal spine and pelvis evaluations are presented in Table 2, which shows the differences between the scoliosis cohort as a whole and the control group. Significant differences ($p < 0.001$) were seen in the thoracic region, with scoliosis patients exhibiting decreased thoracic curvatures as measured by the following: T1–T12 kyphosis (control, $43.4 \pm 12.7°$ vs. AIS $34.1 \pm 17.1°$), T4–T12 kyphosis (control, $37.7 \pm 15.1°$ vs. AIS, $27.1 \pm 18.8°$), and T5–T12 (control $32.9 \pm 15.0°$ vs. AIS $24.9 \pm 15.8°$). No significant difference was found between the lumbar or pelvic regions of control and scoliosis patients when all

scoliosis patients were averaged together, regardless of curve type (p values ranged from 0.290 to 0.830).

Results when patients were stratified by the Lenke curve morphology are presented in Table 3. Thoracic curvature was decreased across T1–T12, T4–T12, and T5–T12 in all groups from Lenke 1–6 compared to the control. T4–T12 kyphosis was found to be significantly lower, with different Lenke types' mean values ranging from 18.5° to 32.6° compared to 37.7° in the control group. However, in T1–T12 kyphosis and T5–T12 kyphosis, differences were only significant in Lenke 1, 3, 5, and 6 groups (T1–T12, AIS 26.5°–38.8° vs. control 43.4°; T5–T12, 20.1°–27.7° vs. control 32.9°). In Lenke 2 and 4, group values were lowered compared to those of controls but were not significant ($p = 0.060, 0.185$). The lumbar and pelvic parameters again were not found to differ significantly from controls.

Pelvic parameters and main sagittal curvature values were compared using linear regression analysis as seen in Table 4. The values of the lumbar lordosis showed significant correlation with PI ($p = 0.035$) and SS ($p < 0.001$) in control and in AIS ($p < 0.001$). Thoracic kyphosis showed a correlation with PT in both groups (control $p = 0.017$, AIS $p < 0.001$) and with PI in AIS ($p < 0.001$).

Discussion

Adolescent idiopathic scoliosis is one of the most common structural spine deformities in childhood, affecting up to 1–4% of the population [26]. Understanding of the natural history, early identification, and proper

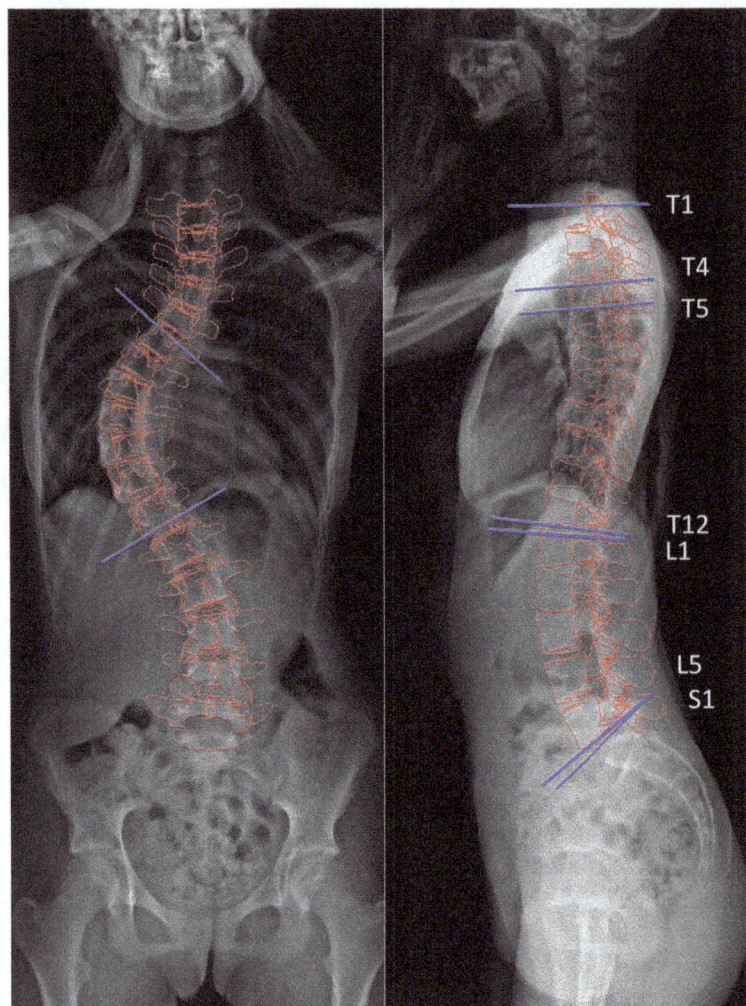

Fig. 2 Measured spine parameters. The left picture shows the line of the superior endplate of the upper vertebra of the scoliotic curve and the line of the inferior end plate of the lower vertebra of the curve; the complementary angle of these lines is the Cobb angle The right picture shows the sagittal parameters. The kyphosis and lordosis parameters are defined as the angle between the superior endplate of the upper vertebra and inferior endplate surface of the lower vertebra

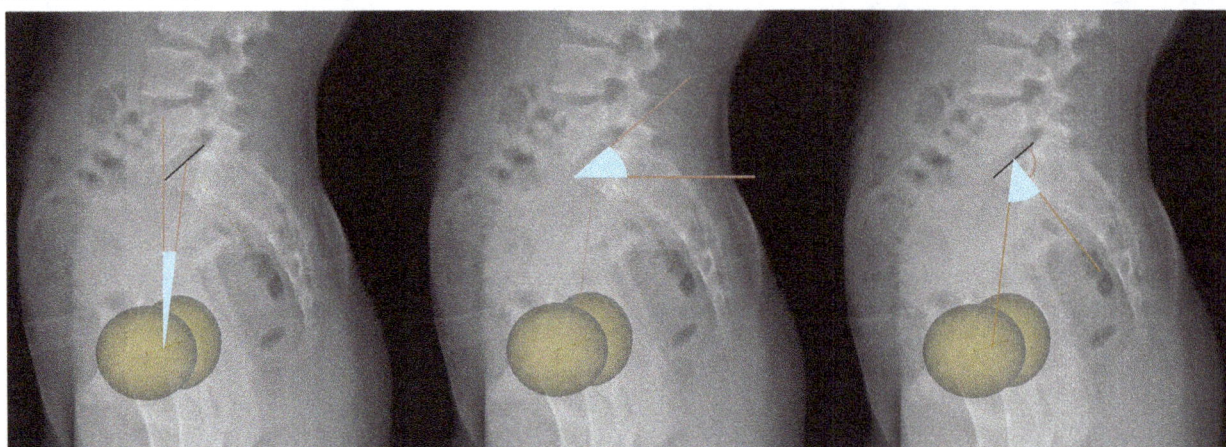

Fig. 3 Measured pelvic parameters. From left to right: pelvic tilt, sacral slope, and pelvic incidence

Table 1 The partition of scoliotic cases based on the Lenke classification and the average Cobb angle values of the subgroups

	n =	L mod			S mod			Cobb angle (°)					
		A	B	C	–	N	+	Prox		MT		TL/L	
								Mean	S.D.	Mean	S.D.	Mean	S.D.
Lenke 1	165	131	28	6	34	108	23	–	–	**36.7**	**20.4**	–	–
Lenke 2	12	6	4	2	3	5	4	**37.3**	**8.8**	**45.5**	**15.5**	–	–
Lenke 3	92	5	30	57	30	55	7	–	–	**57.9**	**22.9**	41.0	15.2
Lenke 4	8	1	3	4	3	3	2	**39.8**	**7.2**	**73.1**	**13.9**	53.9	19.5
Lenke 5	155	–	–	155	9	127	19	–	–	–	–	26.7	13.1
Lenke 6	26	–	–	26	5	20	1	–	–	**41.1**	**13.1**	49.7	14.2
Sum/average	458	143	65	250	84	318	56	**38.4**	**8.5**	**44.8**	**21.0**	34.3	16.5

S.D. standard deviation, Prox proximal curve, MT main thoracic curve, L lumbar curve, TL thoracolumbar curve. In Lenke 1–6, the lumbar modifier (L mod) is based on the lumbar position of the central sacral vertical line (CSVL). The sagittal modifier (S mod) is based on the value of T5–T12 kyphosis
Data in bold are significant values

management may all be aided by high-resolution virtual visualization of the global spino-pelvic complex.

In addition to the changes seen with normal growth [16–18], the sagittal position of the pelvis is known to be altered in spino-pelvic disorders. In spondylolisthesis, for example, the pelvic incidence angle, SS, and lumbar lordosis have been found to be significantly increased, while thoracic kyphosis is decreased [14, 15]. Intervertebral disc pathology on the other hand has been associated with decreased PI values, which leads to reduced lordosis and consequently a "flatter" spine [6, 14]. The changes in scoliosis, however, are not yet clear. Some authors have described significant alterations in pelvic position [9, 10] while others did not find evidence of change [12]. Different authors have examined different ethnicities, using different parameters at various vertebral levels, however.

In the current study, we aimed to evaluate the changes of the sagittal spino-pelvic parameters in adolescent idiopathic scoliosis, in a large population of 458 Central European (Hungarian) Caucasian adolescent and young adult patients using low-distortion EOS 2D/3D reconstructions. We found no significant difference between the sagittal pelvic parameters of those with scoliosis and control individuals, even when divided by the Lenke curve type. These results were similar to those seen by other authors such as Legaye et al. or Yong et al. [12, 27].

We did not see significantly increased pelvic incidence values in scoliosis similar to those reported by Upasani et al. and Mac-Thiong et al. [9, 10]. Although PI was significantly correlated with lumbar lordosis, neither were significantly altered in our scoliosis group. Mac-Thiong et al. and Upasani et al. attributed the changes in PI to be that of a compensatory mechanism, which tries to deepen the lumbar curvature and stabilize the body's global balance. This was especially thought to be true in the case of thoracic curves. Our results did not show a significant change in PI with thoracic curves, but there was a correlation between thoracic kyphosis and pelvic incidence, seen with linear regression analysis, that may still support this theory.

Lumbar sagittal parameters in AIS patients in our study also did not differ statistically from control values, regardless of frontal deformity appearance. This contrasts with Mac-Thiong et al., who saw a decrease of 6.7° between healthy and scoliosis children's mean lordosis values [9, 28], but agreed with Yong et al. and their study of 95 Chinese children with AIS, who found no significant difference [27].

Values for the thoracic kyphosis however showed a large decrease in all groups when measured from T1–T12, T4–T12, and T5–T12, except for the Lenke 2 and Lenke 4 groups. This agrees with the decreased kyphosis seen in the work of Upasani et al. on Lenke curve types

Table 2 Results of the sagittal parameters

	(Degree)	T1–T12 Kyp	T4–T12 Kyp	T5–T12 Kyp[*]	L1–L5 Lord	L1–S1 Lord	PT	PI	SS
Control (n = 69)	Mean	43.4	37.7	32.9	46.0	57.0	7.1	46.2	39.1
	S.D.	12.7	15.1	15.0	9.1	10.4	7.3	8.3	6.7
AIS (n = 458)	Mean	34.1	27.1	24.9	46.4	54.9	7.5	47.3	39.6
	S.D.	17.1	18.8	15.8	13.2	14.8	8.3	12.8	10.3
t test	p	< 0.001	< 0.001	< 0.001	0.830	0.290	0.722	0.564	0.748

S.D. standard deviation, AIS adolescent idiopathic scoliosis, Kyp kyphosis, Lord lordosis, PI pelvic incidence, PT pelvic tilt, SS sacral slope
[*]T5–T12 kyphosis measured manually on sterEOS 2D workstation

Table 3 The partition of sagittal parameters based on the Lenke classification

(Degree)	Control	Lenke 1	C—L1	Lenke 2	C—L2	Lenke 3	C—L3	Lenke 4	C—L4	Lenke 5	C—L5	Lenke 6	C—L6
	$n = 69$	$n = 165$	t test	$n = 12$	t test	$n = 92$	t test	$n = 8$	t test	$n = 155$	t test	$n = 26$	t test
	Mean ± S.D.	Mean ± S.D.	p	Mean ± S.D.	p	Mean ± S.D.	p	Mean ± S.D.	p	Mean ± S.D.	p	Mean ± S.D.	p
T1–T12 Kyp	43.4 ± 12.7	34.0 ± 17.5	< 0.001	36.9 ± 18.3	0.148	28.3 ± 18.1	< 0.001	33.4 ± 19.9	0.060	38.8 ± 14.5	0.039	26.5 ± 16.9	< 0.001
T4–T12 Kyp	37.7 ± 15.1	27.2 ± 20.9	< 0.001	27.7 ± 20.2	0.049	20.4 ± 19.2	< 0.001	23.4 ± 20.0	0.019	32.6 ± 13.8	0.022	18.5 ± 19.6	< 0.001
T5–T12 Kyp	32.9 ± 15.0	25.1 ± 18.3	0.005	26.2 ± 18.8	0.185	21.0 ± 15.9	< 0.001	23.3 ± 16.9	0.102	27.6 ± 12.5	0.012	21.1 ± 11.4	< 0.001
L1–L5 Lord	46.0 ± 9.1	46.8 ± 13.9	0.688	49.4 ± 13.6	0.285	44.5 ± 13.2	0.449	47.5 ± 8.8	0.657	47.1 ± 12.1	0.542	44.6 ± 15.9	0.630
L1–S1 Lord	57.0 ± 10.4	54.5 ± 17.7	0.310	58.3 ± 14.6	0.718	53.0 ± 12.9	0.054	55.6 ± 8.4	0.707	56.4 ± 12.7	0.724	52.9 ± 14.5	0.151
PT	7.1 ± 7.3	7.4 ± 8.0	0.821	5.2 ± 7.8	0.415	8.7 ± 9.9	0.314	6.7 ± 4.5	0.866	7.3 ± 8.1	0.862	7.0 ± 6.7	0.937
PI	46.2 ± 8.3	46.4 ± 11.9	0.934	47.5 ± 13.7	0.690	49.8 ± 14.3	0.095	49.9 ± 3.7	0.227	46.7 ± 13.1	0.822	46.3 ± 11.6	0.913
SS	39.1 ± 6.7	39.0 ± 9.8	0.926	42.3 ± 10.0	0.187	41.1 ± 10.3	0.199	43.2 ± 3.1	0.095	38.9 ± 11.4	0.896	39.5 ± 7.5	0.817

Kyp kyphosis, *Lord* lordosis, *PI* pelvic incidence, *PT* pelvic tilt, *SS* sacral slope, *S.D.* standard deviation. The statistical analysis of Lenke groups is compared to control with independent sample *t* test

1 and 5. Hu et al. and Yong et al. too found decreased thoracic kyphosis in AIS [10, 27, 29].

To our knowledge, we are presenting one of the largest populations of scoliotic individuals with spino-pelvic assessment. However, despite our large sample size, only a few clear trends were observed in our data. Even when divided by Lenke curve type, great variation was present between individuals within each type, such that group mean comparisons did not reveal significant differences in pelvic values. Inter-individual differences in pelvic and spinal parameters are known to exist in normal and scoliosis populations; however, we believe that possible ethnic differences between populations has not been paid sufficient attention. Of the publications produced by other authors that did find significant differences, not only are there distinctly different magnitudes and directions of the pelvic changes in scoliosis, there are marked differences between values for the normal populations (see Table 5). Ethnic differences in sagittal pelvic values we believe have been frequently overlooked, despite numerous publications indicating these differences.

Reports on sagittal alignment in Chinese, Caucasian, and African-American cohorts, for example, have revealed significant differences especially in pelvis orientation. In a study by Zhu et al. of a normal Chinese population, the pelvic incidence was 44.6° (± 11.2°), and in a study by Hu et al. of a scoliotic Chinese population, pelvic incidence was 43.1° (± 10.1) [7, 29]. These values are all lower than those found in Caucasian populations, as reported by Mac-Thiong et al. and Roussouly et al. In their studies in Caucasian populations, the pelvic incidence in normal individuals was much closer to 50°, with values of 49.1° (± 11.0°), 51.9° (± 10.7°), and 52.4° (± 10.8°) (female)–52.7° (± 10.0°) (male) [6, 28, 30]. Caucasian patients with scoliosis had even higher values with mean pelvic incidence of 57.3° (± 10.9°) [9]. Interestingly, in the values reported from the Chinese population, the pelvic incidence was found to fall very slightly in those with scoliosis, in contrast to the notable increase in the Caucasian populations. Furthermore, African-Americans were reported to have higher pelvic incidences than Caucasians in cadaveric specimen and radiological studies, on average 3.5–4.1° higher, although absolute values differed from study to study [13, 31]. To us, this raises questions not only about ethnic diversity in pelvic shape in normal populations, but also about how pelvic compensatory responses to scoliosis-associated imbalances

Table 4 The linear regression analysis

	Control						AIS					
	PI		PT		SS		PI		PT		SS	
	B coef	p	B coef	p	B coef	p	B coef	P	B coef	p	B coef	p
Thoracic kyphosis	− 0.19	0.165	− 0.32	0.017	− 0.11	0.409	− 0.20	< 0.001	− 0.21	< 0.001	0.07	0.142
Lumbar lordosis	0.28	0.035	0.26	0.058	0.63	< 0.001	0.47	< 0.001	− 0.02	0.623	0.57	< 0.001

B coef beta coefficient, *PT* pelvic tilt, *PI* pelvic inclination, *SS* sacral slope, *AIS* adolescent idiopathic scoliosis

Table 5 Table summarizing recent studies of interest of sagittal spino-pelvic position in different ethnicities, in normal and scoliosis populations

	Ethnicity		Type	Subjects	PI	SS	PT	L1–L5 Lord	L1–S1 Lord	Age
Current study	Caucasian		asx	69	46.2 ± 8.3	39.1 ± 6.7	7.1 ± 7.3	46.0 ± 9.1	57.0 ± 10.4	17.1 ± 4.4
			scol	458	47.3 ± 12.8	39.6 ± 10.3	7.5 ± 8.3	46.4 ± 13.2	54.9 ± 14.8	16.8 ± 4.7
Mac-Thiong et al. [28]	Caucasian (N. American)		asx	341	49.1 ± 11.0	41.4 ± 8.2	7.7 ± 8.0	48.0 ± 11.7	x	12.1 ± 3.3
Mac-Thiong et al. [30]	Caucasian (N. American)	F	asx	709	52.4 ± 10.8	39.8 ± 7.9	12.7 ± 7.0	x	x	36.8 ± 14.3
		M			52.7 ± 10.0	39.3 ± 8.0	13.4 ± 6.7			
Roussouly et al. [6]	Caucasian		asx	160	51.9 ± 10.7	39.9 ± 8.2	12.0 ± 6.5	x	61.4 ± 9.7	27 †
Mac-Thiong et al. [8]	Caucasian		scol	160	57.3 ± 13.8	47.8 ± 9.3	9.5 ± 8.7	41.3 ± 10.9	x	13.5 ± 2.0
Lonner et al. [13]	Caucasian		scol	421	52.5 †	42.2 †	10.8 †	x	59.1 †	14.8 †
	African American		scol	115	56.0 †	42.5 †	13.9 †	x	63.6 †	15.0 †
Zárate-K et al. [32]	Mexican		asx	202	56.7 ± 13.4	40.9 ± 10.6	15.8 ± 13.4		60.2 †	46.5 †
Bakouny et al. [33]	Lebanese		asx	92	52.0 ± 11.3	41.2 ± 7.9	10.8 ± 7.0	x	61.6 ± 9.2	21.5 ± 2.2
Yong et al. [27]	Chinese		asx	33	44.6 ± 11.5	33.3 ± 8.2	11.3 ± 10.8	x	49.3 ± 9.9	13.7 †
			scol	95	44.2 ± 10.0	35.1 ± 7.9	9.2 ± 8.5	x	48.5 ± 11.2	14.1 †
Zhu et al. [7]	Chinese		asx	260	44.6 ± 11.2	32.5 ± 6.5	11.2 ± 7.8	x	48.2 ± 9.6	34.3 ± 12.6
Hu et al. [29]	Chinese		scol	184	43.1 ± 10.1	37.5 ± 8.8	5.5 ± 6.9	x	55.8 ± 12.2	15.5 ± 3.3

F female, *M* male, *S.D.* standard deviation, *PT* pelvic tilt, *PI* pelvic inclination, *SS* sacral slope, *Lord* lordosis. Studies were included if they contained data on PI, SS, PV, and lumbar and thoracic curvatures
†Standard deviation information could be found in this paper

may differ due to different pelvic shapes. It must be noted, however, that marked differences between individuals were present too, though the mean group values clearly differ.

We present the data from these 458 AIS patients as a representative sample of a Caucasian Central European population, as this is the largest published radiological spino-pelvic assessment study, to our knowledge.

Recent literature has indicated that for effective treatment and planning, emphasis must be put on the correct evaluation and treatment of the sagittal condition of the spine and pelvis [3]. However, as can be seen by our results and those of other recent studies, uncertainty and controversy still exist over the assessment and definition of the normal values of the spino-pelvic complex. Due to inter-individual differences and possible ethnic differences, we still cannot confidently predict sagittal deformity from frontal images nor predict the sagittal effect of different curve types on other regions of the spine. As a result, individual assessments must be performed on all patients to ensure optimal treatment outcomes.

The main limitations of our study are the relatively low number of individuals in the control group (69 individuals) and the lower patient numbers for Lenke groups 2, 4, and 6, which may have led to a higher likelihood of observing significant differences in these cases. It must also be noted that the step-forward position with raised hands may affect the position of the pelvis and the spine. For this reason, a consistent and strict positioning

protocol was applied in this study in an attempt to keep this potential effect to a minimum.

Conclusions

This study presents the sagittal profile of 458 children with AIS, from a Central European Caucasian population, as assessed by full-body biplanar X-ray scanner. Adolescent idiopathic scoliosis in our population was connected to a significant decrease in thoracic kyphosis but did not show a significant change in pelvic alignment. This study indicates that the spino-pelvic unit sagittal alignment is not uniform. In both healthy individuals and those with spinal disorders such as scoliosis, distinct differences can be shown in different ethnic groups, in addition to inter-individual differences. In spinal deformities, the sagittal appearance cannot be deduced from frontal curvature images, and so, in all cases, an individual, personalized sagittal assessment is recommended.

Abbreviations
2D: Two dimensional; 3D: Three dimensional; AIS: Adolescent idiopathic scoliosis; B coef: Beta coefficient; CSVL: Central sacral vertical line; Kyp: Kyphosis; L mod: Lumbar modifier; L: Lumbar; Lord: Lordosis; MT: Main thoracic curve; PI: Pelvic incidence; Prox: Proximal curve; PT: Pelvic tilt; S mod: Sagittal modifier; S.D.: Standard deviation; SS: Sacral slope; TL: Thoracolumbar curve

Acknowledgements
The present scientific contribution is dedicated to the 650th anniversary of the foundation of the University of Pécs, Hungary.

Funding
The present study was partly supported by the GINOP-2.3.3-15-2016-00031 grant of the Hungarian Government.

Authors' contributions
MB participated in the investigation, study design, manuscript preparation, and submission of the statistical analysis. ATS, IOS, and IM participated in data analysis and manuscript preparation. CSV and MTCS participated in the conception coordination and design of the study and took part in the manuscript preparation. All authors read and approved the final manuscript.

Competing interests
The authors declare that they have no competing interests.

References

1. Berthonnaud E, Dimnet J, Roussouly P, Labelle H. Analysis of the sagittal balance of the spine and pelvis using shape and orientation parameters. J Spinal Disord Tech. 2005;18:40–7.
2. Roussouly P, Pinheiro-Franco JL. Sagittal parameters of the spine: biomechanical approach. Eur Spine J. 2011;20(Suppl 5):578–85.
3. Roussouly P, Nnadi C. Sagittal plane deformity: an overview of interpretation and management. Eur Spine J. 2010;19:1824–36.
4. Boulay C, Tardieu C, Hecquet J, Benaim C, Mouilleseaux B, Marty C, et al. Sagittal alignment of spine and pelvis regulated by pelvic incidence: standard values and prediction of lordosis. Eur Spine J. 2006;15:415–22.
5. Vialle R, Levassor N, Rillardon L, Templier A, Skalli W, Guigui P. Radiographic analysis of the sagittal alignment and balance of the spine in asymptomatic subjects. J Bone Joint Surg Am. 2005;87:260–7.
6. Roussouly P, Gollogly S, Berthonnaud E, Dimnet J. Classification of the normal variation in the sagittal alignment of the human lumbar spine and pelvis in the standing position. Spine. 2005;30:346–53.
7. Zhu Z, Xu L, Zhu F, Jiang L, Wang Z, Liu Z, et al. Sagittal alignment of spine and pelvis in asymptomatic adults: norms in Chinese populations. Spine. 2014;39:1–6.
8. Kobayashi T, Atsuta Y, Matsuno T, Takeda N. A longitudinal study of congruent sagittal spinal alignment in an adult cohort. Spine. 2004;29:671–6.
9. Mac-Thiong JM, Labelle H, Charlebois M, Huot MP, de Guise JA. Sagittal plane analysis of the spine and pelvis in adolescent idiopathic scoliosis according to the coronal curve type. Spine. 2003;28:1404–9.
10. Upasani VV, Tis J, Bastrom T, Pawelek J, Marks M, Lonner B, et al. Analysis of sagittal alignment in thoracic and thoracolumbar curves in adolescent idiopathic scoliosis: how do these two curve types differ? Spine. 2007;32:1355–9.
11. de Jonge T, Dubousset JF, Illés T. Sagittal plane correction in idiopathic scoliosis. Spine. 2002;27:754–60.
12. Legaye J, Duval-Beaupère G, Hecquet J, Marty C. Pelvic incidence: a fundamental pelvic parameter for three-dimensional regulation of spinal sagittal curves. Eur Spine J. 1998;7:99–103.
13. Lonner BS, Auerbach JD, Sponseller P, Rajadhyaksha AD, Newton PO. Variations in pelvic and other sagittal spinal parameters as a function of race in adolescent idiopathic scoliosis. Spine. 2010;35:374–7.
14. Barrey C, Jund J, Noseda O, Roussouly P. Sagittal balance of the pelvis-spine complex and lumbar degenerative diseases. A comparative study about 85 cases. Eur Spine J. 2007;16:1459–67.
15. Labelle H, Roussouly P, Berthonnaud E, Transfeldt E, O'Brien M, Chopin D, et al. Spondylolisthesis, pelvic incidence, and spinopelvic balance: a correlation study. Spine. 2004;29:2049–54.
16. Mac-Thiong JM, Berthonnaud E, Dimar JR, Betz RR, Labelle H. Sagittal alignment of the spine and pelvis during growth. Spine. 2004;29:1642–7.
17. Mangione P, Gomez D, Senegas J. Study of the course of the incidence angle during growth. Eur Spine J. 1997;6:163–7.
18. Szuper K, Schlégl Á, Leidecker E, Vermes C, Somoskeöy S, Than P. Three-dimensional quantitative analysis of the proximal femur and the pelvis in children and adolescents using an upright biplanar slot-scanning X-ray system. Pediatr Radiol. 2015;45:411–21.
19. Vrtovec T, Janssen MM, Likar B, Castelein RM, Viergever MA, Pernuš F. A review of methods for evaluating the quantitative parameters of sagittal pelvic alignment. Spine J. 2012;12:433–46.
20. Illés T, Somoskeöy S. The EOS™ imaging system and its uses in daily orthopaedic practice. Int Orthop. 2012;36:1325–31.
21. Deschênes S, Charron G, Beaudoin G, Labelle H, Dubois J, Miron MC, et al. Diagnostic imaging of spinal deformities: reducing patients radiation dose with a new slot-scanning X-ray imager. Spine. 2010;35:989–94.
22. Schlégl Á, Szuper K, Somoskeöy S, Than P. Three dimensional radiological imaging of normal lower-limb alignment in children. Int Orthop. 2015;39:2073–80.
23. Schlégl Á, O'Sullivan I, Varga P, Than P, Vermes C. Determination and correlation of lower limb anatomical parameters and bone age during skeletal growth (based on 1005 cases). J Orthop Res. 2017;35:1431–41.
24. Winer BJ. Statistical principles in experimental design. 1st ed. New York: McGraw Hill; 1971. p. 283–93.
25. Lenke LG, Betz RR, Harms J, Bridwell KH, Clements DH, Lowe TG, et al. Adolescent idiopathic scoliosis: a new classification to determine extent of spinal arthrodesis. J Bone Joint Surg Am. 2001;83:1169–81.
26. Cheng JC, Castelein RM, Chu WC, Danielsson AJ, Dobbs MB, Grivas TB, et al. Adolescent idiopathic scoliosis. Nat Rev Dis Primers. 2015;1:15030.
27. Yong Q, Zhen L, Zezhang Z, Bangping Q, Feng Z, Tao W, et al. Comparison of sagittal spinopelvic alignment in Chinese adolescents with and without idiopathic thoracic scoliosis. Spine. 2012;37:714–20.
28. Mac-Thiong JM, Labelle H, Berthonnaud E, Betz RR, Roussouly P. Sagittal spinopelvic balance in normal children and adolescents. Eur Spine J. 2007;16:227–34.
29. Hu P, Yu M, Liu X, Zhu B, Liu Z. Analysis of the relationship between coronal and sagittal deformities in adolescent idiopathic scoliosis. Eur Spine J. 2016;25:409–16.
30. Mac-Thiong JM, Roussouly P, Berthonnaud E, Guigui P. Sagittal parameters of global spinal balance: normative values from a prospective cohort of seven hundred nine Caucasian asymptomatic adults. Spine. 2010;35:1193–8.
31. Weinberg DS, Morris WZ, Gebhart JJ, Liu RW. Pelvic incidence: an anatomic investigation of 880 cadaveric specimens. Eur Spine J 2016;25:3589–3595.
32. Zárate-Kalfópulos B, Romero-Vargas S, Otero-Cámara E, Correa VC, Reyes-Sánchez A. Differences in pelvic parameters among Mexican, Caucasian, and Asian populations. J Neurosurg Spine. 2012;16:516–9.
33. Bakouny Z, Assi A, Yared F, Bizdikian AJ, Otayek J, Nacouzi R, et al. Normative spino-pelvic sagittal alignment of Lebanese asymptomatic adults: comparisons with different ethnicities. Orthop Traumatol Surg Res. 2017.

20

When and how to discontinue bracing treatment in adolescent idiopathic scoliosis: results of a survey

Lucas Piantoni*⊙, Carlos A. Tello, Rodrigo G. Remondino, Ida A. Francheri Wilson, Eduardo Galaretto and Mariano A. Noel

Abstract

Background: Currently, there is little consensus on how or when to discontinue bracing in adolescent idiopathic scoliosis (AIS). An expert spine surgeon national survey could aid in elucidate discontinuation of the brace. Few data have been published on when and how to discontinue bracing treatment in patients with AIS resulting in differences in the management of the condition. The aim of this study was to characterize decision-making of surgeons in the management of bracing discontinuation in AIS.

Methods: An original electronic survey consisting of 12 multiple choice questions was sent to all the members of the National Spine Surgery Society (497 surveyed). Participants were asked about their type of medical practice, years of experience in the field, society memberships, type of brace they usually prescribed, average hours of daily brace wearing they recommended, and how and when they indicated bracing discontinuation as well as the clinical and/or imaging findings this decision was based on. Exclusion criteria include brace discontinued because of having developed a curve that warranted surgical treatment.

Results: Of a total of 497 surgeons, 114 responded the survey (22.9%). 71.9% had more than 5 years of experience in the specialty, and 51% mainly treated pediatric patients. Overall, 95.5% of the surgeons prescribed the thoracolumbosacral orthosis (TLSO), indicated brace wearing for a mean of 20.6 h daily. Regarding bracing discontinuation, indicated gradual brace weaning, a decision 93.9% based on anterior-posterior (AP) and lateral radiographs of the spine and physical examination, considered a Risser ≥ IV and ≥ 24 months post menarche.

Conclusions: The results of this study provide insight in the daily practice of spine surgeons regarding how and when they discontinue bracing in AIS. The decision of bracing discontinuation is based on AP/lateral spinal radiographs and physical examination, Risser ≥ IV, regardless of Tanner stage, and ≥ 24 months post menarche. Gradual weaning is recommended.

Keywords: Adolescent idiopathic scoliosis, Brace, Orthosis, Brace discontinuation, Non-operative scoliosis treatment

Background

When and how to discontinue bracing treatment in patients with idiopathic scoliosis who are reaching skeletal maturity and are not candidates for surgery is a historically complex issue in the management of this deformity on which little has been published. Currently, in the literature, there is little consensus either on when or how the spine surgeon should discontinue the bracing treatment in

patients with adolescent idiopathic scoliosis (AIS), the imaging parameters that should be considered, whether weaning should be gradual and progressive, and based on what studies or clinical signs discontinuation should be determined [1–3].

In the absence of an objective and validated protocol, bracing control and discontinuation as well as clinical care of the patient with AIS are subjected to heterogeneous expert opinions without a standardized criteria resulting in a lack of clarity in the management of the condition. Given these limitations, it would be useful to

* Correspondence: lucaspiantoni@hotmail.com
Servicio de Patología Espinal, Hospital de Pediatría Prof. Dr. Juan P. Garrahan, Combate de los Pozos 1881, C1245AAM CABA Buenos Aires, Argentina

establish a series of guidelines with the aim of improving the quality of life of the patient and reducing the cost and social burden of bracing treatment. A better understanding of bracing management based on an academic consensus of members of the National Spine Society may allow for a protocol on bracing discontinuation in AIS focusing on clinical and imaging findings.

The aim of this study was to characterize the management of bracing in AIS from the National Spine Surgery Society (SAPCV), regarding when and how to discontinue the brace in patients who are reaching skeletal maturity but are not candidates for surgical treatment through an electronic survey sent to all the members of the national society in order to evaluate the possibility of developing consensus-based guidelines.

Methods

An original electronic survey consisting of 12 multiple choice questions was sent to all 497 members of the National Spine Surgery Society (SAPCV) (Table 1). Participants could opt for more than one answer, and if required, an additional response could be added. The demographic and clinical features of the patients that were the subject of this survey were (1) patients with idiopathic scoliosis, (2) between 10 years of age and the time of reaching skeletal maturity (adolescents), and (3) regardless of the type of brace used. Participants were asked not to include patients with curves greater than 50° or candidates for surgery or those who develop thoracic lordosis.

The variables considered in the survey were years of experience in the specialty, membership of national and international societies, and type of practice (adults, pediatrics, deformity, etc.) of the respondent, as well as the type of brace they prescribe in patients with AIS, hours of daily brace wearing recommended, and the clinical and imaging findings on which their decision to discontinue bracing treatment is based.

The survey was designed and administered using the online platform surveymonkey.com (Survey Monkey, CA, USA), and the survey was sent through an invitation by e-mail after written approval from the National Spine Society. No incentives were offered for participating in the survey.

Results

Of a total of 497 spine surgeons who were contacted by e-mail, 114 responded the survey, with a response rate of 22.9%. Of the surveyed population, 10.2% were doing a post-residency second fellowship, 18.6% had less than 5 years of experience, and 72.9% had more than 5 years of experience in spine surgery at the moment of the survey.

Overall, 100% of the surveyed population stated to be a member of the National Spine Surgery Society (SAPCV), 81.2% of the National Orthopaedic Surgery

Table 1 Survey on when and how to discontinue bracing treatment in adolescent idiopathic scoliosis

Association (AAOT), 13.3% of the National Pediatric Orthopaedic Surgery Society (SAOTI), and 11.2% of the Scoliosis Research Society (SRS). Seventy-five percent of the surgeons stated to work mainly with adult patients, 50% with children, 47.3% specialized in deformity, 34.8% in trauma, and 20.5% in tumors. Within pediatric deformity, 75.5% of the respondents stated to have more than 5 years of experience in the field.

Overall, 95.5% of the surveyed population prescribed the thoracolumbosacral (TLSO) brace, 13.4% the Milwaukee brace, and 8% the Boston brace. When asked how many hours they recommended the patients to wear the brace, 67.1% stated to prescribe brace wearing for more than 20 h daily, 26.7% for an average of 18 h, 5.3% for an average of 14 h, and 0.9% for less than 12 h daily. Of the surgeons working in pediatric practice, 94.6% indicated wearing of the TLSO brace for an average of 20.6 h daily, without significant differences between those who had more and those who had less than 5 years of experience in the field.

Furthermore, 93.5% of the surgeons stated that, regardless of the type of brace, they discontinue bracing treatment gradually or progressively. Of those mainly working with pediatric patients, 98.2% recommend gradual discontinuation of the brace. Of the surgeons with less than 5 years of experience in the field 98.2% and of those with more than 5 years of experience 90.1% recommend gradual brace weaning from the brace.

A 39% of the respondents recommend their patients to discontinue brace wearing without a fixed time schedule and quantity of hours, until the following control visit; 31% recommend discontinuation by reducing time of brace wearing to only night time bracing until the following visit; 28% indicate their patients to reduce the time of brace wearing by 25% until the following visit; and 6% indicate the patient to reduce the time of brace wearing by 50% until the following visit. Of the surgeons working with pediatric patients, 34.8% indicate their patients to reduce bracing according to their convenience (without a fixed time schedule and quantity of hours) until the following control visit, 30.4% recommend brace wearing only at night time, 28.3% indicate to reduce brace wearing by 25% and 6.5% by 50% until the following visit. Of those with less than 5 years of experience, 54% recommend only night time brace wearing and of those with more than 5 years of experience 34.2% recommend to reduce brace wearing to night time only and 34.2% recommend their patients to discontinue brace wearing according to their own convenience until the following visit.

Regarding clinical and imaging findings on which discontinuation was based, 90.6% of the surveyed population based their decision on posterior-anterior and lateral radiographs, 85.5% on radiographs and clinical findings, and 35.3% on clinical findings only. Of the surgeons who work in pediatric practice, 93.9% based their decision to discontinue bracing treatment on a combination of radiographs and clinical examination. Of the surgeons with less than 5 years of experience in the field, 66.7% based their decision of brace discontinuation on anterior-posterior and lateral radiographs and of those with more than 5 years of experience on both anterior-posterior and lateral radiographs and physical examination.

When evaluating the role of clinical findings in the decision-making on bracing treatment discontinuation, 97.2% of the surveyed population considered the Risser sign, 43.9% menarche, 14.9% the tri irradiate cartilage, and 12.1% Tanner stage, among others, to be important signs. When breaking up these data, 58.8% use a Risser sign ≥ IV. Overall, 70.4% stated they indicated discontinuation of the orthosis regardless of Tanner stage, regardless of menarche 35.2% and 28.4% ≥ 24 months post menarche.

Among surgeons working in pediatric practice, 93.3% recommend brace discontinuation at a Risser ≥ IV, 63.6% regardless of Tanner stage, and 36.5% at 18 months post menarche. Of the surgeons with less than 5 years of experience, 93.6% recommended bracing discontinuation at Risser sign ≥ IV, 42.8% regardless of Tanner stage, 50% ≥18 months post menarche, while of those with more than 5 years of experience, 98.8% recommend discontinuation at Risser ≥ IV, 69.2% regardless of Tanner stage, and 48.8% ≥ 24 months post menarche.

The results of the survey were analyzed, and a final list of recommendations was established (Table 2).

Discussion

To our knowledge, currently there is little consensus in the literature on how and when to discontinue bracing treatment in AIS [2, 3]. In one of the few studies published in the literature, Andersen et al. administered a questionnaire to 136 patients with AIS who underwent bracing treatment and found that daily activities and social contacts were affected during treatment and follow-up. They concluded that brace weaning should be started as early as possible and not later than 36 months post menarche in girls [3].

Table 2 Study variables on which the highest degree of consensus was reached (%) in pediatric spine surgeons

Gradual weaning from the brace	98.2%
AP/L radiographs + physical exam	93.9%
Risser ≥ IV	93.3%
Risser + menarche	87.5%
Use of the brace > 20 h/day	68.7%
Regardless of Tanner stage	63.6%
Weaning (x hours for x time)	54.1%
Brace discontinuation according to menarche > 24 months	48.8%

In another interesting and well-known published paper, Negrini et al. among the SOSORT Society made recommendations about the weaning brace issue in the 2016 SOSORT Guidelines. The stated that "It is recommended that braces are worn until the end of vertebral growth and then the wearing time is gradually reduced…" and the second recommendation was…"It is recommended that the wearing time of the brace is gradually reduced while performing exercises…" [4]. We believe that these treatment guidelines should be taken into account when performing or conducting any spine deformity non-surgical basic study. Take into consideration that there is no straight age correlation about stature growth and bone mass density in published literature. Any kind of aerobic or anaerobic exercises are recommended during brace treatment.

This electronic survey was conducted with the aim to characterize the management of bracing discontinuation among members of the National Spine Society. They were asked for their expert opinion on this issue in an attempt to develop guidelines regarding brace weaning in patients with AIS with a special focus on the variables listed in Table 2.

The opinions of the surgeons, however, cannot be generalized as they develop their activities in different areas within the field of spine surgery. Additionally, it would be difficult to determine whether this expert opinion may modify the decision-making of spine surgeons regarding brace discontinuation in these patients.

One of the weaknesses of our study is the limited number of variables evaluated in the survey as other findings that were not mentioned may have to be included in working guidelines for bracing discontinuation. An additional limitation may be that the surveyed population consisted of spine surgeons from a single country with a relatively low response rate (22.9%). Another weakness of the study is that participants were not asked how much time apart they scheduled control visits and on what parameters they based this decision. Nevertheless, one of the strengths of the study is the large population surveyed—a total of 114 surgeons responded—and the fairly homogeneous nature of their responses. Another strength of the study is that all the members of the National Spine Surgery Society were included, of whom a considerable percentage felt compelled to answer the survey in spite of not specializing in pediatric deformity. The methodology of an electronic survey allowed us to reach all the members of the NSSS while ensuring anonymity and thereby avoiding of bias. The electronic modality of the survey facilitated fast and reliable data collection. It should be taken into account that this methodology provides an overview of expert opinion rather than validated scientific evidence.

Currently, there is no standardized strategy to determine in this extremely crucial matter of how and when to discontinue bracing in AIS and a standardized protocol and algorithm should be developed.

Future validation studies would be necessary to define whether the inclusion of the variables evaluated in this survey are useful in the daily practice of spine surgeons treating patients with AIS, including a larger number of participants with involvement international societies. Clinical and imaging variables are important in the decision-making on bracing discontinuation in AIS. The indication and management of bracing discontinuation should be based on continuous interaction between the opinion of surgeon and the needs and objectives of the patient.

Conclusion

Based on the survey, the main variables considered in the management of bracing discontinuation in AIS were gradual brace weaning, AP-L radiographs together with physical examination, Risser status $\geq$ IV, regardless of Tanner stage, $\geq$ 24 months post menarche, and a weaning method (x hours for x time).

The results of the study help to shed a light on the decision-making in the management of non-surgical treatment of children with AIS by the spine surgeon, which may be useful when outlining consensus-based working guidelines for the management and discontinuation of bracing in patients with AIS.

Authors' contributions
CAT and MN contributed to the design of the study. IAFW contributed to the references. LP, ESB, and CAT recruited the surgeons. LP, IAFW, and MN participated in the drafting of the manuscript. LP carried out questionnaires through surveymonkey.com. IADFW, CAT, ESB, RR, and MN revised the manuscript. All authors read and approved the final manuscript.

Competing interests
The authors declare that they have no competing interests.

References
1. Weinstein SL, Dolan LA, Wright JG, et al. Effects of bracing in adolescents with idiopathic scoliosis. N Engl J Med. 2013;369(16):1512–21.
2. Steen H, Lange JE, Brox JI. Early weaning in idiopathic scoliosis. Scoliosis. 2015;10:32.
3. Andersen MO, Andersen GR, Thomsen K, et al. Early weaning might reduce the psychological strain of Boston bracing: a study of 136 patients with adolescent idiopathic scoliosis at 3.5 years after termination of brace treatment. J Pediatr Orthop B. 2002;11:96–9.
4. Negrini S, Donzelli S, Aulisa AG, et al. 2016 SOSORT guidelines: orthopaedic and rehabilitation treatment of idiopathic scoliosis during growth. Scoliosis Spinal Disord. 2018;13:3. https://doi.org/10.1186/s13013-017-0145-8.

21

Factors influencing adherence to an app-based exercise program in adolescents with painful hyperkyphosis

Karina A. Zapata[1]* (iD), Sharon S. Wang-Price[2], Tina S. Fletcher[3] and Charles E. Johnston[4]

Abstract

Background: Software applications (apps) could potentially promote exercise adherence. However, it is unclear whether adolescents with painful hyperkyphosis will use an app designed for a home exercise program. The purpose of this study is to assess factors regarding adherence to an app-based home exercise program in adolescents with hyperkyphosis and back pain who were provided a one-time exercise treatment.

Methods: Twenty-one participants were instructed in a one-time exercise treatment and asked to complete a home exercise program 3 times a week for 6 months using an app called PT PAL. At a 6-month follow-up, 14 participants completed a survey assessing factors related to their experiences using the app and their treatment engagement.

Results: Although most participants did not use the app, they reported performing their exercises a few times per week. The adolescent participants considered the app to be more of a barrier than a supportive measure for promoting exercise adherence. Most participants still reported bothersome back pain.

Conclusions: Although adherence to the 6-month app-based home exercise program was not successful, adolescents still viewed technology support such as text reminders as a potential solution.

Background

Adolescents with hyperkyphosis have decreased quality-of-life (QOL), particularly the self-image and appearance components [1, 2]. Hyperkyphosis is also associated with back pain in long-term follow-up studies [3, 4]. The standard medical management for kyphosis includes observation with or without exercises, bracing, and surgery. In North America, utilization of physical therapy (PT) for kyphosis varies by institution, and the optimal treatment is controversial. Although PT exercises designed to improve pain and posture are generally recommended for hyperkyphosis, the evidence for the effectiveness of these exercises is very limited [5, 6].

Exercise adherence is problematic in the rehabilitation of adolescents with back pain [7–9]. Numerous factors influence adherence to an exercise program such as personal characteristics, treatment and disease variables, and the patient-to-physical therapist interaction [7, 10].

Specifically, personal characteristics related to patients' behaviors, including enjoyment of the activity, social support, and self-motivation could have a profound impact on exercise adherence [7, 10]. Of these personal characteristics, motivation can be influenced by a patient's self-esteem or perceived competence [7]. Treatment variables, such as the complexity of exercises, may also be factors [10]. Additionally, chronic illnesses and pain experiences are examples of disease variables that can influence exercise adherence [10]. Lastly, exercise adherence factors related to the patient-to-physical therapist interaction include patients' need for more feedback, specifically positive feedback [7, 10].

Software applications (apps) have the potential to play an important role in promoting exercise adherence. Apps can monitor patients remotely, are cheap, can provide reminders, and can enable feedback to patients. Although apps are widely used by adolescents, app-based exercise programs have not been incorporated in rehabilitation for adolescents with musculoskeletal

* Correspondence: karina.zapata@tsrh.org
[1]Therapy Services, Texas Scottish Rite Hospital for Children, 2222 Welborn Street, Dallas, TX 75219, USA
Full list of author information is available at the end of the article

disorders [11]. In addition, a systematic review showed limited evidence regarding the effectiveness of using apps to increase physical activity in adolescents [8]. Furthermore, apps aimed at increasing physical activity in adolescents were not effective [12]. Although app-based exercise programs can provide objective information regarding exercise adherence, it is unclear whether adolescents with painful hyperkyphosis will use an app designed for a home exercise program (HEP). Therefore, the purpose of this study was to assess factors regarding adherence to an app-based exercise program in adolescents with hyperkyphosis and back pain after one-time exercise treatment followed by a 6-month app-based HEP.

Methods
Participants
This study was a prospective pre-post study design. This study was approved by the Institutional Review Board of the primary investigator's affiliated institute and registered with ClinicalTrials.gov. Participants were recruited from a tertiary facility that holds specialty clinics, including spine deformity, and is staffed by a multidisciplinary team including physical therapists. Prior to data collection, each adolescent participant's assent and caregiver's consent to participate in the study were obtained. Eligible participants were adolescents with hyperkyphosis, including Scheuermann's kyphosis, and met the following inclusion criteria: ages 10 to 18 years, Cobb angles at least 50°, and pain > 2 on the numeric pain rating scale (NPRS) during the past week. Participants' pain intensity was evaluated according to the NPRS on a scale of 0 (no pain) to 10 (worst imaginable pain) [13]. Exclusion criteria included scoliosis greater than 25° Cobb angle, conditions preventing understanding and compliance with an exercise schedule, current brace wear, previous spine surgery, and inability to commit to at least 15 min of exercises for 3 days a week for 6 months.

Once eligibility was determined, each participant was asked to complete the Scoliosis Research Society-22 Health-Related Quality-of-Life Questionnaire (SRS-22r) to evaluate participants' QOL. The SRS-22r includes five domains: pain, self-image/appearance, function/activity, mental health, and management satisfaction. Higher scores indicate better scoliosis-related QOL. The SRS-22r is reliable and valid in adolescent idiopathic scoliosis (AIS) [14]. Although it has not been validated for assessing adolescent patients with hyperkyphosis, it is considered well suited [1, 2]. Participants were also asked about their physical activity level, which was defined as the number of hours of organized physical activity per week.

Next, a physical therapist instructed each participant in PT exercise treatment targeting spinal stabilization. The standard PT practice at the investigators' facility is to provide one-time exercise instruction on the same day that patients are seen by the orthopedic surgeon.

Patients also typically prefer this treatment model, as it is less burdensome and more cost-effective, especially because many patients live at least an hour from our facility and come from low socioeconomic backgrounds, thus having difficulty returning for PT on a regular basis. Participants were instructed to perform each exercise for 100 s based on a previous work [9]. Instructions included performing a total of 5 exercises targeting the trunk and core for at least 3 days a week for 6 months. Participants were also asked to refrain from slouching while sitting throughout the day.

In addition, each participant was given access to a software app called Pt Pal (Los Angeles, CA) on their smart phone or tablet. Pt Pal uses a cloud-based platform which sends patients (children or adults) their exercises and exercise prescriptions digitally. The physical therapist can use a web portal to add participants and enter their exercises independently, and the participants can access their prescribed exercises from the app on their phone or tablet. After participants log in to the app, they see their prescribed exercises by image and exercise name. Exercise pictures are in black-and-white. To perform an exercise, they click on the respective exercise, which shows the same picture and written instructions on how to perform the exercise. The prescribed amount of time counts down similar to an interval timer. During the time of this study, Pt Pal did not have the ability to send reminders to participants to do their exercises and to allow participants to give feedback. In addition, exercises adherence was defined by examining each participant's app and averaging the percentage of exercise sessions completed out of 78 sessions (3 sessions per week for 6 months).

Participants were asked to use the app whenever they performed their exercises throughout the 6-month period. The principal investigator (PI), a physical therapist, had administrative access to the app to monitor exercise adherence. Each participant was contacted and instructed to use the app within 2 weeks after study initiation in an attempt to maximize exercise adherence. During this follow-up contact, the PI answered questions regarding their exercises or app use if there was any. In addition, participants were instructed to contact the PI when they had additional questions regarding their exercises or the app. However, most participants still did not use the app. Consequently, the effectiveness of the app on exercise adherence was unable to be assessed. In order to understand the adolescent participants' lack of interest in using the app for their HEP, the investigators developed a survey to obtain information about these participants' experiences using the app and performing the exercises.

Instrumentation: survey
The PI administered a 19-item survey to all participants either in person at a 6-month follow-up or over the phone if they did not return for follow-up. The PI read

Kids have had trouble sticking with our exercise app. We are trying to figure out why. Will you help us by circling an answer to each question? You won't get into trouble or hurt our feelings for being honest with us. We won't let anyone else see your answers. You may receive a follow-up call later. Thanks for your help!

1. My back pain bothers me...	Not true at all	Mostly not true	No opinion	Kind of true	Really true
2. I used the app...	Never	Monthly	Weekly	Few times a week	Daily
3. Using an app will help me to do exercises.	Not true at all	Mostly not true	No opinion	Kind of true	Really true
4. If I have follow-up visits with my therapist, I will be more likely to use the app.	Not true at all	Mostly not true	No opinion	Kind of true	Really true
5. The app was...	Very boring	A little boring	No opinion	Kind of motivating	Really motivating
6. Compared to exercises on paper, the app was...	Much worse	A little worse	The same	A little better	A lot better
7. Using this app was...	Very confusing	A little confusing	No opinion	Kind of easy	Really easy
8. Getting access to this app was...	Very hard	A little hard	No opinion	Kind of easy	Really easy
9. I check my e-mail...	Never	Monthly	Weekly	Few times a week	Daily
10. I text...	Never	Monthly	Weekly	Few times a week	Daily
11. I did my PT exercises...	Never	Monthly	Weekly	Few times a week	Daily
12. The PT exercises were...	Very boring	A little boring	No opinion	Kind of motivating	Really motivating
13. Doing the PT exercises was...	Very hard	A little hard	No opinion	Kind of easy	Really easy
14. After the PT exercises, my back pain was...	Much worse	A little worse	No opinion	A little better	A lot better
15. After the PT exercises, my posture was...	Much worse	A little worse	No opinion	A little better	A lot better
16. My parents encourage me to exercise...	Never	Monthly	Weekly	Few times a week	Daily
17. I am confident I can follow an exercise routine for...	0 months	1 month	2-3 months	4-5 months	6 months or longer
18. I am motivated to exercise...	Never	Monthly	Weekly	Few times a week	Daily
19. The amount of energy I have to exercise is...	Not there at all	Mostly not there	No opinion	Kind of there	Really there

I came to the hospital because...	I was concerned	My parents were concerned	My doctor or nurse was concerned

Please add some comments about your experience with the app, emails, exercises, or pain related to this project.

_____

_____

What will help you exercise?

_____

Fig. 1 Survey

the survey to all participants to ensure their understanding of the instructions and the survey, and wrote down responses to gather details related to their experiences with the app and exercises.

The investigators developed the survey (Fig. 1) based on the previous works that identified factors related to exercise adherence, app usability, and acceptability [7, 10, 12]. Each question was scored on a scale of 1 to 5, with 1 indicating the smallest endorsement or most disagreeable response, and 5 indicating the greatest endorsement or most agreeable response (e.g., better, more agreement, easier). The survey included factors such as motivation, support, the environment, and reinforcing value [7]. In particular, personal characteristics, disease variables, treatment variables, and the patient-to-physical therapist interaction were considered [8, 10, 15–17]. The questions were aimed at understanding participants' views regarding the exercises provided, exercising in general, their back pain, the app, and technological preferences. Two additional open-ended questions offered the participants opportunities to provide more explanation or details (see Fig. 1).

Prior to implementing the survey, six healthy adolescents without any deformity or back pain reviewed the questions to ensure that wording was appropriate for an adolescent patient population. Specifically, reviewers provided feedback to include questions should not appear punitive (e.g., "They need to know they aren't in trouble"), questions should not be similar in tone or formatting to formal testing protocols (e.g., "Don't use Scantron forms or punch cards"), and the survey should be easy to complete (e.g., "Provide some lines, not too many though").

Data analysis

Means, standard deviations, and paired t tests ($P < 0.05$) were used to describe all the survey variables. Two investigators independently analyzed responses to the two open-ended questions. Each response, whether a word, phrase, or sentence, was analyzed to determine whether it contained enough information to become a unit of analysis or node. To ensure rigor of this study, each investigator independently eliminated extraneous words, then created node sets from responses. This resulted in 54 nodes for the request for participants to provide any additional comments, and 14 nodes for "What will help you exercise?" The investigators then independently grouped nodes into agreed-upon categories. In the final phase of analysis, the investigators collaborated to create one categorized data set.

Results

Twenty-one participants were enrolled in the original study, but only 14 either returned for the 6-month post-treatment assessment or responded to phone calls to complete the survey. See Table 1 for participant

Table 1 Characteristics of participants ($n = 14$)

	Pretest
Age (years)*	15.3 ± 2.0
Gender	5 girls
	9 boys
Ethnicity	11 Caucasian
	3 Hispanic
Body mass index (kg/m^2)*	27.0 ± 0.6
Physical activity (hrs/wk)*	1.3 ± 0.2
Risser grade*	3.3 ± 1.7
Curve magnitude*	60.1 ± 0.9°
Days of back pain*	870 ± 64
Pain intensity*	5.2 ± 2.1

*Data are mean ± SD

characteristics at baseline. Participants who were lost to follow-up did not differ by age, BMI, physical activity, curve magnitude, pain intensity, and SRS-22 scores as compared to the participants who completed the survey at the 6-month follow-up ($P > 0.05$). Participants had intermittent back pain for about 2 years and 5 months on average. The participants were mostly sedentary, averaging 1.3 h a week of physical activity at baseline. Lastly, the SRS-22 scores did not significantly improve at the 6-month follow-up (Table 2).

The app usage reports revealed that most participants did not use the app. One participant did not have a Smart phone or tablet. This participant logged exercise adherence on a sheet of paper, which was used to assess exercise adherence, and we could not assess his adherence according to the app. One participant had 100% HEP adherence according to the app usage report. The remaining 12 participants either did not use the app or used it less than once per week. This app usage report was similar to participants' response to question 2 of the survey regarding the app usage, for which most participants indicated that they used the app less than weekly (question 2, Table 3).

Table 2 Average scores and standard deviations (SD) of the Scoliosis Research Society-22 Health-Related Quality-of-Life Questionnaire (SRS-22r) at pretest ($n = 14$) and at posttest ($n = 14$)

Outcome measure	Pretest	Posttest	P value
SRS-22r total	3.3 ± 0.3	3.6 ± 0.4	0.09
Pain	3.2 ± 0.6	3.5 ± 1.0	0.40
Self-image	2.9 ± 0.8	3.1 ± 0.9	0.34
Function	3.9 ± 0.6	4.2 ± 0.9	0.13
Mental Health	3.5 ± 0.9	3.7 ± 0.4	0.13
Satisfaction	3.5 ± 0.9	3.5 ± 0.9	0.39

Table 3 Means and standard deviations of survey responses

Question	Mean ± SD* (n)	Means defined**
1. My back pain bothers me…	3.9 ± 1.6 (n = 14)	Kind of true
2. I used the app…	2.6 ± 1.2 (n = 14)	Weekly
3. Using an app will help me to do exercises.	3.7 ± 1.1 (n = 14)	Kind of true
4. If I have follow-up visits with my therapist, I will be more likely to use the app.	3.5 ± 1.5 (n = 14)	Kind of true
5. The app was…	3.0 ± .6 (n = 11)	No opinion
6. Compared to exercises on paper, the app was…	3.8 ± .8 (n = 12)	A little better
7. Using this app was…	3.4 ± 1.2 (n = 12)	No opinion
8. Getting access to this app was…	3.1 ± 1.7 (n = 13)	No opinion
9. I check my e-mail…	3.6 ± 1.3 (n = 14)	Few times a week
10. I text…	4.7 ± .8 (n = 14)	Daily
11. I did my PT exercises…	3.6 ± .9 (n = 14)	Few times a week
12. The PT exercises were…	2.8 ± .7 (n = 14)	No opinion
13. Doing the PT exercises was…	3.6 ± 1.2 (n = 14)	Kind of easy
14. After the PT exercises, my back pain was…	3.4 ± 1.1 (n = 14)	No opinion
15. After the PT exercises, my posture was…	3.4 ± .7 (n = 14)	No opinion
16. My parents encourage me to exercise…	3.6 ± 1.2 (n = 14)	Few times a week
17. I am confident I can follow an exercise routine for…	3.9 ± 1.5 (n = 14)	4–5 months
18. I am motivated to exercise…	3.8 ± 1.1 (n = 14)	Few times a week
19. The amount of energy I have to exercise is…	3.6 ± 1.4 (n = 14)	Kind of there

*Scale of 1 to 5. *1* smallest endorsement or most disagreeable response,
5 greatest endorsement or most agreeable response
**Means defined according to rounding rules

Participants were largely ambivalent regarding their attitudes regarding the app (questions 3–8, Fig. 1) and regarding the exercises (questions 12–15, Table 3). When asked for more details about the app, participants cited having technical difficulties such as logging in, having limited storage on their phone, and forgetting to use the app when they performed their exercises. Participants suggested that receiving reminders such as text messages or pop-up notifications to use the app might facilitate app use. In addition, participants indicated that they texted almost daily, significantly more than the frequency of checking their e-mail (questions 9–10, Table 3).

Although most participants did not use the app, 10 participants reported that they performed their exercises a few times per week (question 11, Table 3). Nine of them reported that they were motivated to exercise at least a few times a week, and that they were confident that they could follow an exercise routine for at least 4 months (questions 17–18, Table 3). When asked what would help them to perform a HEP, a specific goal like training for marching band was mentioned. Participants also reported that adherence to an exercise program would likely increase if their parents were involved in their HEP or if the app provided exercise reminders. Other responses included that the exercise had to be fun (1 response) and decrease pain (2 responses). However, three participants were not sure what would help them exercise.

Surprisingly, only three participants who reported no back pain at follow-up attributed the exercises to helping their back pain. The remaining 11 participants still reported having back pain and that their back pain bothered them (question 1, Table 3). Eight of these 11 participants reported that the exercises did not help their back pain at all. Although the other 3 of these 11 participants reported that their back pain still bothered them, they considered that the exercises had helped their back pain.

Results from the query for additional comments fell into either barriers (32) or supports (20) for app use and exercise adherence (Fig. 2). Barriers included technology and resources such as technology device limitations, connectivity, and Internet access; personal factors such as forgetfulness, poor posture, and pregnancy; or unchanged or worsening pain. Supportive measures included technology and resources such as help from people (e.g., mother and physical therapist) and equipment (e.g., exercise band and foam roll); personal attributes such as happy disposition, habit of daily exercise, and owning a phone; and exercise belief such as the exercises could cause pain reduction and muscle strengthening (Fig. 2). Further, results from the query asking participants what would help them exercise included pain relief (4 responses), social participation (4 responses, e.g., marching in a band, having fun with friends, and playing basketball), self-improvement (2 responses), receiving support from others (2 responses), or receiving supports from technology devices (1 response) (Fig. 3).

Discussion

A variety of factors contributed to the lack of app use in adolescents with painful hyperkyphosis. Technology-related, connectivity-related, and participant-induced considerations all contributed to app adherence. When the free-text questions were analyzed, adolescents considered that using an app for exercise adherence was more of a barrier than a supportive measure. Specifically, technology and resources were more frequently viewed by the participants as barriers than as supportive measures. Several participants mentioned technical and logistical difficulties using the app, and app-specific troubleshooting may have

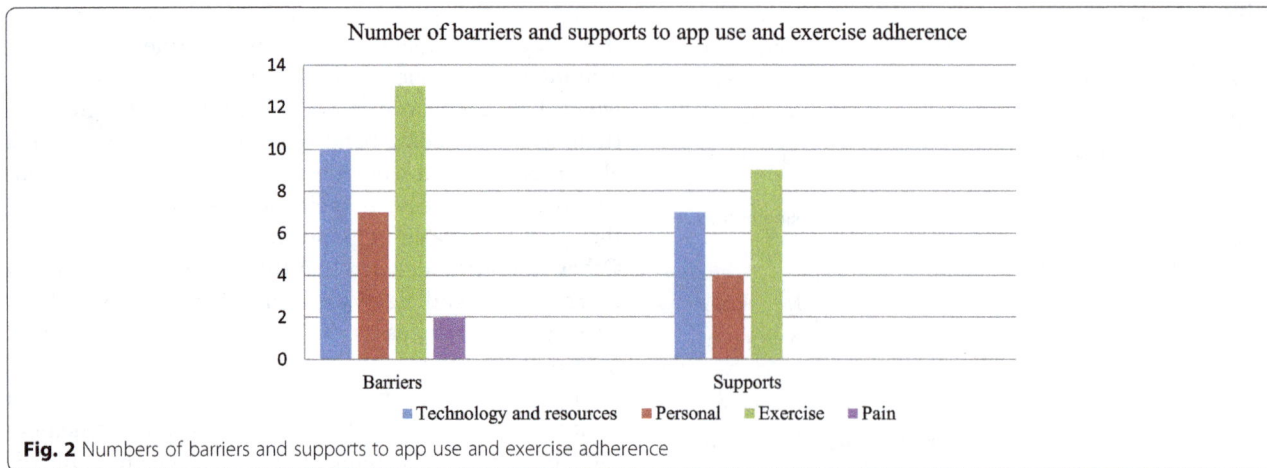

Fig. 2 Numbers of barriers and supports to app use and exercise adherence

been beneficial to improve the app's usability. Similarly, a study which used a mobile phone app to monitor caloric intake found that only 20% of participants consistently used an app, namely, those with higher exercise motivation scores [18]. However, we did not explore participants' initial willingness to use an app-based routine. Therefore, the preferences and feedback from the target users should be included in the early development of an app for its usage. In addition, because the app's look and features may be more important to children than to adults, feedback form children regarding this aspect also should be included in the early stage of an app development. As some participants forgot to use the app, additional social media interaction such as daily text message reminders and individualized feedback may increase motivation for this patient population to perform prescribed exercises and use the app. Perhaps the physical therapist should collaborate with adolescents to determine which

method of communication for a home program support would benefit them. Because many adolescents prefer texting, apps may be more beneficial for exercise adherence if text messages or pop-up alerts are incorporated in the app as another mechanism for therapists to provide feedback.

The most common rationale for participants to perform exercise was social participation and pain relief. Therefore, social participation should be included when designing exercises to improve exercise adherence for this patient population. Social environment, such as parents, friends, neighbors, teachers, and coaches may influence exercise adherence [19]. A systematic review also found strong evidence that multicomponent interventions involving the family or community could increase physical activity in adolescents, although studies referenced were school-based [8]. School social connections have been found to be a more important factor in increasing adolescents' physical activity than the school physical

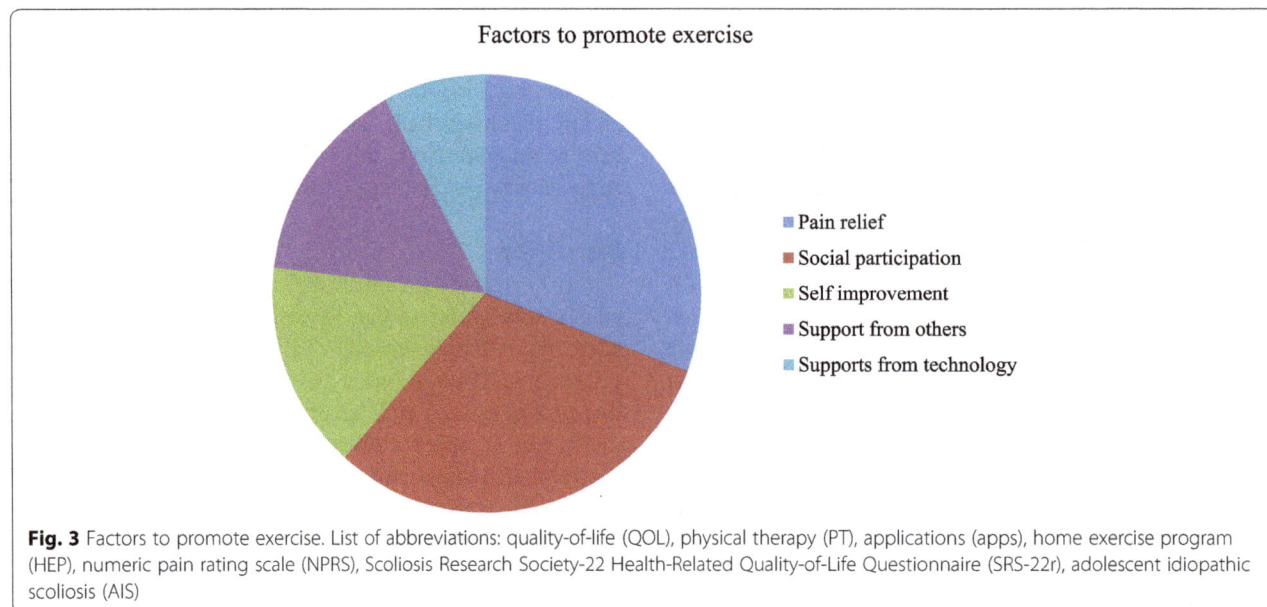

Fig. 3 Factors to promote exercise. List of abbreviations: quality-of-life (QOL), physical therapy (PT), applications (apps), home exercise program (HEP), numeric pain rating scale (NPRS), Scoliosis Research Society-22 Health-Related Quality-of-Life Questionnaire (SRS-22r), adolescent idiopathic scoliosis (AIS)

environment [20]. One example of this can be illustrated by a participant who was motivated to exercise so that he could participate in marching band. Team building interventions also have improved exercise adherence and satisfaction in an adolescent exercise setting [21]. Another systematic review found an association between higher levels of physical activity among friends and higher levels of an individual's physical activity [22]. However, there were mixed results regarding a friend's sedentary behavior and individual sedentary behavior [22].

A family-centered approach could also align personal and technical supportive measures with patients' capabilities and preferences to increase app use and exercise adherence. Strong evidence indicates that poor social or family support is a barrier for treatment adherence [16]. Involving families and social support systems is of particular importance to this patient population given their lower-than-normal QOL scores according to the SRS-22r [23–25]. The low SRS-22r scores indicated that the participants in this study had high-perceived back pain, low self-image, low physical function, and low mental health. Strong evidence has shown that psychological barriers such as depression, anxiety, and stress are barriers for treatment adherence [16].

Some researchers believe that decreased QOL in patients with hyperkyphosis implies increased indications for surgery [26]. However, non-operative management such as PT and psychology has not been adequately explored. We believe that patients with painful hyperkyphosis will benefit from more detailed psychological construct analysis. A more comprehensive treatment approach may also be necessary to address the chronic pain, sedentary lifestyles, obesity, and poor QOL scores that accompany painful hyperkyphosis, as evidence has shown that an intensive inpatient rehabilitation consisting of posture education, psychology, PT exercises, acupuncture, and the rare use of medication improved pain and posture in patients with Scheuermann kyphosis [27, 28].

More frequent in-person follow-ups by physical therapists and psychologists may help to promote behavior-changing strategies and help to evaluate whether an app for exercise may be an appropriate treatment for this patient population. Although most patients reported exercising a few times a week and that they were motivated to exercise to decrease back pain, we cannot be sure that these were not socially desirable answers, especially given that most of the patients were sedentary. Emphasizing physical activity in the context of social participation, a factor found to promote exercise, may be more enjoyable than a formal exercise program.

Although participants were ambivalent regarding whether they would be more likely to use the app if they had follow-up visits with their therapist, we did not objectively evaluate this assertion, as the participants only received a one-time supervised PT treatment only. In addition, the survey administration occurred at the 6-month follow-up with the orthopedic surgeon. Waiting 6 months may have influenced the validity of reported barriers. Earlier and multiple survey administrations may have been preferable so that problems with exercise adherence could be detected earlier. A previous study on adolescents with idiopathic scoliosis and back pain compared patients who were provided a one-time exercise treatment followed by an unsupervised 4-month HEP to patients who received 2 months of weekly supervised PT at 6-month follow-up [29]. Results showed that patients in the supervised PT group had greater improvements in pain and satisfaction compared to the one-time exercise treatment group [29]. Although patients from the abovementioned study had scoliosis, the increased attention and social support received by patients in the supervised group may improve treatment adherence in patients with hyperkyphosis.

One study limitation is the small sample size, which is primarily due to the low return rate of participants at the 6-month follow-up despite efforts to phone and include those who did not return for their follow-up visit. Another study limitation is that we used a standard outcome measure specific to scoliosis rather than one for hyperkyphosis because no standardized outcome measures are available for this patient population. Therefore, the SRS-22r scores may not give a full representation of quality-of-life for the participants of this study. Finally, because most participants did not use the app, we had to rely on self-report measures of exercise adherence, thus introducing the potential for bias.

Future research should focus on examining strategies to improve exercise adherence to an app in adolescents with back pain caused by spinal disorders. Three factors: technology related, connectivity related, and participant induced, all contribute to app adherence and should each be more systematically evaluated so that their unique contribution to connected health therapy programming can be more strategically planned and realistically managed. In addition, because adolescents text frequently, future research should consider using Health Insurance Portability and Accountability Act (HIPAA)-secure text messages instead of e-mails or phone calls as a means of communication for follow-up needs. Finally, kyphosis-specific outcome measures should be developed, as current outcome measures evaluating quality-of-life (SRS-22r) and self-image (Spinal Appearance Questionnaire) have been validated in the AIS population and not in patients with kyphosis [14, 30].

Conclusion

Patients with painful hyperkyphosis who were given a one-time exercise treatment followed by a 6-month app-based HEP did not use the app due to ambivalence regarding the usability and acceptability of the app and the exercises. Understanding a specific population's technology habits is important before assuming potential effectiveness of an app or other electronic measure. Adolescents viewed technology support such as text reminders as a potential solution. A more comprehensive approach with additional research is needed to better understand how to improve app use to promote a successful rehabilitation for this patient population.

Acknowledgements
The authors wish to acknowledge Maria King for assisting with the data analysis.

Authors' contributions
Each author contributed significantly to the design of the study and the writing of the manuscript. KZ conceived of the study, performed the PT treatment, implemented surveys, and drafted the manuscript. SW contributed to the study design and revised the manuscript. TF contributed to the study and survey design, qualitative analysis, and revised the manuscript. CJ conceived of the study, supervised the project, assisted with patient referrals, and revised the manuscript. All authors read and approved the final manuscript.

Competing interests
The authors declare that they have no competing interests.

Author details
[1]Therapy Services, Texas Scottish Rite Hospital for Children, 2222 Welborn Street, Dallas, TX 75219, USA. [2]School of Physical Therapy, Texas Woman's University–Dallas, Dallas, TX, USA. [3]School of Occupational Therapy, Texas Woman's University–Dallas, Dallas, TX, USA. [4]Texas Scottish Rite Hospital for Children, Dallas, TX, USA.

References
1. Petcharaporn M, Pawelek J, Bastrom T, Lonner B, Newton PO. The relationship between thoracic hyperkyphosis and the Scoliosis Research Society outcomes instrument. Spine (Phila Pa 1976). 2007;32(20):2226–31.
2. Lonner B, Yoo A, Terran JS, et al. Effect of spinal deformity on adolescent quality of life comparison of operative Scheuermann's kyphosis, adolescent idiopathic scoliosis and normal controls. Spine (Phila Pa 1976). 2013;38(12):1049–55.
3. Murray P, Weinstein S, Spratt KF. Natural history and long-term follow-up of Scheuermann kyphosis. J Bone Joint Surg Am. 1993;75A(2):236–48.
4. Ristolainen L, Kettunen JA, Heliövaara M, Kujala UM, Heinonen A, Schlenzka D. Untreated Scheuermann's disease: a 37-year follow-up study. Eur Spine J. 2012;21(5):819–24.
5. de Mauroy J, Weiss H, Aulisa A, et al. 7th SOSORT consensus paper: conservative treatment of idiopathic & scheuermann's kyphosis. Scoliosis. 2010;5:9.
6. Zaina F, Atanasio S, Ferraro C, et al. Review of rehabilitation and orthopedic conservative approach to sagittal plane diseases during growth: hyperkpyhosis, junctional kyphosis, and scheuermann disease. Eur J Phys Rehabil Med. 2009;45(4):595–603.
7. Prasad SA, Cerny FJ. Factors that influence adherence to exercise and their effectiveness: application to cystic fibrosis. Pediatr Pulmonol. 2002;34(1):66–72.
8. van Sluijs EMF, McMinn AM, Griffin SJ. Effectiveness of interventions to promote physical activity in children and adolescents: systematic review of controlled trials. BMJ. 2007;335(7622):703.
9. Zapata KA, Wang-Price SS, Sucato DJ, Thompson M, Trudelle-Jackson E, Lovelace-Chandler V. Spinal stabilization exercise effectiveness for low back pain in adolescent idiopathic scoliosis. Pediatr Phys Ther. 2015;27(4):396–402.
10. Bassett SF. The assessment of patient adherence to physiotherapy. New Zeal J Physiother. 2003;31(July):60–6.
11. Madden M, Lenhart A, Cortesi S, Gasser U. Teens and mobile apps privacy. Washington, DC: Pew Internet & American Life Project; 2013. [2015-04-21]. *webcite* http://www.pewinternet.org/2013/08/22/teens-and-mobile-apps-privacy/ [Ref list].
12. Direito A, Jiang Y, Whittaker R, Maddison R. Apps for IMproving FITness and increasing physical activity among young people: the AIMFIT pragmatic randomized controlled trial. J Med Internet Res. 2015;17(8):e210.
13. Williamson A, Hoggart B. Pain: a review of three commonly used pain rating scales. J Clin Nurs. 2005;14(7):798–804.
14. Asher M, Min Lai S, Burton D, Manna B. The reliability and concurrent validity of the scoliosis research society-22 patient questionnaire for idiopathic scoliosis. Spine (Phila Pa 1976). 2003;28(1):63–9.
15. Campbell R, Evans M, Tucker M, Quilty B, Dieppe P, Donovan JL. Why don't patients do their exercises? Understanding non-compliance with physiotherapy in patients with osteoarthritis of the knee. J Epidemiol Community Health. 2001;55(2):132–8.
16. Jack K, McLean SM, Moffett JK, Gardiner E. Barriers to treatment adherence in physiotherapy outpatient clinics: a systematic review. Man Ther. 2010;15(3):220–8.
17. Henry K, Rosemond C, Eckert L. Effect of number of home exercises on compliance and performance in adults over 65 years of age. Phys Ther. 1999;79(3):270–7.
18. Goh G, Tan NC, Malhotra R, et al. Short-term trajectories of use of a caloric-monitoring mobile phone app among patients with type 2 diabetes mellitus in a primary care setting. J Med Internet Res. 2015;17(2):e33.
19. Markward M, McMillan LS, Markward N. Social support among youth. Child Youth Serv Rev. 2003;25(7):571–87.
20. Button B, Trites S, Janssen I. Relations between the school physical environment and school social capital with student physical activity levels. BMC Public Health. 2013;13:1191.
21. Bruner MW, Spink KS. Effects of team building on exercise adherence and group task satisfaction in a youth activity setting. Group Dyn-Theor Res. 2011;15(2):161–72.
22. Sawka KJ, Mccormack GR, Nettel-aguirre A, Hawe P, Doyle-baker PK. Friendship networks and physical activity and sedentary behavior among youth: a systematized review. Int J Behav Nutr Phys Act. 2013;10:130.
23. Daubs MD, Hung M, Neese A, et al. Scoliosis research society-22 results in 3052 healthy adolescents aged 10 to 19 years. Spine (Phila Pa 1976). 2014;39(10):826–32.
24. Verma K, Lonner BS, Hoashi JS, et al. Demographic factors affect Scoliosis Research Society-22 performance in healthy adolescents: a comparative baseline for adolescents with idiopathic scoliosis. Spine (Phila Pa 1976). 2010;35(24):2134–9.
25. Carreon LY, Sanders JO, Diab M, Sucato DJ, Sturm PF, Glassman SD. The minimum clinically important difference in scoliosis research Society-22 appearance, activity, and pain domains after surgical correction of adolescent idiopathic scoliosis. Spine (Phila Pa 1976). 2010;35(23):2079–83.
26. Kuklo TR, Diab M, Richards BS, Sucato DJ, Lenke LG, Spinal Deformity Study Group. Are there SRS preoperative questionnaire differences between kyphosis and scoliosis patients? E-Poster Presentation at: 43rd Annual Meeting of the Scoliosis Research Society. Salt Lake City, UT: Scoliosis Research Society (SRS);2008.
27. Weiss H-R, Dieckmann J, Gerner HJ. The practical use of surface topography: following up patients with scheuermann's disease. Pediatr Rehabil. 2003;6(1):39–45.
28. Weiss H-R, Dieckmann J, Gerner HJ. Effect of intensive rehabilitation on pain in patients with scheuermann's disease. In: Tanguy A, Peuchot B, editors. Research into Spinal Deformities 3, vol. 88. Oxford: IOS Press; 2002. p. 254–7.
29. Zapata KA, Wang-Price SS, Sucato DJ. Six-month follow-up of supervised spinal stabilization exercises for low back pain in adolescent idiopathic scoliosis. Pediatr Phys Ther. 2017;29(1):62–6.
30. Sanders JO, Harrast JJ, Kuklo TR, et al. The spinal appearance questionnaire: results of reliability, validity, and responsiveness testing in patients with idiopathic scoliosis. Spine (Phila Pa 1976). 2007;32(24):2719–22.

22

Evaluation of functional and structural leg length discrepancy in patients with adolescent idiopathic scoliosis using the EOS imaging system

Tatsuhiro Sekiya[1][*] iD, Yoichi Aota[2], Katsutaka Yamada[1], Kanichiro Kaneko[1], Manabu Ide[1] and Tomoyuki Saito[1]

Abstract

Background: To our knowledge, no studies have reported the exact structural leg length discrepancies (LLDs) in patients with adolescent idiopathic scoliosis (AIS). Therefore, this study aimed to evaluate the differences between functional and structural LLDs and to examine the correlations between LLDs and spinopelvic parameters in patients with AIS using an EOS imaging system, which permits the three-dimensional reconstruction of spinal and lower-limb bony structures.

Methods: Eighty-two consecutive patients with AIS underwent whole-body EOS radiography in a standing position between August 2014 and March 2016. Functional LLD, lumbar Cobb angle, thoracic curve Cobb angle, coronal balance, and pelvic obliquity were measured using two-dimensional EOS radiography. Structural LLDs were measured using three-dimensional EOS-reconstructed images. The comparison between LLDs was assessed using paired t test. Pearson's correlation coefficient (r) was used to determine potential correlations between the LLDs and spinopelvic alignment parameters.

Results: Functional LLDs were significantly larger than structural LLDs (5.6 ± 5.0 vs. 0.2 ± 3.6 mm, respectively; $p < 0.001$). Both functional and structural LLDs were significantly correlated with pelvic obliquity ($r = 0.69$ and $r = 0.51$, respectively; $p < 0.001$ for both). Functional LLD, but not structural LLD, was correlated with lumbar Cobb angle ($r = 0.44$, $p < 0.001$; $r = 0.17$, $p = 0.12$, respectively). In addition, functional and structural LLDs were not correlated with thoracic Cobb angle ($r = 0.09$ and $r = -0.05$, respectively; $p \geq 0.68$ for both).

Conclusions: Although patients with AIS often have functional LLDs, structural LLDs tend to be smaller. The correlation between functional LLDs and the lumbar Cobb angle indicates that functional LLDs compensate for the lumbar curve. Thus, the difference between functional and structural LLDs indicates a compensatory mechanism involving extension and flexion of the lower limbs.

Keywords: Adolescent idiopathic scoliosis, Leg length discrepancy, Spinopelvic parameters, EOS radiography

* Correspondence: ts0806@yokohama-cu.ac.jp
[1]Department of Orthopedic Surgery, Yokohama City University, Fukuura 3-9, Kanazawa-ku, Yokohama City, Kanagawa Prefecture 236-0004, Japan
Full list of author information is available at the end of the article

Background

Adolescent idiopathic scoliosis (AIS) is a three-dimensional (3D) spinal deformity consisting of lateral deviation and axial rotation of the spine [1]. Clinical interest in 3D imaging for understanding, quantifying, and predicting the evolution of spinal deformities has long existed [2]. However, the gold standard for the initial diagnosis and longitudinal surveillance of AIS involves two-dimensional (2D) posterior-anterior (PA) full-length spine radiography [3].

In clinical practice, standing PA radiographs often reveal leg length discrepancies (LLDs) in patients with AIS. LLDs can be subdivided into functional LLDs, resulting from altered mechanics, and structural LLDs, which is associated with bony shortening [4]. Measuring the difference in femoral head heights on standing PA radiographs is a simple and reliable method for functional LLD documentation [5]. Unfortunately, limitations in measuring leg length using 3D imaging have been reported [6]. To our knowledge, no study has reported the exact structural LLDs in patients with AIS. In the past decade, a biplanar low-dose X-ray device, the EOS 2D/3D system (Biospace Imaging, Paris, France), was developed [7] to accurately measure leg length three-dimensionally (Fig. 1) [8]. In this study, we aimed to evaluate the differences between functional and structural LLDs and determine whether there are true LLDs in patients with AIS. In addition, we aimed to examine the correlations between LLDs and spinopelvic parameters in patients with AIS using the EOS imaging system.

Methods

Patients

Eighty-two consecutive patients with AIS (age range, 10–18 years; 70 girls and 12 boys) and Cobb angles of > 10° who were admitted to our hospital between August 2014 and March 2016 were surveyed. Patients with a history of scoliosis surgery, congenital scoliosis, secondary scoliosis, neuromuscular primeval scoliosis, scoliosis associated with intellectual disability, and/or congenital heart disease were excluded.

Measurements

Patients underwent whole-body EOS radiography in the upright position during their first visit. We measured the functional LLD, lumbar Cobb angle, thoracic curve Cobb angle, pelvic obliquity, and coronal balance using 2D EOS PA standing radiographs, conducted according to the Spinal Deformity Study Group Radiographic Measurement Manual [9]. The femoral horizontal reference line was defined as a horizontal line tangent to the top of the highest portion of the femoral head. The height between right and left femoral horizontal reference lines was defined as the functional LLD. The angle between the horizontal reference line and the pelvic coronal reference

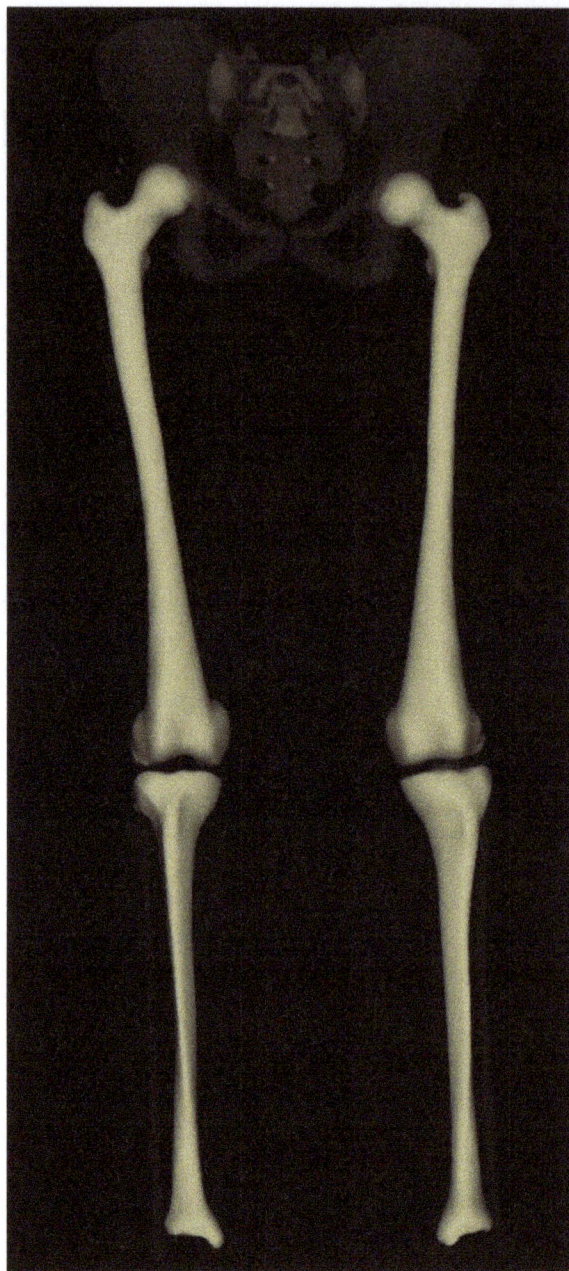

Fig. 1 Three-dimensional imaging of the lower limbs using the EOS system. The EOS system was developed to accurately measure leg length three-dimensionally

line was defined as the pelvic obliquity. The tips of the sacral ala were used to create the pelvic coronal reference line (Fig. 2). Coronal balance was defined as the distance between the C7 plumb line and the center sacral vertical line, and a negative sign denotes a shift to the left. Structural LLD was defined as the difference between the sums of bilateral femoral lengths and tibial lengths obtained from three-dimensional distance using the EOS system. We took points with a front view and a side view and

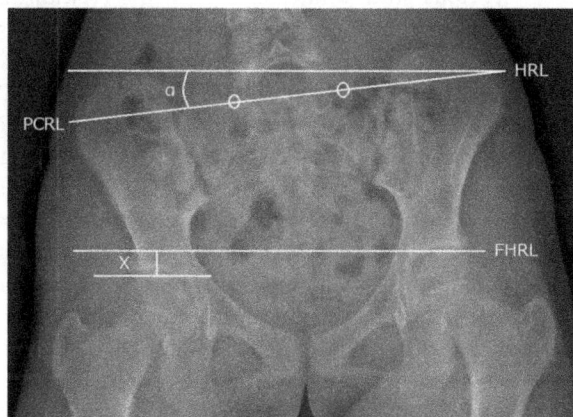

Fig. 2 Functional leg length discrepancy and pelvic obliquity assessed using two-dimensional standing radiograph. Functional leg length discrepancy (X) and pelvic obliquity (α) measured using the two-dimensional posterior-anterior standing radiograph obtained from the EOS imaging system. FHRL femoral horizontal reference line, HRL horizontal reference line, PCRL pelvic coronal reference line

calculated a three-dimensional distance. The femoral length was measured from the femoral head to the inter-condylar fossa, and the tibial length was measured from the intercondylar fossa to the inferior articular surface of the tibia (Fig. 3).

Additionally, the Risser sign, an indirect measure of skel-etal maturity, was used as a bone growth parameter. Risser sign stage (0–5) was determined for each participant.

Statistical analysis

Functional and structural LLDs were compared using a paired t test. Pearson's correlation coefficient was used to investigate the correlations between the LLDs (functional and structural) and spinopelvic alignment parameters (pelvic obliquity, lumbar Cobb angle, and thoracic curve Cobb angle). A p value < 0.05 was considered to be statis-tically significant. Analyses were performed using Statis-tical Package for the Social Sciences, version 16.0 (SPSS, Chicago, IL, USA).

Results

Patient demographics are presented in Table 1. Ten patients were classified according to Risser sign staging as stage 0, 5 as stage 1, 14 as stage 2, 15 as stage 3, 33 as stage 4, and 5 as stage 5. Of 58 female patients who experienced menarche, the mean age at menarche was 12.1 ± 1.2 years. According to the Lenke classification of AIS [10], type 1 AIS was noted in 50 patients, type 2 in 7 patients, type 3 in 9 patients, type 4 in 0 patients, type 5 in 16 patients, and type 6 in 0 patients.

Functional LLD (mm) was significantly greater than structural LLD (5.6 ± 5.0 vs. 0.2 ± 3.6 mm; $p < 0.001$).

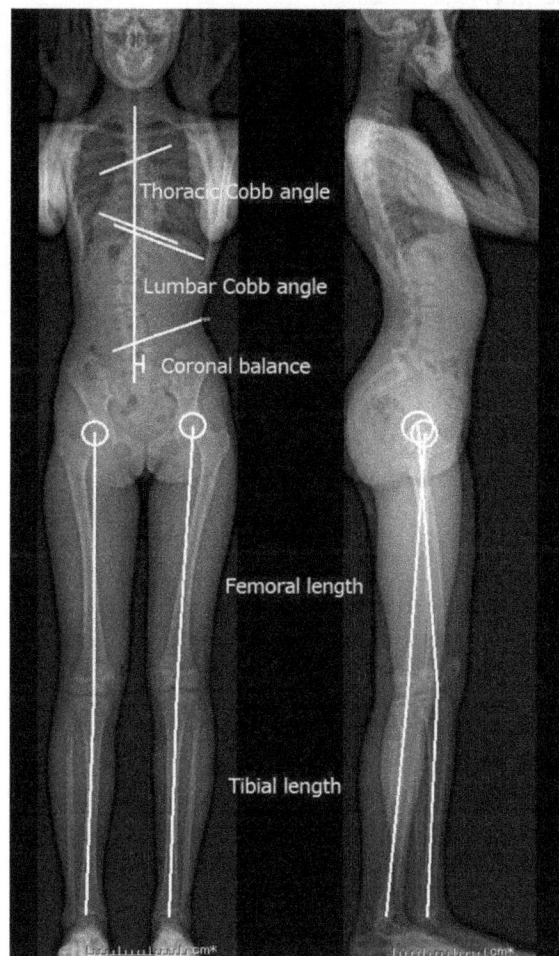

Fig. 3 Measurements obtained using whole-body EOS radiography in the upright position. Thoracic Cobb angle, lumbar Cobb angle, and coronal balance were assessed in the coronal plane obtained from whole-body EOS radiography. Structural leg length discrepancy was defined as the difference between the sums of the bilateral femoral and tibial lengths obtained from three-dimensional distance using the EOS system

Additionally, no patients had a structural LLD ≥ 10 mm although 18 patients had a functional LLD ≥ 10 mm.

Functional and structural LLDs were significantly corre-lated with pelvic obliquity ($p < 0.001$ for both; Table 2). Functional LLD, but not structural LLD, was significantly correlated with the lumbar Cobb angle ($p < 0.001$ and $p = 0.12$, respectively). In addition, both functional and structural LLDs were not significantly correlated with thoracic Cobb angle ($p = 0.43$ and $p = 0.68$, respectively). Further, the mean coronal balance was − 9.0 ± 13.5 mm, and only one patient had a coronal balance > 40 mm.

Discussion

It is necessary to measure 3D leg length in the standing position in order to compare functional and structural LLDs under the same conditions. However, lower limb

Table 1 Demographic data

Characteristic	Value
Sex	
Male	12
Female	70
Age (years)	13.7 ± 1.9
Height (cm)	157.0 ± 7.4
Weight (kg)	45.4 ± 6.7
Seated height (cm)	84.5 ± 9.3
Arm span (cm)	158.6 ± 8.3
Risser sign (stage)	2.9 ± 1.1
Pelvic obliquity (°)	4.1 ± 3.0
Lumbar Cobb angle (°)	22.8 ± 12.5
Thoracic curve Cobb angle (°)	24.6 ± 11.6
Coronal balance (mm)	− 9.0 ± 13.5

Data are presented as frequency or mean ± standard deviation

analyses rely on conventional radiography (2D view) or computed tomography in the decubitus position in clinical practice. Unfortunately, these modalities do not allow 3D analyses in the standing position [11]. Recently, an EOS 2D/3D system was developed that allows simultaneous PA and lateral 2D images of the whole body to be obtained in a calibrated environment, permitting the 3D reconstruction of spinal and lower limb bony structures via stereoradiography [7]. Guenoun et al. found that the EOS 3D modeling technique showed excellent inter- and intra-observer reliabilities, which were better than the reliabilities for 2D measurements [12]. In addition, several reports found that EOS is more accurate than both computed tomography scanography and conventional radiography [13, 14]. Therefore, the present study capitalized on this recent technological advancement to measure 3D structural LLDs, as well as functional LLDs, in patients with AIS. We revealed that a difference exists between functional LLDs and structural LLDs in patients with AIS. Furthermore, a functional LLD ≥ 10 mm was noted in 18 patients, while no patients had a structural LLD > 10 mm. Thus, although standing PA radiographs often show significant LLDs in patients with AIS at our clinical practice, the results of the present study revealed only a small amount of true LLDs in patients with AIS.

Furthermore, we assessed the correlations between LLDs and spinopelvic parameters in patients with AIS.

Several previous studies have examined the relationship between the pelvis and the lower limbs/spine in terms of both anthropological and clinical problems [15]. There is evidence of pelvic abnormalities in patients with AIS. For example, Qiu et al. noted that standing PA radiographs show that the concave and convex ilia are not always symmetrical in patients with AIS in clinical practice [16]. The authors concluded that this phenomenon may be due to transverse pelvic rotation. In addition, Jones et al. reported that LLDs are more common in individuals with Marfan syndrome than in the general population and are associated with increased structural scoliosis [17]. The authors also stated that correlations between LLDs and scoliosis severity and convexity suggest that the two entities are related, although no causal relationship is clear.

Several studies have reported that structural LLDs cause pelvic obliquity in the frontal plane and lumbar scoliosis with convexity toward the shorter extremity [18, 19]. Scoliosis that develops due to LLDs is included within functional scoliosis. This type of scoliosis regresses completely or partially when its cause (i.e., LLD) is removed. Raczkowski et al. reported that minor LLDs cause pelvic obliquity in the frontal plane, which in turn causes scoliosis in the lumbar region [19]. These changes are believed to result from asymmetry of the spinal static and dynamic loads, as well as from intervertebral disc dislocation. However, in the present study, the structural LLD was very slight. Thus, it is considered that functional LLDs were caused by scoliosis. Recently, Pasha et al. reported a 3D analysis of spinopelvic alignment in patients with AIS. The authors concluded that the pelvic coronal tilt is significantly correlated with functional LLD. Relative spinopelvic alignment was suggested as a compensatory mechanism to maintain trunk equilibrium [20]. These conclusions are consistent with the present results regarding structural LLD and coronal balance.

In this study, functional and structural LLDs were significantly correlated with pelvic obliquity. However, the structural LLDs were so small that the correlations between structural LLD and pelvic obliquity can be ignored. Furthermore, functional LLD, but not structural LLD, was correlated with lumbar curve. Given that functional LLD was greater than structural LLD in AIS patients, structural LLDs probably do not influence scoliosis and pelvic obliquity. Rather, it seems likely that scoliosis affects functional LLD and pelvic obliquity. Since coronal balance was within the normal range in almost all patients, the difference

Table 2 Pearson's correlation coefficients between leg length deficiencies and spinopelvic alignment parameters

	Pelvic obliquity (r)	Lumbar Cobb angle (r)	Thoracic curve Cobb angle (r)
Functional LLD	0.69*	0.44*	0.09
Structural LLD	0.51*	0.17	− 0.05

LLD leg length discrepancy
*Statistically significant at $p < 0.05$

between the functional and structural LLDs is suggestive of a compensatory mechanism for poor coronal balance in scoliosis through extension and flexion of the lower limbs.

Our study has a few limitations, including a small sample size. In addition, we did not add the length of the ankle joints or the hip joints to the leg length. However, we considered that the subjects are young and we think that the deformity changes of ankle joints and hip joints are almost negligible. Finally, to accurately measure leg length, the subjects stood by shifting the left and the right feet by several centimeters during EOS radiography. We thought that the difference is small and the measured value is not affected, but it is necessary to investigate in the future.

Conclusions

This study revealed that patients with AIS have functional (apparent) LLD, but not significant structural (true) LLD. The correlation between lumbar Cobb angle and functional LLD indicates that the lumbar curve contributes to functional LLD; thus, the difference between functional and structural LLDs represents a compensatory mechanism involving extension and flexion of the lower limbs.

Abbreviations
2D: Two-dimensional; 3D: Three-dimensional; AIS: Adolescent idiopathic scoliosis; LLDs: Leg length discrepancies; PA: Posterior-anterior

Authors' contributions
YA made substantial contributions to the conception and design of the study, acquisition of data, and analysis and interpretation of data. KY contributed to the analysis and interpretation of data and assisted in the preparation of the manuscript. KK participated in the design of the study and helped to revise the manuscript. MI performed the statistical analysis and helped to revise the manuscript. TS conceived of the study and participated in its design and coordination and helped to draft the manuscript. All authors approved the final version of the manuscript and agreed to be accountable for all aspects of the work in ensuring that questions related to the accuracy or integrity of any part of the work are appropriately investigated and resolved.

Competing interests
The authors declare that they have no competing interests.

Author details
[1]Department of Orthopedic Surgery, Yokohama City University, Fukuura 3-9, Kanazawa-ku, Yokohama City, Kanagawa Prefecture 236-0004, Japan.
[2]Department of Orthopedic Surgery, Yokohama City Brain and Spine Center, Takigasira 1-2-1, Isogo-ku, Yokohama City, Kanagawa Prefecture 235-0012, Japan.

References
1. Perdriolle R, Vidal J. Morphology of scoliosis: three-dimensional evolution. Orthopedics. 1987;10:909–5.
2. Humbert L, De Guise JA, Aubert B, Godbout B, Skalli W. 3D reconstruction of the spine from biplanar X-rays using parametric models based on transversal and longitudinal inferences. Med Eng Phys. 2009;31:681–7.
3. Raso VJ, Lou E, Hill DL, Mahood J, Moreau MJ, Durdle NG. Trunk distortion in adolescent idiopathic scoliosis. J Pediatr Orthop. 1998;18:222–6.
4. Gurney B. Leg length discrepancy. Gait Posture. 2002;15:195–206.
5. Sabharwal S, Zhao C, McKeon JJ, McClemens E, Edgar M, Behrens F. Computed radiographic measurement of limb-length discrepancy. Full-length standing anteroposterior radiograph compared with scanogram. J Bone Joint Surg Am. 2006;10:2243–51.
6. Terry MA, Winell JJ, Green DW, Schneider R, Peterson M, Marx RG, et al. Measurement variance in limb length discrepancy: clinical and radiographic assessment of interobserver and intraobserver variability. J Pediatr Orthop. 2005;25:197–201.
7. Dubousset J, Charpak G, Dorion I, Skalli W, Lavaste F, Deguise J, et al. A new 2D and 3D imaging approach to musculoskeletal physiology and pathology with low-dose radiation and the standing position: the EOS system. Bull Acad Natl Med. 2005;189:287–97. discussion 297-300. [Article in French]
8. Gheno R, Nectoux E, Herbaux B, Baldisserotto M, Glock L, Cotten A, et al. Three-dimensional measurements of the lower extremity in children and adolescents using a low-dose biplanar X-ray device. Eur Radiol. 2012;22:765–71.
9. O'Brien MF, Kuklo TR, Blanke KM, Lenke LG. The spinal deformity study group radiographic measurement manual. Memphis, TN: Medtronic Sofamor Danek USA, Inc.; 2004.
10. Lenke LG, Betz RR, Harms J, Bridwell KH, Clements DH, Lowe TG, et al. Adolescent idiopathic scoliosis: a new classification to determine extent of spinal arthrodesis. J Bone Joint Surg Am. 2001;83-A:1169–81.
11. Chaibi Y, Cresson T, Aubert B, Hausselle J, Neyret P, Hauger O, et al. Fast 3D reconstruction of the lower limb using a parametric model and statistical inferences and clinical measurements calculation from biplanar X-rays. Comput Methods Biomech Biomed Engin. 2012;15:457–66.
12. Guenoun B, Zadegan F, Aim F, Hannouche D, Nizard R. Reliability of a new method for lower-extremity measurements based on stereoradiographic three-dimensional reconstruction. Orthop Traumatol Surg Res. 2012;98:506–13.
13. Escott BG, Ravi B, Weathermon AC, Acharya J, Gordon CL, Babyn PS, et al. EOS low-dose radiography: a reliable and accurate upright assessment of lower-limb lengths. J Bone Joint Surg Am. 2012;95:e1831–7.
14. Garner MR, Dow M, Bixby E, Mintz DN, Widmann RF, Dodwell ER. Evaluating length: the use of low-dose biplanar radiography (EOS) and tantalum bead implantation. J Pediatr Orthop. 2016;36:e6–9.
15. Boulay C, Tardieu C, Bénaim C, Hecquet J, Marty C, Prat-Pradal D, et al. Three-dimensional study of pelvic asymmetry on anatomical specimens and its clinical perspectives. J Anat. 2006;208:21–3.
16. Qiu XS, Zhang JJ, Yang SW, Lv F, Wang ZW, Chiew J, et al. Anatomical study of the pelvis in patients with adolescent idiopathic scoliosis. J Anat. 2012;220:173–8.
17. Jones KB, Sponseller PD, Hobbs W, Pyeritz RE. Leg-length discrepancy and scoliosis in Marfan syndrome. J Pediatr Orthop. 2002;22:807–12.
18. Papaioannou T, Stokes I, Kenwright J. Scoliosis associated with limb-length inequality. J Bone Joint Surg Am. 1982;64:59–62.
19. Raczkowski JW, Daniszewska B, Zolynski K. Functional scoliosis caused by leg length discrepancy. Arch Med Sci. 2010;6:393–8.
20. Pasha S, Aubin CE, Sangole AP, Labelle H, Parent S, Mac-Thiong JM. Three-dimensional spinopelvic relative alignment in adolescent idiopathic scoliosis. Spine (Phila Pa 1976). 2014;39:564–70.

Permissions

The contributors of this book come from diverse backgrounds, making this book a truly international effort. This book will bring forth new frontiers with its revolutionizing research information and detailed analysis of the nascent developments around the world.

We would like to thank all the contributing authors for lending their expertise to make the book truly unique. They have played a crucial role in the development of this book. Without their invaluable contributions this book wouldn't have been possible. They have made vital efforts to compile up to date information on the varied aspects of this subject to make this book a valuable addition to the collection of many professionals and students.

This book was conceptualized with the vision of imparting up-to-date information and advanced data in this field. To ensure the same, a matchless editorial board was set up. Every individual on the board went through rigorous rounds of assessment to prove their worth. After which they invested a large part of their time researching and compiling the most relevant data for our readers.

The editorial board has been involved in producing this book since its inception. They have spent rigorous hours researching and exploring the diverse topics which have resulted in the successful publishing of this book. They have passed on their knowledge of decades through this book. To expedite this challenging task, the publisher supported the team at every step. A small team of assistant editors was also appointed to further simplify the editing procedure and attain best results for the readers.

Apart from the editorial board, the designing team has also invested a significant amount of their time in understanding the subject and creating the most relevant covers. They scrutinized every image to scout for the most suitable representation of the subject and create an appropriate cover for the book.

The publishing team has been an ardent support to the editorial, designing and production team. Their endless efforts to recruit the best for this project, has resulted in the accomplishment of this book. They are a veteran in the field of academics and their pool of knowledge is as vast as their experience in printing. Their expertise and guidance has proved useful at every step. Their uncompromising quality standards have made this book an exceptional effort. Their encouragement from time to time has been an inspiration for everyone.

The publisher and the editorial board hope that this book will prove to be a valuable piece of knowledge for researchers, students, practitioners and scholars across the globe.

List of Contributors

Manuel Rigo
Elena Salvá Institute (Rigo Quera Salvá S.L.P.), Vía Augusta 185, 08021 Barcelona, Spain

Mina Jelačić
Specijalističa Ordinacija za fizikalnu medicine I rehabiliraciju "Ledja I vrat", Stojana Protića 48, Belgrade, Republic of Serbia

Angelo G. Aulisa, Vincenzo Guzzanti, Francesco Falciglia and Paolo Pizzetti
U.O.C. of Orthopedics and Traumatology, Children's Hospital Bambino Gesù, Institute of Scientific Research, P.zza S. Onofrio 4, 00165 Rome, Italy

Vincenzo Guzzanti
University of Cassino, 03043 Cassino, FR, Italy

Marco Galli and Lorenzo Aulisa
Department of Orthopedics, University Hospital "Agostino Gemelli", Catholic University of the Sacred Heart School of Medicine, 00168 Rome, Italy

Steven Kyriacou, Matthew Shaw and Kia Rezajooi
Spinal Deformity Unit, Royal National Orthopaedic Hospital, Stanmore, UK

Yuen Man and Karen Plumb
The Royal National Orthopaedic Hospital, Stanmore, UK

Elisabetta D'Agata
Vall d'Hebron Research Institut, Passeig Vall d'Hebron, 119-129, 08035 Barcelona, Spain

Judith Sánchez-Raya and Juan Bagó
Vall d'Hebron Hospital, Passeig Vall d'Hebron, 119-129, 08035 Barcelona, Spain

Kenny Yat Hong Kwan, Hui Yu Koh and Kenneth Man Chee Cheung
Department of Orthopaedics and Traumatology, Li Ka Shing Faculty of Medicine, The University of Hong Kong, Pokfulam, Hong Kong

Aldous C.S. Cheng and Alice Y.Y. Chiu
Department of Physiotherapy, Duchess of Kent Children's Hospital, Sandy Bay, Hong Kong

Xiaoyu Wang and Carl-Eric Aubin
Department of Mechanical Engineering, Polytechnique Montréal, Downtown Station, Montreal, Quebec H3C 3A7, Canada

Xiaoyu Wang, Stefan Parent, Hubert Labelle and Carl-Eric Aubin
Sainte-Justine University Hospital Center, 3175, Cote Sainte-Catherine Road, Montreal, Quebec H3T 1C5, Canada

A. Noelle Larson
Department of Orthopedic Surgery, Mayo Clinic, 200 1st Street SW, Rochester, MN 55905, USA

Dennis G. Crandall
Sonoran Spine Center and Research Foundation, 1255 W Rio Salado Pkwy, Suite 107, Tempe, AZ 85281, USA

Charles G. T. Ledonio
Department of Orthopaedic Surgery, University of Minnesota, 2450 Riverside Avenue South, Suite R200, Minneapolis, MN 55454, USA

Sayf S.A. Faraj, Tsjitske M. Haanstra, Hugo Martijn and Barend J. van Royen
Department of Orthopaedic Surgery, VU University Medical Center, De Boelelaan 1117, 1081HV Amsterdam, The Netherlands

Marinus de Kleuver
Department of Orthopedics, Radboud University Medical Center, Huispost 611, 6500HB Nijmegen, The Netherlands

Christian Wong and Stig Sonne-Holm
Department of Orthopaedics, University Hospital of Hvidovre, Kettegaard Allé 30, 2650 Hvidovre, Denmark

Kasper Gosvig
Department of Radiology, University Hospital of Hvidovre, Kettegaard Allé 30, 2650 Hvidovre, Denmark

James Cheshire
Institute of Metabolism and Systems Research (IMSR), University of Birmingham, Birmingham, UK

Adrian Gardner and Fiona Berryman
The Royal Orthopaedic Hospital NHS Foundation Trust, Birmingham, UK

Adrian Gardner and Paul Pynsent
Department of Anatomy, Institute of Clinical Science, University of Birmingham, Birmingham, UK

Brian Degenhardt, Zane Starks, Shalini Bhatia and Geoffroey-Allen Franklin
A.T. Still University, 800 W. Jefferson St, Kirksville 63501, Missouri, USA

Miriam K. Minsk, Kristen D. Venuti and Paul D. Sponseller
Department of Orthopaedic Surgery, The Johns Hopkins University, Baltimore, MD, USA

Gail L. Daumit
Division of General Internal Medicine, The Johns Hopkins University School of Medicine, Baltimore, MD, USA
Welch Center for Prevention, Epidemiology, and Clinical Research, The Johns Hopkins University, Baltimore, MD, USA
Department of Epidemiology, The Johns Hopkins Bloomberg School of Public Health, Baltimore, MD, USA
Department of Health Policy and Management, The Johns Hopkins Bloomberg School of Public Health, Baltimore, MD, USA

Paul D. Sponseller
Bloomberg Children's Center, 1800 Orleans Street, 7359A, Baltimore, MD 21287, USA

J-C. Bernard, E. Berthonnaud, J. Deceuninck and E. Chaleat-Valayer
Croix Rouge française – CMCR des Massues, 92, rue Edmond Locard, 69322 Lyon Cedex 05, France

E. Berthonnaud
Hôpital Nord Ouest de Villefranche sur Saône, Gleizé 69400, France
Laboratoire de Physiologie de l'Exercice, Saint Etienne, France

L. Journoud-Rozand and G. Notin
Etablissements Lecante, Lyon, France

Larry Cohen, Sarah Kobayashi, Milena Simic, Sarah Dennis, Kathryn Refshauge and Evangelos Pappas
Faculty of Health Sciences, Discipline of Physiotherapy, The University of Sydney, 75 East Street, Lidcombe, NSW 2141, Australia

Masayuki Ishikawa, Shinichi Ishihara, Makoto Nishiyama and Yasuyuki Fukui
1Spine and Spinal Cord Center, Mita Hospital, International University of Health and Welfare, 1-4-3 Mita, Minato-ku, Tokyo 108-8329, Japan

Kai Cao, Long Pang, Nobuyuki Fujita, Masaya Nakamura, Morio Matsumoto and Kota Watanabe
Department of Orthopedic Surgery, School of Medicine, Keio University, 35 Shinanomachi, Shinjuku-ku, Tokyo 160-8582, Japan

Mitsuru Yagi and Masafumi Machida
Department of Orthopedic Surgery, Murayama Medical Center, 2-37-1 Gakuen, Musashimurayama-shi, Tokyo 208-0011, Japan

Naobumi Hosogane
Department of Orthopedic Surgery, National Defense Medical College, 3-2 Namiki, Tokorozawa-shi, Saitama 359-8513, Japan

Takashi Tsuji
Department of Orthopedic Surgery, Kitasato University, Kitasato Institute Hospital, 5-9-1 Shirokane, Minato-ku, Tokyo 108-8642, Japan

Masayuki Ishikawa, Nobuyuki Fujita, Mitsuru Yagi, Naobumi Hosogane, Takashi Tsuji, Shinichi Ishihara, Yasuyuki Fukui, Masaya Nakamura, Morio Matsumoto and Kota Watanabe
Keio Spine Research Group, 35 Shinanomachi, Shinjuku-ku, Tokyo 160-8582, Japan

D.A. Jason Black, Christine Pilcher and Erika Maude
Scoliosis SOS Clinic, 63 Mansell Street, London E1 8AN, UK

Shawn Drake
Arkansas State University, Jonesboro, AR 72467, USA

David Glynn
Independent, York, UK

Nikita Cobetto, Carl-Éric Aubin, Stefan Parent, Soraya Barchi, Isabelle Turgeon and Hubert Labelle
Department of Mechanical Engineering, Polytechnique Montreal, Downtown Station, Montreal, Quebec H3C 3A7, Canada

Michele Romano and Matteo Mastrantonio
ISICO (Italian Scientific Spine Institute), Via Bellarmino 13/1, Milan, Italy

Balaji Zacharia, Dhiyaneswaran Subramaniyam and Sadiqueali Padinharepeediyekkal
Department of Orthopedics, Government Medical College, Kozhikode, Kerala 673008, India

Máté Burkus, Ádám Tibor Schlégl, Ian O'Sullivan, István Márkus, Csaba Vermes and Miklós Tunyogi-Csapó
Department of Orthopedics, Medical School, University of Pécs, Akác st. 1, Pécs H-7623, Hungary

Máté Burkus
Department of Traumatology and Hand Surgery, Petz Aladár County Teaching Hospital, Vasvári Pál st. 2-4, Győr H-9023, Hungary

Lucas Piantoni, Carlos A. Tello, Rodrigo G. Remondino, Ida A. Francheri Wilson, Eduardo Galaretto and Mariano A. Noel
Servicio de Patología Espinal, Hospital de Pediatría Prof. Dr. Juan P. Garrahan, Combate de los Pozos 1881, C1245AAM CABA Buenos Aires, Argentina

Karina A. Zapata
Therapy Services, Texas Scottish Rite Hospital for Children, 2222 Welborn Street, Dallas, TX 75219, USA

Sharon S. Wang-Price
School of Physical Therapy, Texas Woman's University–Dallas, Dallas, TX, USA

Tina S. Fletcher
School of Occupational Therapy, Texas Woman's University–Dallas, Dallas, TX, USA

Charles E. Johnston
Texas Scottish Rite Hospital for Children, Dallas, TX, USA

Tatsuhiro Sekiya, Katsutaka Yamada, Kanichiro Kaneko, Manabu Ide and Tomoyuki Saito
Department of Orthopedic Surgery, Yokohama City University, Fukuura 3-9, Kanazawa-ku, Yokohama City, Kanagawa Prefecture 236-0004, Japan

Yoichi Aota
Department of Orthopedic Surgery, Yokohama City Brain and Spine Center, Takigasira 1-2-1, Isogo-ku, Yokohama City, Kanagawa Prefecture 235-0012, Japan

Index